EPIDEMIOLOGY

BIOSTATISTICS
AND
PREVENTIVE MEDICINE

SAUNDERS TEXT AND REVIEW SERIES

EPIDEMIOLOGY

BIOSTATISTICS

AND

PREVENTIVE MEDICINE

JAMES F. JEKEL, M.D., M.P.H.

Professor of Epidemiology and Public Health
C.-E. A. Winslow Professor of Public Health
Yale University School of Medicine
New Haven, Connecticut

in collaboration with

JOANN G. ELMORE, M.D., M.P.H.

Assistant Professor of Medicine
Yale University School of Medicine
New Haven, Connecticut

and

DAVID L. KATZ, M.D., M.P.H.

Assistant Clinical Professor of Medicine
Lecturer in Epidemiology and Public Health
Yale University School of Medicine
New Haven, Connecticut

W.B. SAUNDERS COMPANY
A Division of Harcourt Brace & Company
Philadelphia London Toronto Montreal Sydney Tokyo

W.B. SAUNDERS COMPANY
A Division of Harcourt Brace & Company

The Curtis Center
Independence Square West
Philadelphia, Pennsylvania 19106

Library of Congress Cataloging-in-Publication Data

Jekel, James F.
    Epidemiology, biostatistics, and preventive medicine / James F.
Jekel; with the collaboration of Joann G. Elmore and David L. Katz.
—1st ed.

       p.   cm.

    ISBN 0–7216–5258–1

    1. Epidemiology. 2. Medical statistics. 3. Medicine, Preventive.
I. Elmore, Joann G.   II. Katz, David L.   III. Title.
    [DNLM: 1. Epidemiologic Methods.   2. Biometry.   3. Preventive
Medicine.   WA 950 J25e 1996]

RA652.J45   1996   614.4'4—dc20

DNLM/DLC   95–42002

Epidemiology, Biostatistics, and Preventive Medicine   ISBN 0–7216–5258–1

Printed in the United States of America.

Last digit is the print number: 9   8   7   6   5   4   3   2   1

PREFACE

Epidemiology is the basic science of preventive medicine and public health, and biostatistics is the quantitative foundation of epidemiology. To separate these fields—as is usually done in texts for students of medicine, public health, and related disciplines—incurs the risks of providing incomplete coverage of each field and failing to integrate the subject matter.

In developing this book, the goal was to present a comprehensive view of the fields of epidemiology, biostatistics, preventive medicine, and public health by showing their interrelationships and emphasizing their relevance to clinical practice, research, and public health policy. In particular, the objectives were to combine theory and application in a manner that enables readers to interpret the scientific literature with understanding; to approach clinical practice with an emphasis on prevention; and to understand the social, organizational, financial, and governmental environments in which physicians and other health professionals must practice today.

Section I, Epidemiology, reviews the many ways in which epidemiology contributes to the medical sciences; discusses the sources of health data; incorporates numerous figures and graphs to illustrate how epidemiologic measurements are made and used; outlines the steps in epidemiologic surveillance, outbreak investigation, and assessment of causation and risks; and discusses common research designs used by epidemiologists.

Section II, Biostatistics, builds on the concepts introduced in the first section and emphasizes that an understanding of biostatistics is important not only for analyzing the results of research but also for understanding and reducing errors in clinical medicine. Biostatistical tests and equations are clearly explained and easy to follow, with special "boxes" used to illustrate the steps in calculating standard errors, t values, chi-square values, and other measurements.

Section III, Preventive Medicine and Public Health, focuses on methods of primary, secondary, and tertiary prevention; provides tables with up-to-date information on immunization schedules, available vaccines and antitoxins, screening recommendations, effects of toxic exposures, and similar topics; and discusses the nutritional, environmental, and behavioral factors that have an impact on health, as well as the socioeconomic and political climate that influences health care policy.

In addition to being a textbook for medical students and others taking courses in epidemiology, biostatistics, preventive medicine, and public health, this book is a source of information for health care professionals who wish to study these topics on their own or to review them for medical board examinations. The approach taken in this book evolved from my experiences in teaching a variety of courses to both students and professionals at Yale University School of Medicine, where the Department of Epidemiology and Public Health is an accredited school of public health and also serves as a department of epidemiology, biostatistics, and preventive medicine for the medical school. As a result, I have had the privilege of teaching many of these topics to public health students for 28 years, biostatistics to medical students for 13 years, public health to medical students for 8 years, and biostatistics and related topics to specialist physicians in the Robert Wood Johnson Clinical Scholar Program for 19 years, and directing the Yale Residency Program in General Preventive Medicine and Public Health for 17 years. These varied groups of outstanding individuals, from different backgrounds and levels of training and experience, have given me the best education a teacher could obtain. Any strengths this book may have are due in significant measure to the challenges put forth by these students, who have numbered in the thousands during my three decades of university work.

I owe a tremendous debt to my collaborators, Dr. Joann Elmore and Dr. David Katz, both of whom are general internists with public health degrees and an orientation toward prevention. At first among my best students ever, they soon became trusted colleagues in teaching medical students and in research. They have achieved outstanding reputations at Yale University and are in considerable demand as teachers of medical and public health students and as research consultants. Dr. Elmore and Dr. Katz not only offered valuable suggestions regarding the book's general outlines but also provided extensive critiques of each chapter. Whenever we had differences, we resolved them in conference. For some chapters, the process of reviewing and revising was repeated several times. The final product was, therefore, a true collaboration. Any deficiencies, however, must be laid at my door alone.

Special thanks are also due to Dr. David Lane, a family practitioner and clinical epidemiologist, and to Michael Fischer, a medical student, for their insightful reviews of the epidemiology and biostatistics sections of the book. Dr. William Beckett, who has been a valued colleague for years in teaching public health to medical students, reviewed and made helpful suggestions about the information dealing with occupational health and exposure to toxins. Sharon Maddox, the book's developmental editor, made major contributions to the organization, clarity, and accuracy of the text. William Schmitt of W. B. Saunders has been a patient and supportive editor from the time he first suggested this effort.

My intellectual debts to others are countless, and unfortunately, they cannot all be acknowledged here. The late Dr. Alexander Langmuir was the inspiration for me (as for hundreds of others) to enter epidemiology and public health as a career. Dr. Steven Helgerson, another student of Dr. Langmuir, was an inspiring colleague in efforts to improve the teaching of epidemiology, particularly the investigation of acute disease outbreaks. The late Dr. Edward M. Cohart first saw that I might make an academician and persisted until I agreed to give an academic career a try. Dr. Alvan Feinstein has been a continuous inspiration by his tireless and brilliant efforts to improve clinical epidemiology and biostatistics. His 1975 request for me to assist in the Robert Wood Johnson Clinical Scholar Program at Yale University was a major stimulus to become more involved in teaching biostatistics. Dr. Lowell Levin has consistently helped me to take a wide perspective regarding the sources of health and ways to improve health. Dr. David Allen was a coinvestigator in our research into the crack cocaine problem, and he has helped me to see the mental and spiritual aspects of many health problems.

I cannot count the lessons I have learned from my parents, who at this writing are preparing to celebrate their sixty-ninth wedding anniversary, and from my wife, Jan, who has been my loving and supportive companion for 37 years. They have taught me what it means to live in an environment filled with wholeness, peace, and health, perhaps best described by the Hebrew word *shalom*.

JAMES F. JEKEL

CONTENTS

SECTION II

BIOSTATISTICS

SECTION III

PREVENTIVE MEDICINE AND PUBLIC HEALTH

CHAPTER SIXTEEN

CHAPTER SEVENTEEN

CHAPTER EIGHTEEN

CHAPTER NINETEEN

CHAPTER TWENTY

CHAPTER TWENTY-ONE

EPIDEMIOLOGY

CHAPTER ONE

EPIDEMIOLOGIC APPROACHES, CONTRIBUTIONS, AND ISSUES

BASIC EPIDEMIOLOGIC CONCEPTS

Epidemiology has been defined in many ways. The word comes from the Greek language, in which *epi* means upon, *dēmos* denotes the population, and the combining form *-logy* means the study of. Thus, epidemiology is the study of something that afflicts (affects) a **population.** Usually, epidemiology is defined as the study of factors that determine the occurrence and distribution of disease in a population.

Epidemiology can be thought of as one of the ways in which disease is studied. In general, there are four levels at which the scientific study of disease can be approached: (1) the submolecular or molecular level (e.g., cell biology, biochemistry, and immunology); (2) the tissue or organ level (e.g., anatomic pathology); (3) the level of individual patients (e.g., clinical medicine); and (4) the level of populations (e.g., epidemiology). Perspectives gained from these four levels are related, and research should be coordinated among the various disciplines to maximize the scientific understanding of disease.

Some people distinguish between classical epidemiology and clinical epidemiology. **Classical epidemiology,** which is population-oriented, studies the community origins of health problems, particularly those related to nutrition, the environment, human behavior, and the psychologic, social, and spiritual state of a population. Classical epidemiologists are interested in discovering risk factors that might be altered in a population to prevent or delay disease or death.

Investigators involved in **clinical epidemiology** often use similar research designs and statistical tools. However, clinical epidemiologists study patients in health care settings in order to improve the diagnosis and treatment of various diseases and the prognosis for patients already affected by a disease. Because clinical epidemiologists usually study people who are ill and are receiving medical care, they must take special care to adjust for the presence of other diseases (comorbidity) and for any clinical interventions (Sackett 1969; Sackett, Haynes, and Tugwell 1991; Feinstein 1985). Because the primary goal of clinical epidemiology is to improve clinical decisions, some prefer to call clinical epidemiology **clinical decision analysis** (Last 1988), but usually this latter term has a more limited meaning.

The epidemiology section of this book is generally oriented toward classical epidemiology, although clinical examples are sometimes used. Chapters 7 and 8 in the biostatistics section present several concepts of special interest to clinical epidemiology. The more highly statistical parts of epidemiology are found in the biostatistics section, so that the basic concepts and methods of epidemiology can be introduced without undue complexity.

Epidemiology can also be divided into **infectious disease epidemiology** and **chronic disease epidemiology.** The former is more heavily dependent on laboratory support (especially microbiology and serology), and the latter is more dependent on complex sampling and statistical methods. This distinction is becoming less valid as molecular laboratory markers (genetic and otherwise) are being used increasingly in chronic disease epidemiology and also as complex statistical analyses are being used more frequently in infectious disease epidemiology (Longini et al. 1988). Moreover, some illnesses, such as tuberculosis and acquired immunodeficiency syndrome (AIDS), may be thought of as both infectious and chronic diseases.

The "BEINGS" Model

The acronym BEINGS serves as a helpful device for remembering the major groups of etiologic factors for disease, as shown in Table 1–1. Some of these factors are easier to change than others. Currently, genetic factors are the most difficult to change, and immunologic factors are often the least difficult to change because of effective immunization programs.

Host, Agent, and Environment

The natural history of a disease is normally described under a triad of factors: the host, the agent, and the environment. For many diseases, it is useful to add a fourth factor, the vector. In measles, the host is a human being who is susceptible to measles infection, the agent is a highly infectious virus that can produce serious disease in human beings, and the environment enables susceptible people to be exposed. In malaria, the host, agent, and environment are all important, but the vector, the *Anopheles* mosquito, is also critical.

Host factors are responsible for the degree to which the individual can adapt to the stressors produced by the agent. Host resistance is influenced by a person's genotype, nutritional status, immune system, and social behavior. General resistance in people without immunodeficiency depends partly on good nutrition. This is evident in the fact that measles is seldom fatal in well-nourished children, even in the absence of measles immunization and modern medical care. In contrast, up to 25% of children with marasmus (starvation) or kwashiorkor (protein-calorie malnutrition, usually related to weaning) die from complications of measles. That social behavior has an effect on disease spread is seen in the case of dysentery caused by the organism *Shigella.* This type of dysentery is seldom spread by person-to-person contact where personal hygiene is good but can spread rapidly via this method in a home for retarded individuals.

TABLE 1–1. "BEINGS": An Acronym for Remembering the Categories of Preventable Causes of Disease

Biologic factors and **B**ehavioral factors
Environmental factors
Immunologic factors
Nutritional factors
Genetic factors
Services, **S**ocial factors, and **S**piritual factors

Biologic agents of disease or illness not only include infectious organisms (bacteria, viruses, fungi, etc.) but also include allergens and even, under certain circumstances, vaccines, antibiotics, and foods (such as a high-fat diet). **Chemical agents** include chemical toxins (e.g., lead) and dusts, which can cause either acute or chronic illness. **Physical agents** include kinetic energy (e.g., in cases involving bullet wounds, blunt trauma, and vehicular injuries), radiation, heat, cold, and noise. Epidemiologists are now studying the extent to which **social and psychologic stressors** can be considered agents in the production of health problems.

The **environment** influences the probability and circumstances of contact between the host and the agent. For example, poor restaurant sanitation increases the probability of patrons being exposed to *Salmonella* infections. Poor roads and bad weather conditions increase the number of automobile collisions and airplane crashes. But the environment also includes social, political, and economic factors: crowded homes and schools make exposure to measles and other infectious diseases more likely, and the political structure and economic health of a society partly determine the nutritional status of the members of that society.

Vectors of disease commonly include insects (e.g., mosquitoes associated with the spread of malaria), arthropods (e.g., the ticks associated with Lyme disease), and animals (e.g., raccoons associated with rabies in the eastern USA). The concept of the vector, however, can be applied more widely to include groups of human beings (e.g., vendors of heroin and cocaine) and even objects (e.g., contaminated needles associated with hepatitis and AIDS). A vector may be considered part of the environment, or it may be treated separately, as shown in Fig. 1–1. To be an effective transmitter of disease, the vector must have a specific relationship to the agent, the environment, and the host.

In the case of human malaria, mentioned briefly above, the vector is a mosquito of the genus *Anopheles;* the agent is a parasitic organism of the genus *Plasmodium;* the environment is warm and enables the mosquito to breed; and the host is a human being.

Specifically, the parasitic organism must go through part of its life cycle in the mosquito; the climate must be relatively warm and have standing water in which the mosquito can breed; the mosquito must be willing to bite human beings and must be able to spread the disease; the host must be bitten by an infected mosquito (in the case of malaria, usually the biting is done in houses at night); and the host must be susceptible to the disease.

In the case of Lyme disease, human beings are an accidental host. The agent is the spirochete *Borrelia burgdorferi,* which is normally found in the deer mouse. The spirochete is spread by the vector, an *Ixodes* tick, from mouse to mouse in the spring and early summer and is spread to deer by the mature ticks. The environment is usually a wooded area that permits all of these animals to coexist.

As mentioned above, the factors involved in the natural history of disease can be remembered by the acronym BEINGS (see Fig. 1–1 and Table 1–1). Behavioral, biologic, genetic, and immunologic factors are usually associated with the host. Nutritional and biologic factors are commonly considered under the agent, and the vector may be classified with the environment.

CONTRIBUTIONS OF EPIDEMIOLOGISTS TO THE MEDICAL SCIENCES

Investigating the Modes of Transmission of a New Disease

Using the surveillance and investigative methods discussed in detail in Chapter 3, epidemiologists have often provided the initial hypotheses for others to test in the laboratory. Since 1975, epidemiologic methods have suggested the probable type of agent and modes of transmission for the diseases listed in Table 1–2, usually within months of their recognition as new or emergent diseases. Knowledge of the modes of transmission in turn led epidemiologists to suggest ways to prevent each of these diseases before the causative agents were determined or extensive laboratory results were available. Laboratory work to identify the causal agents, clarify the pathogenesis, and develop vaccines or treatments for most of these diseases still continues many years after this basic epidemiologic work was done.

Concern about the many recently discovered and resurgent diseases, although not new, is at a peak because of a variety of newly emerging disease problems (see Jekel 1972; Institute of Medicine 1992; Gibbons 1993). The rapid growth in population, increased travel and contact with new areas such as jungles, declining effectiveness of antibiotics and insecticides, and many other factors appear to be encouraging the development of new diseases or the resurgence of older ones.

Determining Preventable Causes of Disease

Preventable causes of disease, particularly life-threatening diseases such as cancer, have been the

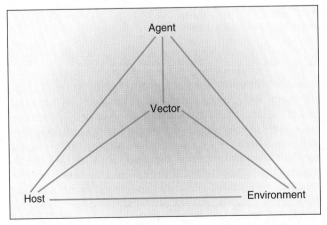

FIGURE 1–1. Factors involved in the natural history of disease.

TABLE 1–2. Six Recent Diseases Whose Natural History and Methods of Prevention Were the Subjects of Early Hypotheses by Epidemiologists

Disease	Date of Appearance	Epidemiologic Hypotheses	
		Agent and Route of Spread	Methods of Prevention
Lyme disease	1975	Infectious agent, spread by ticks.	Avoid ticks.
Legionnaires' disease	1976	Small infectious agent, spread via air-conditioning systems.	Treat the water in air-conditioning systems.
Toxic shock syndrome	1980	Staphylococcal toxin, associated with the use of tampons, especially the Rely brand of tampons.	Avoid using long-lasting tampons.
Acquired immuno-deficiency syndrome (AIDS)	1981	Viral agent, spread via sexual activity, especially male homosexual activity, and via sharing of needles and exchange of blood and blood products during intravenous drug use and transfusions.	Use condoms; avoid sharing needles; and institute programs to exchange needles and screen blood.
Eosinophilia-myalgia syndrome	1989	Toxic contaminant, associated with the use of dietary supplements of L-tryptophan.	Change methods of product manufacturing.
Hantavirus pulmonary syndrome	1993	Hantavirus, spread via contact with the contaminated droppings of deer mice.	Avoid contact with excreta of deer mice.

subject of much epidemiologic research. In 1964, an expert committee of the World Health Organization (WHO) estimated that "the majority" of cancer cases were potentially preventable and were due to "extrinsic factors." In the same year, the US Surgeon General released a report that indicated that the risk of death from lung cancer among smokers was almost 11 times that among nonsmokers (US Surgeon General 1964).

In their 1981 book entitled *The Causes of Cancer*, two leading epidemiologists, Richard Doll and Richard Peto, praised the 1964 WHO report and made the following argument (p. 1197):

> In the years since that report was published, advances in knowledge have consolidated these opinions and few if any competent research workers now question its main conclusion. Individuals, indeed, have gone further and have substituted figures of 80 or even 90% as the proportion of potentially preventable cancers in place of the 1964 committee's cautious estimate of "the majority."

Unfortunately, the phrase "extrinsic factors" (or the phrase "environmental factors" which is often substituted for it) has been misinterpreted by many people to mean only "man-made chemicals," which was certainly not the intent of the WHO committee. The committee included, in addition to man-made or natural carcinogens, viral infections, nutritional deficiencies or excesses, reproductive activities and a variety of other factors determined wholly or partly by personal behavior.

Given the many cell types of cancer and the fact that there are many causal factors to be considered, how do epidemiologists estimate the percentage of deaths caused by cancer?

According to one method, the first step is to look at each type of cancer and determine (from epidemiologic studies) the percentage of cases due to an identifiable and preventable cause. These percentages are then added up in a weighted manner to determine the total percentage due to identifiable causes.

A second method requires the use of annual age- and sex-specific cancer incidence rates from countries which have the lowest rates of a given cell type of cancer and which also have good medical care to ensure a reasonable level of accuracy in detecting the presence of disease. For a particular cell type of cancer, a low rate in such a country presumably is due to a low prevalence of the risk factors for that type of cancer. After epidemiologists have gathered the necessary data concerning other countries, they could calculate the number of cases of each type of cancer that would be expected to occur annually in each age and gender group in the USA if the lowest observed rates had been true for the US population. Next, they would add up the expected numbers for the various cancer types and groups in the USA. Finally, they would compare this total number of expected cases with the total number of cases actually diagnosed in the US population. Using this method, epidemiologists have found that the USA has about five times as many cancer cases as would be expected. Presumably, the excess cancer cases in the USA are due to a high prevalence of risk factors for cancer, such as smoking.

Behavioral Factors

Human behavior is a central factor in health and disease. The most obvious example is cigarette smoking and its contribution to a variety of health problems, including lung, esophageal, and nasopharyngeal cancer; myocardial infarction; and chronic obstructive pulmonary disease. In the USA, cigarettes cause approximately 90% of the cases of lung cancer and about 50% of the cases of myocardial infarction among smokers. Despite these percentages, cigarettes are responsible for more deaths due to heart disease than to lung cancer, because many more people die of heart disease than of lung cancer. In 1992, for example, 480,051 deaths were attributed to ischemic heart disease and 151,269 to lung and related cancers (Kochanek and Hudson 1995).

Multiple behavioral factors also are associated with the spread of some diseases. In the case of AIDS, for instance, the spread of type 1 human immunodeficiency virus (HIV-1) can result from male homosexual activity and from intravenous drug abuse, which are the two predominant routes of transmission in the USA. It can also result from heterosexual activity, which is apparently the predominant route of spread in Africa and is becoming more important in the USA.

Although epidemiologic studies were the first to suggest how to prevent both cigarette-related diseases and HIV-1 infection, satisfactory clinical treatments for these health problems are still lacking.

Among the many other examples of behavior that can lead to disease, injury, or premature death (i.e., death before the age of 65 years) are excessive intake of alcohol, abuse of illegal drugs, driving while intoxicated, and homicide and suicide. In each of these cases, as in cigarette smoking and HIV-1 infection, changes in behavior could prevent the untoward outcomes.

Environmental Factors

To everyone's surprise, early epidemiologic studies suggested that the outbreak of sometimes-fatal pneumonia among members of the American Legion who were attending a 1976 conference in Philadelphia was caused by an agent distributed through the air-conditioning and ventilation systems of the primary hotels hosting the conference. Only later, after *Legionella pneumophila* was identified, was the discovery made that this small bacterium actually thrives in air-conditioning cooling towers and in warm water systems. It was also shown that respiratory therapy equipment that is merely rinsed with water can become a reservoir for *Legionella*, causing hospital-acquired legionnaires' disease.

Early epidemiologic research concerning an illness that was first reported in 1975 in Old Lyme, Connecticut, suggested that the arthritis, rash, and other symptoms of the illness were caused by infection with an organism transmitted by a tick. This was enough information to enable preventive methods to be started. By 1977, it was clear that so-called Lyme disease was spread by *Ixodes* ticks, and this opened the way for more specific prevention and research. Not until 1982, however, was the causative agent, *Borrelia burgdorferi*, discovered and shown to be spread by the *Ixodes* tick.

As a "first responder" in the investigation of new health problems such as legionnaires' disease and Lyme disease, epidemiologists are involved in describing the patterns of disease in the population, developing hypotheses about causal factors, and introducing methods to prevent further cases of disease.

Immunologic Factors

Smallpox is the first infectious disease known to have been eradicated from the globe. The eradication was possible because vaccination against smallpox conferred individual immunity and also produced herd immunity. Discussed in greater detail later in this chapter, **herd immunity** results when a vaccine not only prevents the vaccinated person from contracting the disease but also prevents him or her from spreading the disease. A reduction in the number of people able to spread disease results in reduced disease transmission.

Most people now think of AIDS when they hear of a deficiency of the immune system, but **immunodeficiency** also may be caused by genetic abnormalities or by other factors. For example, transient immune deficiency has been noted following some infections and after the administration of certain vaccines. An important example concerns measles and live measles vaccine, both of which produce a temporary immune deficiency that is potentially serious in malnourished children.

Nutritional Factors

In the 1950s, it was shown that Japanese-Americans living in Hawaii had a much higher rate of myocardial infarction than did persons of similar age and sex in Japan, and Japanese-Americans in California had a still higher rate of this disease than did similar persons in Japan (Keys 1966, 1970; Gordon 1957; Reed 1990). The investigators believed that a difference in diet was the single most important factor producing these differences in disease, and their beliefs generally have been supported by subsequent research.

Before his death, Denis Burkitt, the physician after whom Burkitt's lymphoma was named, spent many years doing epidemiologic research on the critical role that dietary fiber plays in good health. During a lecture at Yale University in 1989, he made some stunning statements that included the following: (1) "By world standards, the entire United States is constipated." (2) "Don't diagnose appendicitis in Africa unless the patient speaks English." (3) "African medical students go through 5 years of training without seeing coronary heart disease or appendicitis." (4) "Populations with large stools have small hospitals. Those with small stools have large hospitals."

Based on his cross-cultural studies, Burkitt observed that many of the diseases commonly seen in the USA were rarely encountered in indigenous populations of tropical Africa (Table 1–3). This observation was true even of areas with good medical care, such as Kampala, Uganda, at the time Burkitt was there—a fact suggesting that these diseases were not being missed due to lack of diagnosis. Nor were these differences primarily genetic in origin, because African-Americans in the USA suffer from these diseases at roughly the same rate as other groups in the USA. If the diseases listed in Table 1–3 suddenly disappeared, most US hospitals and many US physicians

TABLE 1–3. **Diseases That Are Rare in the Indigenous Populations of Tropical Africa**

Appendicitis
Breast cancer
Colon cancer
Coronary heart disease
Diabetes mellitus
Diverticulitis
Gallstones
Hemorrhoids
Hiatal hernia
Varicose veins

Source of data: Burkitt, D. Lecture at Yale University School of Medicine, New Haven, Conn., April 28, 1989.

would be at risk of bankruptcy, unless these diseases were quickly replaced by others. The cross-cultural differences suggest that the current heavy burden of these diseases in the USA is *not* inevitable. Indeed, Burkitt proposed mechanisms by which a high intake of dietary fiber could prevent these diseases or markedly reduce their incidence (Kellock 1985).

The Framingham Heart Study showed that an elevated blood cholesterol level was associated with an elevated risk for myocardial infarction (for a description of the study's inception, see Dawber, Meadors, and Moore 1951). This and other studies led to laboratory research into the behavior of blood lipids, and now, decades later, much of the pathogenesis of atherosclerosis and coronary artery disease has been worked out. Only recently have effective medical interventions to prevent myocardial infarction been developed, yet the death rates from this health problem have been falling for two decades, partly because of societal improvements in diet and exercise and the reduction of cigarette smoking, all of which had been suggested by epidemiologic studies in the past.

Genetic Factors

It is well established that the genetic inheritance of individuals interacts with diet and environment in complex ways to promote or protect against a variety of illnesses, including heart disease and cancer. Genetic epidemiology is a growing field of research. Population genetics and genetic epidemiology are concerned with, among other things, the distribution of normal and abnormal genes in the population and whether or not these are in equilibrium. According to experts, population gene frequencies appear to be stable (Scriver 1988). Genetic epidemiology is also concerned with gene mutation rates, which do not appear to be changing either. Considerable research involves studying the possible interaction of various genotypes with environmental, nutritional, and behavioral factors and investigating the extent to which environmental adaptations can reduce the burden of genetic disease.

Genetic disease now accounts for a higher proportion of disease than in the past, not because the incidence of genetic disease is rising but instead because the incidence of noninherited disease is falling. This point is illustrated in the following discussion by Scriver (1988):

Heritability refers to . . . the contribution of genes relative to all determinants of disease. Rickets, a genetic disease, recently showed an abrupt fall in incidence and an increase in heritability in Quebec. The fall in incidence followed universal supplementation of dairy milk with calciferol. The rise in heritability reflected the disappearance of a major environmental cause of rickets (vitamin D deficiency) and the persistence of Mendelian disorders of calcium and phosphate homeostasis without a change in their incidence.

Scriver lists other genetic problems for which the environmental-nutritional-behavioral component has been reduced, with little or no fall in the genetic disease in the same area. For example, as a result of the control of paralytic poliomyelitis through immunization, juvenile musculoskeletal disorders show an increased **heritability**—that is, an increased proportion of cases due to genetic causes.

Genetic screening is important to identify a few problems in newborns for which rapid therapy can be extremely beneficial (such as phenylketonuria and congenital hypothyroidism) and to identify other genetic disorders for which genetic counseling can be beneficial. Nevertheless, the greatest future possibilities for improvement in health in the genetic area may be a better understanding of how identification of individual genotypes can lead to special protection for people who are particularly susceptible to environmental problems at home and at work or for those who cannot tolerate certain foods, medicines, or behaviors. Major screening efforts for "susceptibility genes" will undoubtedly increase in the future, but there are ethical concerns about potential problems, such as insurers hesitating to insure individuals with known genetic risks.

Services, Social Factors, and Spiritual Factors

Medical care services may be quite beneficial to health, but they can also be dangerous. One of the important tasks of epidemiology is to determine the value of medical care in different settings. Approximately 5% of hospitalized patients acquire a hospital infection (Inlander, Levin, and Weiner 1988), and 3.7% of hospitalized patients suffer "adverse events" (medical errors) other than infection (Leape et al. 1991). Other medical care–related causes of illness include unnecessary and inappropriate diagnostic or surgical procedures.

The effects that **social and spiritual factors** have on disease and health have been less intensively studied than have the effects of other causal factors. However, evidence is accumulating that personal beliefs concerning the meaning and purpose of life, access to forgiveness, and the support received from members of a social network are powerful influences on health. Studies have shown that both experimental animals and human beings are better able to resist noxious stressors when they are in the presence of other members of the same species. Social support may be achieved through the family, friendship networks, and membership in various groups such as churches and clubs.

Many investigators have explored factors related to health and disease in Mormons and Seventh-Day Adventists. Both groups have been shown to have lower than average age-adjusted death rates from all types of disease and specifically from heart disease, cancer, and respiratory diseases (Berkman and Breslow 1983). Part of their protection undoubtedly arises from the behaviors proscribed or prescribed by these groups. For example, Mormons prohibit the use of coffee, tea, alcohol, and tobacco. Seventh-Day Adventists likewise tend to avoid alcohol and tobacco, and in addition they strongly encourage (but do not require) their members to eat a vegetarian diet. However, as Berkman and Breslow (1983:62) indicated, it is not clear that these behaviors are solely responsible for the health differences: "It is difficult . . . to separate the effects of health practices from other aspects of life-style common among those belonging to such religions, for example, differing social stresses and network systems."

In an earlier study, Berkman and Syme (1979) showed that for all age groups, the greater one's participation in churches and other groups and the stronger one's social networks, the lower the mortality that was observed.

The work of the psychiatrist Frankl (1963) also documented the importance of a person's having a meaning and purpose in life, which can be useful in the treatment of distressed persons and in promoting a reduction of emotional problems. Such factors are increasingly being studied as important in understanding the web of causation of diseases.

Determining the Natural History of Disease

The name of a medical discipline indicates both a method of research into health and disease and the body of knowledge acquired by using that method of research. Thus, pathology is a field of medical research with its own goals and methods, but investigators and clinicians can also speak of the "pathology of lung cancer." Similarly, epidemiology refers to a field of research that uses particular methods, but it can also be used to denote the resulting body of knowledge about the natural history of disease—that is, about the nutritional, behavioral, and environmental sources of disease as identified through epidemiologic studies.

When discussing the etiology of disease, epidemiologists make a distinction between the biologic **mechanisms of disease** and the social and environmental **causes of disease.** In a study of osteomalacia, for example, investigators might explore the mecha-nisms of this bone disease, as well as its causes and consequences in a specific social context, such as among women who observe the custom of purdah. In keeping with this custom, which is generally observed among Muslims and some Hindus in countries such as India, women who have reached puberty avoid public observation by spending most of their time indoors and by wearing clothing that covers virtually all of the body when they go outdoors. Purdah prevents these growing women from getting vitamin D through the action of the sun's radiation on the skin to produce irradiated ergosterol, which is one of the D vitamins. If, as often happens, the diet of these women is also deficient in vitamin D during the rapid growth period of puberty, they may develop osteomalacia as a result of insufficient calcium absorption. Osteomalacia can cause the pelvis to become distorted (more pear-shaped), and this may cause the pelvic opening to be too small for the infant. If such problems should arise, a female surgeon or obstetrician must be available, because it would be unthinkable under purdah for a male physician to attend the birth. In this example, the social and nutritional causes set in motion the biochemical and other biologic mechanisms that may lead to maternal and infant mortality.

Likewise, excessive fat intake, smoking, and lack of exercise are social factors that contribute to biologic mechanisms of atherogenesis, such as elevated blood levels of low-density lipoprotein cholesterol (LDL), very low density lipoprotein cholesterol (VLDL), and triglycerides, as well as reduced blood levels of high-density lipoprotein cholesterol (HDL).

Epidemiologists attempt to go as far back as possible to discover the societal causes of disease, which offer clues to methods of prevention. Hypotheses introduced by epidemiologists frequently guide laboratory scientists as they seek biologic mechanisms of disease, which may suggest methods of treatment.

Studying the Biologic Spectrum of Disease

The first identified cases of a new disease are often fatal or severe, which leads observers to conclude that the disease is always severe. However, as more becomes known, less severe (and even asymptomatic) cases of an infectious or noninfectious disease are generally discovered. If it is an infectious disease, asymptomatic infection may be uncovered either by finding elevated antibody titers to the organism in clinically well people or by culturing the organism from them.

This variation in severity of a disease process is referred to as the **biologic spectrum of disease,** or the **iceberg phenomenon** (Morris 1967). The latter term is appropriate because most of an iceberg remains unseen, below the surface, as do most asymptomatic and mild cases of disease. An outbreak of diphtheria will illustrate the point. In 1962 and 1963, when the author (JFJ) worked with the US Centers for Disease Control, he and a colleague were

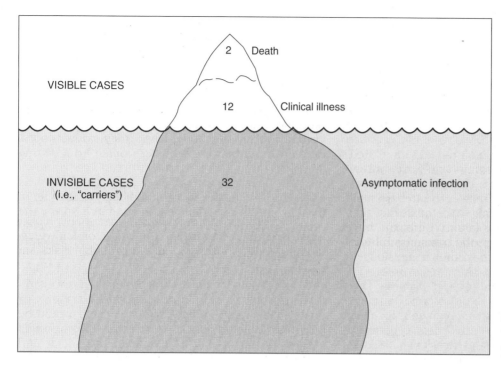

FIGURE 1-2. **The iceberg phenomenon, as illustrated by a diphtheria epidemic in Alabama.** In epidemics, the number of people with severe forms of the disease (the tip of the iceberg) may be much smaller than the number of people with mild or asymptomatic clinical disease. (Source of data: Jekel, J. F., G. S. Zatlin, and O. F. Gay. *Corynebacterium diphtheriae* survives in a partly immunized group. Public Health Reports 85:310, 1970.)

assigned to investigate an epidemic of diphtheria in a county in Alabama. In addition to causing 2 deaths, the diphtheria caused symptoms of clinical illness in 12 children who recovered with or without sequelae. It also caused asymptomatic infection in 32 children, some of whom had even been immunized against diphtheria. The 32 cases of asymptomatic infection were discovered by an extensive campaign of culturing the throats of the school-age children in the outbreak area as well as the home contacts of any infected child. In this "iceberg" (see Fig. 1-2), 14 infections were visible, but the 32 asymptomatic carriers would have remained invisible without the extensive use of culturing and epidemiologic surveillance (Jekel, Zatlin, and Gay 1970).

The iceberg phenomenon is extremely important to epidemiology, because studying only symptomatic individuals may produce a misleading picture of the disease pattern and severity (Evans 1987).

Evaluating Community Health Interventions

Field trials are an important phase of evaluating a new vaccine before it is given to the community at large, but field trials are only one phase of the evaluation of immunization programs. After the introduction of a vaccine, ongoing surveillance of the disease is essential to ensure the continued safety and effectiveness of the vaccine.

The importance of continued surveillance can be illustrated in the case of immunization against poliomyelitis. In 1954, large-scale field trials of the Salk inactivated polio vaccine were done, and these confirmed the value and safety of the vaccine (Francis et al. 1955). In 1955, the polio surveillance program of the Centers for Disease Control discovered an outbreak of vaccine-associated poliomyelitis, which was

linked to vaccine from Cutter Laboratories (Langmuir 1963). Ultimately, 79 vaccinated individuals and 105 family members of the vaccine-associated cases were found to have developed poliomyelitis. Apparently, a slight change from the recommended procedure for producing the vaccine had allowed clumping of the poliovirus to occur, and this enabled some of the virus particles in the center of the clumps to avoid being killed by formaldehyde during production. Because of this faulty processing, some people were vaccinated with a vaccine containing live virus. It was only because of the vaccine surveillance program that the problem was detected quickly and the dangerous vaccine removed from use.

Likewise, ongoing surveillance programs were responsible for detecting outbreaks of measles that occurred in 1971, 1977, and 1990, after impressive initial progress against the disease. Epidemiologists were able to show that much of the unexpected disease occurred in college students and other people who had received only one dose of measles vaccine, which had been administered before the 12th month of life, when the persistence of maternal antibody may have reduced the antigenicity of the vaccine (Marks, Halpin, and Orenstein 1978). Such findings have led to the current recommendations to give measles vaccine initially at 15 months of age, to give a booster dose of measles vaccine before primary school entry, and to ensure that students entering college have had at least two doses of measles vaccine (see American Academy of Pediatrics 1991).

Setting Disease Control Priorities

Disease control priorities should be based not only on the currently existing size of the problem but also on the potential of a disease to spread to others, its likelihood of causing death and disability, and its cost to individuals, families, and society (Jekel 1972). Unfortunately, legislatures often fund disease control efforts inappropriately, by considering only the number of cases reported (Jekel 1968).

In the mid-1980s, the potential threat that AIDS posed to society was recognized as being far greater than was suggested by the absolute numbers and costs involved at that time. Because of this, a much larger portion of national resources was allocated to the study and control of AIDS than to efforts focused on other diseases affecting similar numbers of patients. Special concerns with AIDS included the rapid increase in the number of cases reported during such a brief period, the high case fatality ratio, the huge medical care and social costs, the transmissibility of the disease, and the fact that known methods of prevention were not being well applied.

Improving the Diagnosis, Treatment, and Prognosis of Clinical Disease

The application of epidemiologic methods to clinical questions has improved research concerning the diagnosis, therapy, and prognosis of disease (Feinstein 1985). This application is the domain of clinical epidemiology.

Epidemiologic methods are used to improve disease **diagnosis** through the selection of the best diagnostic tests, the determination of the best cutoff points for diagnostic tests, and the development of strategies to use in screening for disease (Sackett, Haynes, and Tugwell 1991). These issues are discussed later in the biostatistics and preventive medicine sections of this book.

Epidemiologic methods are frequently used to determine the most effective **treatment** in a given situation. For example, Bracken et al. (1990) used a randomized controlled clinical trial in many centers around the USA to test the hypothesis that methylprednisolone reduced spinal cord damage and improved residual motor function following acute spinal cord injury. The hypothesis was confirmed.

Epidemiologic methods also help improve **prognosis.** For example, Horwitz, Cicchetti, and Horwitz (1984) used a case-control study to compare two different coronary prognostic indices, analyze their weaknesses, and suggest ways in which prognostication could be enhanced. Individual patients want to know their prognoses, and such knowledge also helps investigators stratify patients into groups with similar disease severity in clinical trials and other research to evaluate treatments.

Improving Health Services Research

The principles as well as the methods of epidemiology are used in health services research (Spitzer, Feinstein, and Sackett 1975). In health planning, epidemiologic measures are employed to determine the level of community health needs, both present and future. Demographic projection techniques enable good estimations to be made of the size of different age groups in the future, and the analysis of patterns of disease frequency and services use can estimate the level of services that will be required in the future (see Connecticut Hospital Association 1978). Both in health program evaluation and in the broader field of cost-effectiveness analysis and cost-benefit analysis, epidemiologic methods are used to determine the effects of medical care. It is usually more difficult to determine the effect of a program or a policy than to determine its cost.

Providing Expert Testimony in Courts of Law

Increasingly, epidemiologists are being called upon to testify regarding the state of knowledge about product hazards and the probable risks and effects of various environmental exposures. Among the many kinds of lawsuits that may rely on epidemiologic data are those involving claims of damage from general environmental exposures (e.g., the possible association of magnetic fields and brain cancer); occupational illness claims (e.g., occupational lung damage from workplace asbestos); medical liability (e.g., adverse effects from vaccines); and product liability (e.g., lung cancer associated with tobacco use; toxic shock syndrome associated with tampon use; and various disorders associated with silicone breast implants).

ECOLOGIC ISSUES IN EPIDEMIOLOGY

An important characteristic of epidemiology is its ecologic perspective. People are seen not only as individual organisms but also as members of communities, in a social context. The world is understood as a complex ecosystem in which disease patterns vary greatly from one country to another. In fact, the types and rates of diseases in a country are a kind of "fingerprint," which indicates the per capita income (a proxy for the standard of living), the life-style, the predominant occupations, and the climate, among other things. Some epidemiologists see their field as "human ecology," "medical ecology," or "geographic medicine" (Kilbourne and Smillie 1969).

The Solution and Unintended Creation of Problems

One of the most important insights of ecologic thinking is that as people change one element in a system, they inevitably change other parts, and not always for the good. Thus, an epidemiologist will constantly be alert for possible negative side effects that a medical or health intervention might produce. For example, in the USA, the reduction of mortality in infancy and childhood has increased the prevalence of chronic degenerative diseases, because now the majority of people live to retirement age. Medically, nobody would want to go back a hundred years, but still the control of infectious diseases has produced another set of problems. Table 1–4 shows some of the new health and societal problems introduced by the solution of earlier health problems.

TABLE 1–4.   Examples of Negative Ecologic Side Effects from the Solution of Earlier Health Problems

Initial Health Problem	Solution	Negative Ecologic Side Effects
Childhood infections	Vaccination.	Decrease in the level of immunity during adulthood, owing to a lack of repeated exposures to infection.
High infant mortality rate	Improved sanitation.	Increase in the population growth rate; appearance of epidemic paralytic poliomyelitis; and appearance of epidemic hepatitis A infection.
Sleeping sickness in cattle	Control of the tsetse fly (the disease vector).	Increase in the area of land subject to overgrazing and drought, owing to an increase in the cattle population.
Malnutrition and the need for larger areas of tillable land	Erection of large river dams (e.g., on the Aswan and Senegal Rivers).	Increase in the rates of some infectious diseases, owing to water system changes that favor the vectors of disease.

Vaccination and Patterns of Immunity

Understanding **herd immunity** is essential to thinking about the ecologic problems in immunization today. If herd immunity is present, not only will an immunized individual be protected, but he or she will not be able to transmit the disease to others, and this will cause the prevalence of the organism in the population to decline.

Herd immunity is illustrated in Fig. 1–3, where it is assumed that each person comes into sufficient contact with two other persons to expose both of them to the disease if the first person is infected. Under this assumption, if there is no herd immunity against the disease and everyone is susceptible, the number of cases will double every "disease generation" (Fig. 1–3A). If there is 50% herd immunity against the disease, the number of cases will be small and will remain approximately constant (Fig. 1–3B). If

there is greater than 50% herd immunity, as would be true in a well-immunized population, the infection should eventually die out. Obviously, the degree of immunity necessary to eliminate a virus from a population varies depending on the type of virus, the time of year, and the density and social patterns of the population.

It may seem that immunization is simple: immunize essentially everybody in childhood, and there will be no problems from the targeted diseases. Although there is some truth to this way of thinking, in reality the control of diseases by immunization is more complex. In this section, the examples of diphtheria, smallpox, poliomyelitis, and syphilis are used to illustrate some of the current issues concerning vaccination programs and population immunity.

Diphtheria.   Vaccine-produced immunity in individuals tends to decrease over time. This phenom-

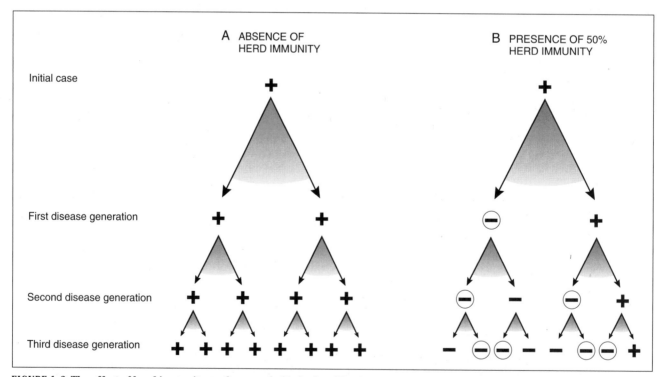

FIGURE 1–3. The effect of herd immunity on the spread of infection. The diagrams illustrate how an infectious disease, such as measles, could spread in a susceptible population if each infected person were exposed to two other persons. In the absence of herd immunity (diagram A), the number of cases doubles each disease generation. In the presence of 50% herd immunity (diagram B), the number of cases remains constant. The plus sign represents an infected person; the minus sign represents an uninfected person; and the circled minus sign represents an immune person who will not pass the infection to others.

enon has a different impact today, when infectious diseases such as diphtheria are less common, than it did in the past. When diphtheria was a more common disease, people who had been vaccinated against it were exposed more frequently to the causative agent, and this exposure could result in a mild reinfection. The reinfection would produce a "natural booster effect" and maintain a high level of immunity. As diphtheria became less common because of immunization programs, fewer people were exposed and there were fewer subclinical "booster" infections. Today, the less recently immunized people tend to be more susceptible to infection.

This is demonstrated by events in the Russian Federation, where despite the wide availability of diphtheria vaccine, many adults who had not recently been in the military were found to be susceptible to the diphtheria organism (Rappuoli, Perugini, and Falsen 1988). Beginning in 1990, a major epidemic of diphtheria appeared in the Russian Federation, producing over 12,000 cases by the late summer of 1993 (see Centers for Disease Control and Prevention 1993). In 1992, 72% of the reported cases were among people over 14 years of age. This was not due to lack of initial immunization, because more than 90% of the adults in the Russian Federation were fully immunized against diphtheria when they were children. The disease in older people apparently has been due to a decline in the adult immunity levels. The solution has been a massive reimmunization of adults with diphtheria toxoid.

Smallpox. As mentioned earlier in this chapter, the goal of worldwide eradication of smallpox has been met by immunizing people against the disease. There were some potential risks in the attempt to eradicate the disease, however. The dominant form of smallpox in the 1970s was variola minor (alastrim). This was a relatively mild form of smallpox which, although often disfiguring, had a low mortality rate. Yet alastrim provided individual and herd immunity against the much more disfiguring and fatal variola major form of the disease (classical smallpox). If the immunization program were to eradicate variola minor but not variola major, in time some populations might become susceptible to the more severe form of the disease. To eliminate alastrim and instead get variola major would have been a poor exchange. Fortunately, the smallpox vaccine was effective against both forms of smallpox, and the immunization program was successful in eradicating variola minor and variola major.

Poliomyelitis. The need for herd immunity was also demonstrated by poliomyelitis. The Salk (injected) polio vaccine, which became available in 1955, provided protection to the immunized individual but did not produce herd immunity. Although it stimulated the production of blood antibodies against poliovirus, it did not produce cell-mediated immunity in the intestine, where the polioviruses multiplied. Because of this, it did little to interrupt viral replication in the intestine. Declining rates of

paralytic poliomyelitis lulled many people into lack of concern, and immunization rates for newborn children dropped. Unfortunately, this led to recurrent cases and periodic small epidemics of poliomyelitis in the late 1950s and early 1960s.

The live, attenuated Sabin oral polio vaccine (OPV) was approved in the early 1960s. The OPV produced cell-mediated immunity, thus preventing the poliovirus from replicating in the intestine, and therefore it provided herd immunity. After the widespread use of OPV in the USA, the prevalence of all three types of the wild poliovirus declined rapidly, as monitored in waste sewage. As the wild polioviruses became scarce in the environment, even children who were not given polio vaccine usually were protected, because they were not exposed to the virus. Poliovirus now appears to have been eradicated from the Western Hemisphere. The last known case of paralytic poliomyelitis caused by a wild poliovirus was confirmed in Peru in August 1991 (see Centers for Disease Control and Prevention 1994).

It might appear from this information that the OPV is always superior, but that is not true. Currently, most of the infrequent cases of paralytic poliomyelitis in the USA appear to be linked to the administration of the live, attenuated OPV itself. These cases usually occur in inadequately immunized parents of infants who have recently been given the OPV, and the parents acquire the virus from contact with their infants' stool.

When the health department for the Gaza Strip used only the oral polio vaccine in its polio immunization efforts, many cases of paralytic poliomyelitis occurred among Arab children. Because of inadequate sanitation, the children often had other intestinal infections when they were given the OPV, and these infections interfered with the OPV infection in the gut. Because the oral vaccine often did not "take," many children were still unprotected (Lasch 1979). The health department subsequently switched to an immunization program in which children are first injected with Salk vaccine to produce adequate blood immunity. Later, they are given OPV as a booster vaccine to achieve herd immunity.

Syphilis. Syphilis has several stages. In the primary and secondary stages, the lesions are highly contagious, but they subside spontaneously. Next is a latent period, after which a tertiary stage may occur. The immunity that develops from an untreated infection is not absolute. It does not protect the individual from progressive damage to his or her own body. It does, however, provide herd immunity by making the infected person unlikely to develop another highly infectious primary chancre (the initial ulcer of syphilis infection, which is filled with spirochetes) if he or she is exposed to syphilis again (Jekel 1968). When penicillin came into general use, syphilis infections were killed so quickly that "chancre immunity" did not develop, and high-risk persons continued to reacquire and spread the disease.

Effects of Sanitation

In the 19th century, diarrheal diseases were the biggest killer of children, and tuberculosis was the leading cause of adult mortality. The sanitary revolution, which began in England about the middle of the century, was the most important single factor in reducing the infant mortality rate. However, the reduction of infant mortality contributed in a major way to increasing the effective birth rate and, hence, the rate of population growth. The sanitary revolution was therefore one of the causes of today's worldwide population problem.

In discussing this phenomenon, care must be taken to avoid oversimplifying the relationships among the factors involved. On the one hand, the reduction of the infant mortality rate temporarily helps to produce a big difference between the birth and death rates of a society and results in rapid population growth (the so-called **demographic gap**). On the other hand, the control of infant mortality also appears to be necessary for cultures to accept population control. In a time when the infant mortality rate is high, a family needs to have a large number of children to ensure that one or two will survive to adulthood. This is not true in a time when the infant mortality rate is low. Therefore, although it may seem to be contradictory, the reduction of the infant mortality appears to be both a cause of the population problem and a necessity for population control.

In addition to affecting population growth, the sanitary revolution during the 19th century affected disease patterns in unexpected ways. The improvement in sanitation also was a fundamental cause of the appearance of epidemic paralytic poliomyelitis late in the 19th century. Before polio vaccine was introduced, epidemics of paralytic poliomyelitis tended to appear as a nation's infant mortality rate dropped, usually to about 70 or 80 deaths per 1000 live births. The relationship of paralytic poliomyelitis to improvement in sanitation seems counterintuitive, but it illustrates the importance of an ecologic perspective and offers another example of the iceberg phenomenon discussed earlier in this chapter.

The three polioviruses are enteric viruses transmitted by the fecal-oral route. People who have developed antibodies to all three types of poliovirus are immune to their potentially paralytic effects and thus show no symptoms or signs of clinical disease if they are exposed. Newborn infants have passive antibodies from their mothers, and these maternal antibodies normally prevent polioviruses from invading the central nervous system early in an infant's first year of life. Thus, exposure of a young infant to polioviruses rarely results in paralytic disease but instead leads to a subclinical (largely asymptomatic) infection, which causes the infant to produce his or her own active antibodies and cell-mediated immunity.

Although improved sanitation reduced the proportion of people who were infected with polioviruses, it also delayed, on the average, the time when an infant or child was exposed to the polioviruses. More children were exposed after they were no longer protected by maternal immunity, with the result that a higher percentage of them suffered from the paralytic form of the disease. *Epidemic* paralytic poliomyelitis, therefore, can be seen as an unwanted side effect of the sanitary revolution. Because members of the upper socioeconomic groups had the best sanitation, they were hit first and hardest, at least until polio vaccine became available.

A similar phenomenon occurred with hepatitis A, another virus spread by the fecal-oral route. In young children, hepatitis A is normally mild or asymptomatic. In adults, hepatitis A infection usually causes symptoms; rarely, it even causes death. Improved sanitation caused a delay in exposure to the hepatitis A virus, so that epidemic hepatitis A can also be seen as a side effect of improved sanitation.

Vector Control and Land Use Patterns

Sub-Saharan Africa is one of the more disturbing examples of how negative side effects can come from an attempt to do good. A successful effort was made to control the tsetse fly, which is the vector of African sleeping sickness in cattle and sometimes in people. Control of the vector enabled herders to keep larger numbers of cattle, and this in turn led to overgrazing. The overgrazed areas have been subjected to frequent droughts, and some have become dust bowls (Ormerod 1976).

River Dam Construction and Patterns of Disease

For a time, it was fashionable for western nations to build large river dams for developing countries to enable them to increase the amount of available farmland. During this period, the warnings of epidemiologists about potential negative side effects went unheeded, and as they predicted, the number of cases of schistosomiasis increased in the areas supplied by the Aswan High Dam after it was erected in Egypt. There was an increase in the number of cases of mosquito-borne diseases (malaria, Rift Valley fever, and dengue fever) after the main dam and several tributary dams of the Senegal River Project were built in western Africa, and cases of schistosomiasis also developed. Before the dams were erected in Senegal, during the dry season the sea would move far inland and mix with the fresh water, making the water too salty to support the larvae of the blood flukes responsible for schistosomiasis or the mosquitoes that transmit malaria, Rift Valley fever, and dengue fever (Patton 1992).

Synergism of Factors Predisposing to Disease

There may be a synergism between diseases or between factors predisposing to disease, so that each makes the other worse or more easily acquired.

Sexually transmitted diseases, especially those which produce open sores, predispose to the spread of type 1 human immunodeficiency virus (HIV-1). This is thought to be a major factor in countries where HIV-1 is usually spread through heterosexual activity.

AIDS, in turn, predisposes to the reactivation of previously latent infections, such as tuberculosis, and this is partly responsible for the current resurgence of tuberculosis in the USA.

The relationship between malnutrition and infection is also complex. Not only does malnutrition make infections worse, but infections make malnutrition worse. A malnourished child has more difficulty making antibodies and repairing tissue damage, and this makes him or her less resistant to infectious diseases and their complications. This is seen, for example, in the case of measles. In isolated societies without medical care or measles vaccine, if the children were well nourished, fewer than 1% of them would die from measles, whereas as many as 25% of malnourished children may die from measles infection or its complications.

There are several reasons why infection can make malnutrition worse. First, infection puts greater demands on the body, so the relative deficiency of nutrients becomes greater. Second, infection tends to reduce the appetite, and this, in turn, reduces the intake. Third, in the presence of infection, the diet is frequently changed to emphasize bland foods, which often are deficient in proteins and vitamins. And, finally, in cases of gastrointestinal infection, the food is rushed through the irritated bowel at a faster pace (causing diarrhea), and this allows fewer nutrients to be absorbed.

The final example of synergism concerns how ecologic and genetic factors can interact to produce new strains of influenza virus. Many people wonder why most of the new, epidemic strains of influenza virus have names from China (Hong Kong flu, Beijing flu, etc.). In rural China, pigs are in close contact with both ducks and people. Both the duck and human strains of influenza infect pigs, and in the pigs the genetic material of the two influenza strains may mix, producing a new variant of influenza. The new strains produced in the pigs can then infect human beings (Shope 1992). If the genetic changes in the influenza virus are major, this is called an **antigenic shift,** and the new virus may produce a worldwide outbreak (pandemic) of influenza. If the genetic changes in the influenza virus are minor, the phenomenon is called an **antigenic drift,** but this can still produce major regional outbreaks of influenza.

SUMMARY

Epidemiology is a branch of medical science that relates what is happening in the lives of individuals and society to the occurrence and distribution of diseases, injuries, and other health problems. As such, it is concerned with all of the biologic, social, behavioral, spiritual, and psychologic factors that may increase the frequency of disease or offer opportunities for prevention. Epidemiologic methods are often the first scientific methods applied to a new health problem in order to define its pattern in the population and to develop hypotheses about its causes and methods of transmission.

The contributions of epidemiologists to the medical sciences include the following: (1) investigating the modes of transmission of a new disease; (2) determining preventable causes of disease or injury; (3) determining the natural history of disease; (4) studying the biologic spectrum of disease; (5) evaluating community public health interventions; (6) setting disease control priorities; (7) improving the diagnosis, treatment, and prognosis of clinical disease; (8) improving health services research; and (9) providing expert testimony in courts of law.

Epidemiologists generally describe the natural history of a disease in terms of the host, agent, and environment, sometimes adding the vector as a fourth factor for consideration. In exploring the means to prevent a given disease, they look for possible behavioral, genetic, and immunologic causes, which are usually associated with the host. They also look for biologic and nutritional causes, which are usually considered under the agent. And they consider the environment in which the disease occurs. The acronym BEINGS is useful in remembering these categories of preventable causes of disease (see Table 1–1).

Epidemiology is concerned with human ecology and, in particular, the impact that health interventions have on disease patterns and on the environment. Knowing that the solution of one problem tends to create new problems, epidemiologists are particularly concerned to look for undesirable side effects of medical and public health interventions.

References Cited

American Academy of Pediatrics. Report of the Committee on Infectious Disease, 22nd ed. Elk Grove Village, Ill., American Academy of Pediatrics, 1991.

Berkman, L. F., and L. Breslow. Health and Ways of Living: The Alameda County Study. New York, Oxford University Press, 1983.

Berkman, L. F., and L. S. Syme. Social networks, host resistance, and mortality: a nine-year follow-up of Alameda County residents. American Journal of Epidemiology 109:186–204, 1979.

Bracken, M. B., et al. A randomized controlled trial of methylprednisolone or naloxone in the treatment of acute spinal cord injury. New England Journal of Medicine 322:1405–1411, 1990.

Burkitt, D. Lecture at Yale University School of Medicine, New Haven, Conn., April 28, 1989.

Centers for Disease Control and Prevention. Diphtheria outbreak: Russian Federation, 1990–1993. Morbidity and Mortality Weekly Report 42:840–841, 1993.

Centers for Disease Control and Prevention. Progress toward global eradication of poliomyelitis, 1988–1993. Morbidity and Mortality Weekly Report 43:499–503, 1994.

Connecticut Hospital Association. Impact of an aging population on utilization and bed needs of Connecticut hospitals. Connecticut Medicine 42:775–781, 1978.

Dawber, T. R., G. F. Meadors, and F. E. Moore, Jr. Epidemiologic approaches to heart disease: the Framingham Study. American Journal of Public Health 41:279–286, 1951.

Doll, R., and R. Peto. The Causes of Cancer. Oxford, Oxford University Press, 1981.

Evans, A. S. Subclinical epidemiology. American Journal of Epidemiology 125:545–555, 1987.

Feinstein, A. R. Clinical Epidemiology: The Architecture of Clinical Research. Philadelphia, W. B. Saunders Company, 1985.

Francis, T., Jr., et al. An evaluation of the 1954 poliomyelitis vaccine trials. American Journal of Public Health, April supplement, 1955.

Frankl, V. E. Man's Search for Meaning: An Introduction to Logotherapy. New York, Washington Square Press, 1963.

Gibbons, A. Where are "new" diseases born? Science 261:680–681, 1993.

Gordon, T. Mortality experience among the Japanese in the United States, Hawaii, and Japan. Public Health Reports 72:543–553, 1957.

Horwitz, R. I., D. V. Cicchetti, and S. M. Horwitz. A comparison of the Norris and Killip coronary prognostic indices. Journal of Chronic Disease 37:369–375, 1984.

Inlander, C., L. S. Levin, and E. Weiner. Medicine on Trial. Englewood Cliffs, New Jersey, Prentice-Hall, 1988.

Institute of Medicine. Emerging Infections. Washington, D. C., National Academy Press, 1992.

Jekel, J. F. Communicable disease control and public policy in the 1970s: hot war, cold war, or peaceful coexistence? American Journal of Public Health 62:1578–1585, 1972.

Jekel, J. F. Role of acquired immunity to *Treponema pallidum* in the control of syphilis. Public Health Reports 83:627–632, 1968.

Jekel, J. F., G. S. Zatlin, and O. F. Gay. *Corynebacterium diphtheriae* survives in a partly immunized group. Public Health Reports 85:310, 1970.

Kellock, B. The Fiber Man: The Life Story of Dr. Denis Burkitt. Belleville, Mich., Lion Publishing Corporation, 1985.

Keys, A. The peripatetic nutritionist. Nutrition Today 13(4):19–24, 1966.

Keys, A. Summary: coronary heart disease in seven countries. Circulation 42 (supplement 1): 186–198, 1970.

Kilbourne, E. D., and W. G. Smillie. Human Ecology and Public Health, 4th ed. London, Macmillan Company, 1969.

Kochanek, K. D., and B. L. Hudson. Advance report of final mortality statistics, 1992. Morbidity and Mortality Weekly Report 43 (supplement 6), 1995.

Langmuir, A. D. The surveillance of communicable diseases of national importance. New England Journal of Medicine 268: 182–192, 1963.

Lasch, E. [Former health officer in the Gaza Strip.] Personal communication, 1979.

Last, J. M. What is "clinical epidemiology"? Journal of Public Health Policy 9:159–163, 1988.

Leape, L. L., et al. Adverse events and negligence in hospitalized patients. Iatrogenics 1:17–21, 1991.

Longini, I. M., Jr., et al. Statistical inference for infectious diseases. American Journal of Epidemiology 128: 845–859, 1988.

Marks, J. S., T. J. Halpin, and W. A. Orenstein. Measles vaccine efficacy in children previously vaccinated at 12 months of age. Pediatrics 62:955–960, 1978.

Morris, J. N. The Uses of Epidemiology. Edinburgh, E. and S. Livingstone Ltd., 1967.

Ormerod, W. E. Ecological effect of control of African trypanosomiasis. Science 191:815–821, 1976.

Patton, C. L. [Professor of Epidemiology, Yale University School of Medicine, New Haven, Conn.] Personal communication, 1992.

Rappuoli, R., M. Perugini, and E. Falsen. Molecular epidemiology of the 1984–1986 outbreak of diphtheria in Sweden. New England Journal of Medicine 318:12–14, 1988.

Reed, D. The paradox of high risk of stroke in populations with low risk of coronary heart disease. American Journal of Epidemiology 131:579–588, 1990.

Sackett, D. L. Clinical epidemiology. American Journal of Epidemiology 89:125–128, 1969.

Sackett, D. L., R. B. Haynes, and P. Tugwell. Clinical Epidemiology: A Basic Science for Clinical Medicine, 2nd ed. Boston, Little, Brown, and Company, 1991.

Scriver, C. R. Human genes: determinants of sick populations and sick patients. Canadian Journal of Public Health 79:222–224, 1988.

Shope, R. [Professor of Epidemiology, Yale University School of Medicine, New Haven, Conn.] Personal communication, 1992.

Spitzer, W. O., A. R. Feinstein, and D. L. Sackett. What is a health care trial? Journal of the American Medical Association 233:161–163, 1975.

US Surgeon General. Smoking and Health. Public Health Service publication No. 1103. Washington, D. C., US Government Printing Office, 1964.

Selected Readings

Feinstein, A. R. Clinical Epidemiology: The Architecture of Clinical Research. Philadelphia, W. B. Saunders Company, 1985. [Complex, research-oriented clinical epidemiology.]

Fletcher, R. H., S. W. Fletcher, and E. H. Wagner. Clinical Epidemiology: The Essentials, 2nd ed. Baltimore, Williams and Wilkins Company, 1988. [Simple, clinically oriented epidemiology.]

Hennekens, C. H., and J. E. Buring. Epidemiology in Medicine. Boston, Little, Brown, and Company, 1987. [Classical epidemiology.]

Institute of Medicine. Emerging Infections. Washington, D. C., National Academy Press, 1992. [Medical ecology.]

Kelsey, J. L., W. D. Thompson, and A. S. Evans. Methods in Observational Epidemiology. New York, Oxford University Press, 1986. [Classical epidemiology.]

Levine, S., and A. Lilienfeld. Epidemiology and Health Policy. New York, Tavistock Publications, 1987. [Epidemiology and health services.]

Sackett, D. L., R. B. Haynes, and P. Tugwell. Clinical Epidemiology: A Basic Science for Clinical Medicine, 2nd ed. Boston, Little, Brown, and Company, 1991. [Moderately complex, clinically oriented epidemiology.]

CHAPTER TWO

EPIDEMIOLOGIC

DATA SOURCES AND

MEASUREMENTS

SOURCES OF HEALTH DATA

Epidemiologists rely on a variety of sources for obtaining data to analyze health-related rates and risks. Data for the rates used in epidemiologic studies can be discussed in terms of **denominator data,** which define the population at risk, and **numerator data,** which define the events or conditions of concern. Census statistics are generally used in the denominator, and statistics gathered from a wide range of health and disease surveys and registries are used in the numerator.

International Census and Health Data

Most nations collect vital statistics and census data, although the quality varies from country to country. Not all nations have effective disease reporting systems. Data regarding births and deaths usually come from national vital statistics reporting systems, which use recent census data for the denominators of rates. The collection of these data is a national responsibility, but most countries also report their data to the United Nations, which then publishes large compendia of national statistics, such as the *Demographic Yearbook* and the *World Health Statistics Annual.* These permit an investigator, for example, to compare the infant mortality rate in the USA with that in other countries. Ordinarily, these should be among the first sources sought for international health data.

US Census and Health Data

In the USA, most of the birth and death data, as well as many other types of health-related statistics, come from public data systems. The collection of data frequently involves **local, state, and national agencies.** For example, data on births, deaths, causes of death, fetal deaths, marriages, and divorces are initially collected locally by the registrar of vital statistics for the municipality or county involved. Birth certificates are completed by a physician or other birth attendant, and death certificates are completed by a physician, medical examiner, or coroner. The local jurisdiction then sends the original birth and death certificates to the state government, which is responsible for maintaining the permanent records. The state governments (often the state health departments) prepare summaries of these data. The states then send copies of the birth and death certificates to the **National Center for Health Statistics (NCHS),** a federal agency that prepares national summaries.

US Census

In the USA, the census is undertaken by the federal government. A complete population census, effective the first day of April, is done every year ending in 0. Thus, the most recent US census was for the year 1990. Population projections are used to estimate the size of the population between censuses and beyond the most recent census.

US Health Data Bases

In clinical epidemiology, health-related data usually come from examination of the patient, from clinical records, or from special questionnaires containing indexes that the investigator creates to answer specific research questions. In monitoring the health of large populations, however, as much use as possible is made of existing data bases, because this reduces the costs. The following are some of the most important ongoing US health data bases.

US Vital Statistics System. The federal government collates data on births, deaths, causes of death, fetal deaths, marriages, and divorces in the USA and its territories. These data are initially obtained by local and state representatives, as discussed above. Because analyses are, at best, only as good as the data on which they are based, great care is used to make the vital statistics system as accurate as possible. Nevertheless, there are many potential sources of error in these data, including unreported births and deaths, inaccurate death certificate diagnoses, and erroneous demographic and clinical data on the birth and death certificates. This is illustrated in the following discussion of the process followed to record the causes of death on death certificates in the USA.

When the numbers of deaths in the USA are categorized by cause of death and reported in government publications, the cause of death given is the **underlying cause of death,** not necessarily the **immediate cause of death.** If a person dies without medical attention or if foul play is suspected, a medical examiner or coroner decides what the cause of death is. Otherwise, the attending physician is responsible for completing the information on the cause of death.

The cause-of-death portion of the death certificate is shown in Fig. 2–1. If a person dies of pneumonia following a cerebral hemorrhage, the physician probably would put "pneumonia" on line (a) and "cerebral hemorrhage" on line (b). The cerebral hemorrhage would then be considered the underlying cause of death. If, however, the physician decided that the person's coexistent hypertension caused the cerebral hemorrhage, then "hypertension" would be put on line (c), and that would now become the underlying cause of death. On the other hand, the physician might decide that the hypertension was too mild to cause the stroke and enter "hypertension" under "Other Significant Conditions," in which case the cerebral hemorrhage would be the underlying cause of death.

The complications of deciding and recording the underlying cause of death do not end here. There are also complex rules used by the people who make the final determination about which numbered codes will be used for each death and about how to proceed with the coding if what they see does not fit certain

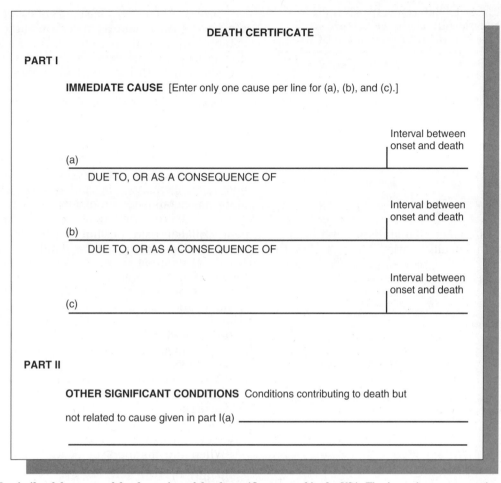

FIGURE 2–1. Facsimile of the cause-of-death portion of death certificates used in the USA. The form also requests information regarding autopsy, referral to a medical examiner or coroner, homicide investigation, and so forth.

expectations. In hospitals, death certificates are often completed at night by sleepy residents who are not the patients' primary physicians.

The death certificate data concerning the underlying cause of death are sufficiently accurate for purposes of setting many national priorities, but there is serious doubt about whether they are good enough for most epidemiologic research. Studies in the USA have suggested that 80–85% of diagnoses were either probably correct or at least were reasonable, while serious questions remained about the other 15–20% of diagnoses on death certificates (Moriyama 1966).

US Disease Reporting System.   Physicians, hospitals, clinics, and laboratories are required to report all cases of many types of infectious diseases to local and state health departments, who in turn report them to the Centers for Disease Control and Prevention (CDC), the federal agency in Atlanta, Georgia. Epidemiologic investigation is done, as needed, by representatives of the local, state, or federal public health agencies. Reporting requirements also apply to some noninfectious diseases, such as lead poisoning in children. Although there is considerable agreement among states regarding the diseases to be reported, some variation exists from state to state. Table 2–1 shows the infectious diseases which the

CDC monitors and which must be reported in most states.

Only a fraction of the disease cases are actually reported, but this fraction tends to vary with the seriousness of the disease. Most of the extremely serious diseases, such as paralytic poliomyelitis, tend to be recognized and reported, but even here epidemiologists must be wary of the numbers reported. For example, one study indicated that only about 58% of the cases of acquired immunodeficiency syndrome (AIDS) in South Carolina were reported (Conway et al. 1989). Part of the problem may be underdiagnosis, and part may be hesitancy to report something that could bring social isolation if discovered by others. Underreporting also applies to other serious infectious diseases, including tuberculosis.

Underreporting is even more frequent for the common and less serious diseases, such as chickenpox. This does not mean that the statistics on chickenpox have no value. As long as the proportion of cases reported remains constant, the pattern revealed by the reporting is useful, because it may reflect actual trends in the occurrence and distribution of the disease.

Studies of the National Center for Health Statistics (NCHS).   The NCHS carries out many important studies in the USA on topics such as the current levels

TABLE 2–1. Infectious Diseases That Are Reportable to the Centers for Disease Control and Prevention (CDC)

Acquired immunodeficiency syndrome (AIDS)	Pertussis (whooping cough)
Amebiasis	Plague
Aseptic meningitis	Poliomyelitis, paralytic
Botulism	Psittacosis
Brucellosis	Rabies, human
Chancroid	Rheumatic fever
Cholera	Rubella (German measles)
Diphtheria	Acquired rubella
Encephalitis	Congenital rubella syndrome
Primary	Salmonellosis
Postinfectious	Shigellosis
Gonorrhea	Syphilis
Granuloma inguinale	Total cases
Hepatitis	Primary and secondary cases
Hepatitis A	Congenital cases
Hepatitis B	Tetanus
Hepatitis C	Toxic shock syndrome
Hepatitis non-A, non-B	Trichinosis
Legionellosis	Tuberculosis
Leprosy	Tularemia
Leptospirosis	Typhoid fever
Lymphogranuloma venereum	Typhus fever
Malaria	Flea-borne (endemic, murine)
Measles (rubeola)	Tick-borne (Rocky Mountain spotted fever)
Meningococcal infections	Varicella (chickenpox)
Mumps	

Source: Centers for Disease Control and Prevention. Summary of notifiable diseases, United States, 1991. Morbidity and Mortality Weekly Report 40:57–63, 1991.

of illness and disability, the practice of preventive health services, the population's use of preventive measures and medical care, and the ways in which sampling methods and instrument design for health surveys can be improved. In addition, the NCHS is responsible for the following surveys that are done on an ongoing basis: (1) the **National Health Interview Survey (NHIS)** to determine yearly changes in acute and chronic illness and disability in the USA; (2) the **National Health and Nutrition Examination Surveys (NHANES),** in which a large probability sample of people in the USA participate in health interviews and physical examinations; (3) the **National Health Care Survey** to monitor the use of medical care in the USA; and (4) the **National Nursing Home Survey** of the numbers and types of people in nursing homes and their illnesses and disabilities (Jekel 1984).

Behavioral Risk Factor Surveillance System (BRFSS). In this system, ongoing surveys of behavioral risk factors in the US population are carried out by state health departments in cooperation with the CDC. When the BRFSS was begun in 1981 by the CDC, only a few states participated. By 1990, however, 45 states and the District of Columbia, which together account for 90% of the US population, were participating. In the behavioral surveys, a random sample of the population is interviewed by telephone and questioned about a variety of behaviors that have an effect on health and well-being, including exercise, smoking, obesity, alcohol consumption, drinking and driving, and use of automobile seat belts and child restraints.

Disease Registries. In some states and regions of the USA, government agencies or authorities have established special registries to record information concerning specific diseases, such as cancer, tuberculosis, and birth defects. For example, the oldest population-based cancer registry in the USA is the **Connecticut Tumor Registry,** which is maintained by the Connecticut State Department of Health and Addiction Services. The name of every Connecticut resident in whom cancer has been diagnosed since 1935 has been reported to the registry, and data have been collected from patient records, including extensive clinical, pathologic, and risk factor data. The state has established an extensive surveillance program to ensure complete reporting of cancers.

The Connecticut Tumor Registry and other such registries have been used for detailed studies of the trends of different types of cancer over time. They also have been employed to determine whether new practices are linked with cancer. For example, the Connecticut Tumor Registry was used to study whether the introduction of alum-adsorbed allergenic extracts used in "allergy shots" was associated with the subsequent occurrence of soft tissue sarcomas or other cancers at the injection sites (Jekel, Freeman, and Meigs 1978). Registries can be used to determine the effectiveness of preventive screening programs, because the rate of subsequent cancer deaths can be determined both in those who are screened and those who are not screened.

EPIDEMIOLOGIC MEASUREMENTS

Clinical phenomena must be measured accurately in order to develop and test hypotheses. Because epidemiologists study phenomena in populations, they need measures that summarize what has happened in populations. The fundamental epidemiologic measure is the frequency with which the events of interest, usually disease or death, occur in the population to be studied.

Frequency

Frequency can be measured in different ways, and it can be related to different denominators, depending on the purpose of the research and the availability of data. The concepts of incidence and prevalence are of fundamental importance to all of epidemiology.

Incidence (Incident Cases)

Incidence is the frequency (number) of new occurrences of disease, injury, or death—that is, the number of transitions from well to ill, from uninjured to injured, or from alive to dead—in the study population *during the time period being examined.* The term *incidence* is sometimes incorrectly used to mean incidence rate, so that to avoid confusion, it is sometimes better to use the term *incident cases* rather than incidence. Fig. 2–2 shows the annual

FIGURE 2–2. Incident cases of acquired immunodeficiency syndrome (AIDS) in the USA, by year of report, 1981–1992. The full height of a bar represents the number of incident cases of AIDS in a given year. The darkened portion of a bar represents the number of patients diagnosed with AIDS in a given year but known to be dead by the end of 1992. The clear portion represents the number of patients diagnosed in a given year and still living at the end of 1992. Statistics include cases from Guam, Puerto Rico, the US Pacific Islands, and the US Virgin Islands. (Source: Centers for Disease Control and Prevention. Summary of notifiable diseases, United States, 1992. Morbidity and Mortality Weekly Report 41:55, 1993.)

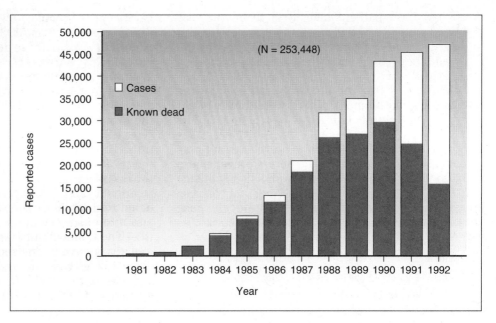

number of incident cases of AIDS by year of report for the USA, beginning in 1981.

Prevalence (Prevalent Cases)

Prevalence (sometimes called point prevalence) is the number of persons in a defined population who have a specified disease or condition *at a point in time,* usually the time a survey is done. The term *prevalence* is sometimes incorrectly used to mean prevalence rate, so to avoid confusion, the somewhat awkward term *prevalent cases* usually is preferable to the term *prevalence.*

Difference between Point Prevalence and Period Prevalence

In this text, when the term *prevalence* is used, **point prevalence** is meant (i.e., prevalence at a point in time). Some articles in the literature will discuss **period prevalence,** which refers to the number of persons who had the disease at any time during the specified time interval. Period prevalence is the sum of the point prevalence at the beginning of the interval plus the incidence during the interval. Because period prevalence is a mixed measure, composed of both point prevalence and incidence, it is not recommended for scientific work.

Illustration of Morbidity Concepts

The concepts of incidence (incident cases), point prevalence (prevalent cases), and period prevalence are illustrated in Fig. 2–3, based on a method devised by Dorn (1957). The figure provides data concerning eight persons who have a given disease in a defined population in which there is no emigration or immigration. Each person is assigned a case number (case no. 1 through case no. 8). A line begins when a person becomes ill and ends when that person either recovers or dies. The

symbol t_1 is the beginning and t_2 is the end of the study period (i.e., a calendar year).

In case no. 1, the patient was ill when the year began and was still alive and ill when it ended. In case nos. 2, 6, and 8, the patients were ill when the year began but recovered or died during the year. In case

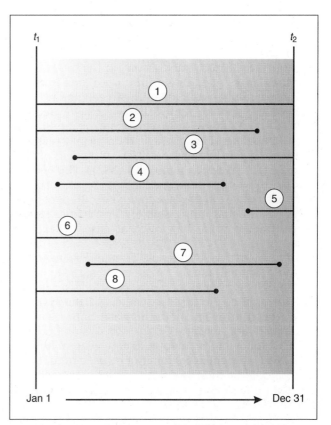

FIGURE 2–3. Illustration of several concepts in morbidity. Lines indicate when eight persons became ill (start of a line) and when they recovered or died (end of a line) between the beginning of a year (t_1) and the end of the same year (t_2). Each person is assigned a case number, which is circled in this figure.

nos. 3 and 5, the patients became ill during the year and were still alive and ill when the year ended. And in case nos. 4 and 7, the patients became ill during the year, and both of them either recovered or died during the year.

On the basis of this illustration, the following calculations can be made: There were four incident cases during the year (case nos. 3, 4, 5, and 7). The point prevalence at t_1 was four (the prevalent cases were nos. 1, 2, 6, and 8). The point prevalence at t_2 was three (case nos. 1, 3, and 5). The period prevalence is equal to the point prevalence at t_1 plus the incidence between t_1 and t_2, or here $4 + 4 = 8$. Note that whereas a case could only be an incident case once, a case could be a prevalent case at both time intervals (as with case no. 1 in this figure).

The Relationship between Incidence and Prevalence

Fig. 2–2 provides data concerning the incidence and prevalence of AIDS. In this figure, the full height of each bar shows the total number of new AIDS cases reported to the CDC each year from the time the disease was identified through 1992. The darkened part of each bar is the number of patients diagnosed with AIDS in a given year but known to be dead by December 31, 1992. The difference between the number diagnosed in a given year and the number known to be dead is shown in the clear part of the bars. Therefore, the clear part represents the prevalent cases.

The total number of incident cases of AIDS reported nationally to the CDC during the years since the appearance of the disease in 1981 is the **cumulative incidence.** According to reported data from the CDC, the cumulative incidence by December 31, 1991, was 206,392, and the number known to have died was 133,232 (see Centers for Disease Control and Prevention 1992). Therefore, if these data are correct, the number of prevalent cases of AIDS at the end of 1991 was 73,160 (206,392 minus 133,232). This is the number of people who were diagnosed with AIDS and were still alive. If people could be cured of AIDS (which is thus far not possible), they would have to be subtracted from the prevalent cases when they were cured.

Prevalence is the result of many factors: the periodic (annual) number of new cases, the immigration and emigration of persons with the disease, and the **duration of the disease,** which is defined as the time from the onset of the disease until death or healing occurs.

The following is an approximate general formula for prevalence which seldom can be used for detailed scientific estimation but which is conceptually important for understanding and predicting the **burden of disease** on a society:

$$\text{Prevalence} = \text{Incidence} \times (\text{Average}) \text{ Duration}$$

This simplified formula only works well if the incidence of the disease and its duration in individual persons are stable for an extended time. The impli-

cation of the formula, however, is that the prevalence of a disease, such as AIDS, could increase as a result of either (1) an increase in the yearly numbers of new cases or (2) an increase in the length of time that symptomatic patients survive before dying (or recovering, if that becomes possible). Note that AIDS is a clinical syndrome, and the discussion here is about the prevalence of AIDS rather than the prevalence of type 1 human immunodeficiency virus (HIV-1) infection. The incidence of AIDS continues to rise, the duration of life of persons with AIDS is increasing with the use of antiviral agents and other new methods of treatment and prophylaxis, and cases are being diagnosed earlier. Therefore, it is reasonable to expect an increase in the prevalent cases of AIDS in the USA. In fact, it appears from Fig. 2–2 that this has already occurred. The rapid increase in AIDS prevalence has led to an increase in the **burden of care** of patients, both in terms of demand on the medical care system and in terms of the dollar cost to society.

Risk
Definition of Risk

Epidemiologically, risk is the proportion of persons who are unaffected at the beginning of a study period but who undergo the risk event during the study period. The **risk event** may be death, disease, or injury, and the persons at risk for the event are called a **cohort,** which is a clearly defined group of persons studied over time. If an investigator follows all of the persons in a cohort over a several-year period, the denominator for the risk of an event will not change (unless persons are lost to follow-up). This means, for example, that in a cohort, the denominator for a 5-year risk of death or disease is the same as for the 1-year risk, because in both situations it is the number of persons entered at the beginning of the study.

Care is needed when applying actual risk estimates (which are derived from populations) to an individual patient. If death, disease, or injury occurs to an individual patient, for that person the risk is 100%. The best way to approach patients' questions regarding, say, the risk related to surgery is probably not to give them a number (e.g., "Your chances of survival are 99%"). They will worry about whether they will be the 1% or the 99%. Rather, it is better to put the risk of surgery in the context of the many other risks they may take frequently, such as those related to long automobile trips. The real issue is whether they are willing to take any risk in order to achieve the potential benefit of surgery. In other cases as well, it is generally better to interpret the risks of a negative outcome in terms other than numbers.

Limitations of the Concept of Risk

Often it is difficult to be sure of the correct denominator for a measure of risk. Who is truly at risk? This may be especially difficult to know for infectious diseases, unless the number of people in the population who lack protective antibodies is known. Ideally, in a risk or rate, only the **susceptible population**—i.e., those without antibody protection—would be counted in the denominator, but antibody levels are usually unknown. Therefore, as a compromise, the denominator will usually consist of either the total population of an area or those in an age group who probably lack antibodies.

The risk of death from an infectious disease, although appearing simple, is actually quite complex. This is because it is the product of many different proportions, as can be seen in Fig. 2–4. There are numerous **subsets of the population** to consider. Those who **die** of an infectious disease are a subset of those who are **ill,** who in turn are a subset of those who are **infected,** who are a subset of those who are **exposed** to the infection, who are a subset of those who are **susceptible,** who are a subset of the **total population.**

The proportion of the clinically ill persons who die is called the **case fatality ratio.** The higher the case fatality ratio, the more virulent the infection is. The proportion of infected persons who are clinically ill is often called the **pathogenicity** of the organism. The proportion of exposed persons who become infected is sometimes called the **infectiousness** of the organism, but this is also influenced by the condi-

tions of exposure. A full understanding of the epidemiology of an infectious disease would require knowledge of all the ratios shown in Fig. 2–4.

The concept of risk has other limitations. For example, assume that three different populations of the same size have the same overall risk of death (say, 10%) in the same year (e.g., from January 1 to December 31, 1994). Yet the deaths in the three populations may occur in very different patterns. Suppose that population A suffered a bad influenza epidemic in January (the beginning of the study year) and that most of those who died during the year died in the first month of the year. Suppose that the influenza epidemic did not hit population B until December (the end of the study year) so that most of the deaths occurred during the last month of the year. Finally, suppose that population C was not hit with the epidemic and that its deaths occurred (as usual) somewhat evenly throughout the year. The 1-year risk (10%) would be the same in all three populations, but the **force of mortality** would not be the same. The force of mortality would be strongest in population A, weakest in population B, and intermediate in population C. Because the measure of risk cannot distinguish between these three patterns, a more precise measure—namely, the rate—is usually used instead. After a brief description of rates, the discussion will return to this example.

Rates

Definition of Rate

A rate is the frequency (number) of events that occur in a defined time period, divided by the average population at risk. Because the midperiod population usually can be considered a good estimate of the average number of people at risk for the outcome during the time period, the midperiod population is often used as the denominator of a rate. The formal structure of a rate is described in the following equation:

$$\text{Rate} = \frac{\text{Numerator}}{\text{Denominator}} \times \text{Constant multiplier}$$

Risks and rates usually have values less than 1, and decimals are awkward to think about and discuss. It is particularly awkward to talk about fractions of a death (e.g., "one one-thousandth of a death per year"). Therefore, rates are usually multiplied by a **constant multiplier,** either 100 (to make a percentage) or else 1000, 10,000, or 100,000, in order to make the numerator larger than 1 and therefore easier to discuss (e.g., "one death per thousand people per year"). When a constant multiplier is used, both the numerator and the denominator are multiplied by the same number, so the value of the ratio is not changed.

An example in which a constant multiplier is customarily used is in the calculation of the crude death rate. In 1990, this rate in the USA was about

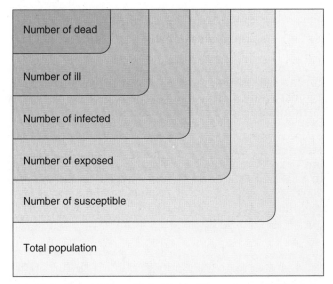

FIGURE 2–4. Illustration of why the death rate from an infectious disease is the product of many proportions. The formula may be thought of as follows:

$$\frac{\text{Number of dead}}{\text{Total population}} = \frac{\text{Number of dead}}{\text{Number of ill}} \times \frac{\text{Number of ill}}{\text{Number of infected}} \times \frac{\text{Number of infected}}{\text{Number of exposed}} \times \frac{\text{Number of exposed}}{\text{Number of susceptible}} \times \frac{\text{Number of susceptible}}{\text{Total population}}$$

If each of the five fractions to the right of the equal sign were 0.5, the persons who were dead would represent 50% of those who were ill; 25% of those who were infected; 12.5% of those who were exposed; 6.25% of those who were susceptible; and 3.125% of the total population.

0.0087 per year, but it is easier to multiply this by 1000 and express it as 8.7 deaths per 1000 individuals in the population per year. The general form for calculating the rate in this case is as follows:

$$\text{Crude death rate} = \frac{\substack{\text{Number of deaths} \\ \text{(defined place and time period)}}}{\substack{\text{Midperiod population} \\ \text{(same place and time period)}}} \times 1000$$

Rates can be thought of somewhat in the same way as velocity. It is possible to talk about **average rates** or average velocity for a period of time. The average velocity is obtained by dividing the miles traveled (e.g., 55) by the time required (e.g., 1 hour), in which case the car averaged 55 miles per hour. This does not mean that the car was traveling at exactly 55 miles per hour for every instant during that hour. In a similar manner, an average rate of an event (e.g., death) is the total number of events divided by the time (e.g., 1 year), but the population exposed to that event also has to be included (e.g., 12 deaths per 1000 people per year).

A rate, like a velocity, also can be thought of as describing reality at an instant in time, when it is sometimes called an **instantaneous death rate** or **hazard rate.** However, because death is a discrete event rather than a continuous function, instantaneous rates cannot be measured at an instant of time; they can only be estimated. The rates discussed in this book will be average rates unless otherwise mentioned.

The Relationship between Risk and Rate

In an example presented in an earlier section (see Limitations of the Concept of Risk), populations A, B, and C each had a 10% overall risk of death in the same year, but their patterns of death differed greatly. Fig. 2–5 shows the three different patterns and illustrates how in this example the concept of rate is superior to the concept of risk in demonstrating the differences.

Because most of the deaths in population A occurred before July 1, the midyear population of the cohort would be the smallest of the three, and the resulting death rate would be the highest (because the denominator is the smallest and the numerator is the same size for all three populations). In contrast, because most of the deaths in population B occurred at the end of the year, the midyear population of the cohort would be the largest of the three and the death rate would be the lowest. The number of deaths before July 1, and therefore the death rate for population C, would be intermediate between those of A and B. Thus, although the 1-year risk did not demonstrate differences in the **force of mortality,** rates were able to do so by reflecting more accurately the mortality experience of the three populations.

A rate is often used to estimate risk. A rate is a good approximation of risk if (1) the event in the numerator occurs only once per individual during the study interval; (2) the proportion of the population affected by the event is small, e.g., less than 5%; and (3) the time interval is relatively short. If the time interval is long or the percentage who die is large, the rate will be noticeably larger than the risk. If the event in the numerator occurs more than once during the study period—as can occur, for example, with ear infections or with asthmatic attacks—a related statistic called **incidence density** (see below) should be used instead of a rate.

Note that although the denominator for the 5-year risk is the same as for the 1-year risk in a cohort study, that would not be true for a rate. The denominator for a rate is constantly changing. It will

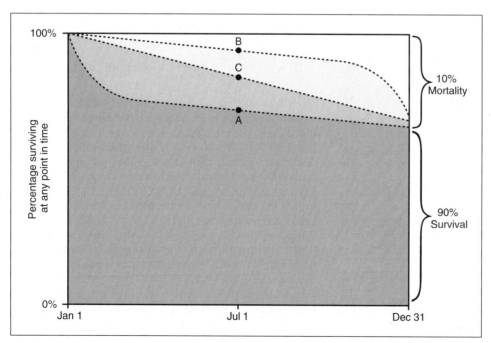

FIGURE 2–5. Illustration of circumstances under which the concept of rate is superior to the concept of risk. Assume that populations A, B, and C are three different populations of the same size; that 10% of each population died in a given year; and that most of the deaths in population A occurred early in the year, most of the deaths in population B occurred late in the year, and the deaths in population C were fairly evenly distributed throughout the year. In all three populations, the risk of death would be the same—that is, 10%—even though the patterns of death differed greatly. However, the rate of death, which is calculated using the midyear population as the denominator, would be the highest in population A, the lowest in population B, and intermediate in population C, reflecting the relative magnitude of the force of mortality in the three populations.

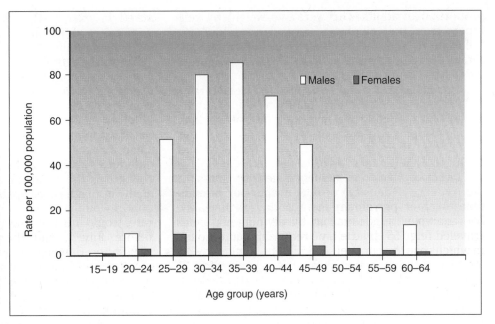

FIGURE 2–6. Incidence rate of acquired immunodeficiency syndrome (AIDS) per 100,000 adult population in the USA, by age and gender groups, 1992. Denominators for computing rates are based on 1992 population estimates from the US Bureau of Census. (Source: Centers for Disease Control and Prevention. Summary of notifiable diseases, United States, 1992. Morbidity and Mortality Weekly Report 41:55, 1993.)

decrease as some people die and others emigrate from the population. The denominator will increase as some immigrate and others are born into the population. In most real populations, all four of these changes are occurring at the same time. The rate reflects these changes by using the midperiod population as an estimate of the average population at risk.

Criteria for the Valid Use of the Term *Rate*

To be valid, a rate must meet certain criteria with respect to the correspondence between numerator and denominator. First, all the events counted in the numerator must have happened to persons in the denominator. Second, all of the persons counted in the denominator must have been at risk for the events in the numerator.

Before comparisons of rates can be made, the following must be true: The numerators for all groups being compared must be defined or diagnosed in the same way; the constant multipliers being used must be the same; and the time intervals must be the same. These criteria may seem obvious, but it is easy to overlook real problems related to comparisons over time and comparisons between populations.

Numerators may not be easy to compare if the quality of medical diagnosis differs over time. For example, in the late 1800s there was no diagnostic category called myocardial infarction, but many persons were dying of acute indigestion. By 1930, the situation was reversed: almost nobody died of acute indigestion, but many died of myocardial infarction. It might be tempting to say that the acute indigestion of the late 1800s was really myocardial infarction, but there is no proof that this is true.

Another example of problems in studying causes of disease over time relates to changes in the classification systems commonly used. In 1948, there was a major revision in the *International Classification of Diseases* (ICD), the international coding manual for

classifying diagnoses. This revision of the ICD was followed by sudden, major changes in the reported numbers and rates of many diseases.

Not only is it difficult to track changes in causes of death over time, but it is difficult to make fair comparisons of cause-specific rates of disease between populations, especially between countries. Different nations have different degrees of access to medical care and different levels in the quality of medical care available to most of those who are dying, as well as different styles of diagnosis. It is not easy to determine how much of any apparent difference in reported causes of death is real and how much of the difference is due to variation in diagnostic styles and quality of care around the time of death.

Definitions of Specific Types of Rates

Earlier in the chapter, the concepts of incidence (incident cases) and prevalence (prevalent cases) were discussed. Now that the concept of a rate has also been reviewed, it is appropriate to define different types of rates.

Incidence Rate. The incidence rate is calculated as the number of incident cases over a defined study period, divided by the population at risk at the midpoint of that study period. An incidence rate is usually expressed per 1000, per 10,000, or per 100,000 population. Fig. 2–6 shows the incidence rate of AIDS per 100,000 adult population in the USA, by age and gender groups, in 1992.

Prevalence Rate. The so-called prevalence rate is actually a proportion and not a rate. However, the term is in common use and will be used here to indicate the proportion (usually the percentage) of persons with a defined disease or condition at the time they are studied. For example, the 1990 Behavioral Risk Factor Survey reported that the prevalence rate of overweight status in adults—that is, the proportion of adults who were overweight by self-report over the telephone—ranged from 16.3% in Colorado to 27.4% in the District of Columbia, with the median state estimate being 22.7% (see Centers for Disease Control 1991).

Prevalence rates can be applied to risk factors as well as to diseases or other conditions. For example, in the USA in 1990, the prevalence rate of smoking among people who were 18 years of age or older varied from 16.8% in Utah to 29.1% in Kentucky and Michigan (see Centers for Disease Control 1991).

Incidence Density. Incidence density refers to the frequency (density) of new events per **person-time** (such as per person-months or person-years). For example, suppose that three patients were followed after tonsillectomy and adenoidectomy for recurrent ear infections. If one patient were followed for 13 months, one for 20 months, and one for 17 months and if 5 ear infections occurred to these three patients during this time, the incidence density would be 5 infections per 50 person-months of follow-up, or 10 infections per 100 person-months.

Incidence density is especially useful when the event of interest (such as colds, otitis media, or myocardial infarction) can occur in a person more than once during the period of study. For example, in a study of the impact of breast feeding versus formula feeding on the rate of infections in normal newborns in Copenhagen, Denmark, Rubin et al. (1990) recorded monthly data on the occurrence of infectious diseases and then compared them by month for the first year. Because infections often occurred more than once per month in infants and certainly more than once over the study year, the authors used incidence density to measure the frequency of the target events. Based on the results, they concluded that breast feeding made no apparent difference.

Special Issues Concerning the Use of Rates

Rates or risks are usually used to make one of three types of comparison. The first is a comparison of an observed rate (or risk) with a target rate (or risk). For example, the USA has set national health goals for the year 2000, including expected rates of various types of death, such as the infant mortality rate (see US Department of Health and Human Services 1990). When the final year 2000 statistics are published, the observed infant mortality rates for the nation and for subgroups will be compared with the target objectives set by the government.

A second type is the comparison of two different populations at the same time. This is probably the most common type. One approach involves comparing the rates of death or diseases in two different countries, states, or ethnic groups for the same year. Another approach involves comparing the results in treatment and control groups participating in randomized clinical trials (e.g., in trials of thrombolytic therapy versus a placebo following a myocardial infarction). A major research concern is to make sure that the two populations are similar and are mea-sured in exactly the same way, especially when comparing different countries, where diagnostic styles and quality may differ.

The third type consists of a comparison of the same population at two different time periods. This is used for studying time trends. Because there are also trends over time in the composition of a population (such as the increasing proportion of older people in the US population), adjustments must be made for such changes before concluding that there are real differences over time in the disease rates. Another concern is the change over time (usually improvement) in diagnostic capabilities.

Use of Crude Rates versus Specific Rates

There are three broad categories of rates: crude, specific, and standardized. Rates that apply to an entire population, without reference to any characteristics of the individuals in it, are **crude rates.** When a population is divided into more homogeneous subgroups based on a particular characteristic of interest (e.g., age, sex, race, risk factors, or comorbidity) and rates are calculated within these groups, the rates are called **specific rates** (age-specific rates, sex-specific rates, etc.). Standardized rates are discussed in the next section.

Crude rates are valid rates, but they are often misleading, which may be why they were named "crude." Here is a quick challenge: Try to guess which of the following three countries—Sweden, Colombia, and the USA—has the highest and which has the lowest crude death rate. Those who guessed that Colombia has the highest and Sweden the lowest crude death rate have the sequence exactly backward. The actual crude death rates and the corresponding life expectancy at birth are found in Table 2–2. Colombia has the lowest crude death rate and Sweden the highest, even though Colombia has the highest age-specific mortality rates and the shortest life expectancy, and Sweden has just the reverse.

This seeming anomaly occurs primarily because the crude death rates do not take age into account. For a population with a young age distribution, such as Colombia, the birth rate is likely to be relatively high and the crude death rate is likely to be relatively low, even though the age-specific death rates (ASDRs) for each age group may be fairly high. In contrast, for an older population, such as Sweden, a low crude birth rate and a high crude death rate would be expected. This is because age has such a profound

TABLE 2–2.   Crude Death Rate and Life Expectancy for Three Countries

Country (Year)	Crude Death Rate	Life Expectancy at Birth
Colombia (1985–1989)	7.4 per 1000	63.4 years
USA (1988)	8.8 per 1000	71.3 years
Sweden (1989)	10.8 per 1000	74.2 years

Source: United Nations. Demographic Yearbook. New York, United Nations, 1990.

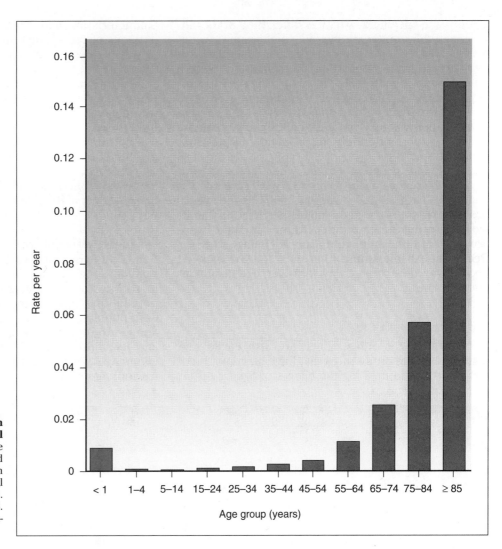

FIGURE 2–7. Age-specific death rates (ASDRs) for deaths from all causes in the USA, 1991. The figure illustrates the profound impact that age has on death rates. (Source of data: National Center for Health Statistics. Health, United States, 1993. Washington, D. C., US Government Printing Office, 1994.)

influence upon the force of mortality that an old population, even if it is relatively healthy, will inevitably have a high overall death rate, and vice versa. The huge impact that age has on death rates can be seen in Fig. 2–7, which shows data on ASDRs in the USA. As a general principle, investigators should never make comparisons of the risk of death or disease between populations without controlling for age. Sometimes other characteristics must be controlled for as well.

Why not avoid crude rates altogether and just use specific rates? There are many circumstances when it is not possible to use specific rates: (1) if the frequency of death or disease (i.e., the numerator) is not known for the subgroups of the population; (2) if the size of the subgroups (i.e., the denominator) is not known; or (3) if the number of persons at risk is too small to provide a stable estimate of the specific rate. However, if the number of persons at risk is large in each of the subgroups of interest, specific rates provide the most information, and they should be sought whenever possible.

Although the biasing effect of age can be controlled in several ways, the simplest (and usually the best) method is to calculate the ASDRs, so that the rates can be compared in similar age groups. The formula is as follows:

Age-specific death rate =
$$\frac{\substack{\text{Number of deaths to people} \\ \text{in a particular age group} \\ \text{(defined place and time period)}}}{\substack{\text{Midperiod population} \\ \text{(same age group, place, and} \\ \text{time period)}}} \times 1000$$

Crude death rates are the result of the ASDRs in each of the age groups, weighted by the relative size of each age group. The underlying formula for any summary rate is as follows:

$$\text{Summary rate} = \Sigma w_i r_i$$

where w_i represents the individual weights (proportions) of each age-specific group, and r_i represents the rates for the corresponding age group.

This formula is useful for understanding why crude rates can be misleading. In studies involving two populations, if the relative weights for the high and low age-specific death rates differ, the ASDRs will be mixed differently, and no fair comparison can be made. This general principle not only applies to demography and population epidemiology, where investigators are interested in comparing the rates of large groups, but also to clinical epidemiology, where investigators may wish to compare the risks or rates of two patient groups that have different proportions of severely ill, moderately ill, and mildly ill patients (Chan et al. 1988).

A similar problem occurs when investigators interested in measuring the quality of care try to compare death rates in various hospitals. To make fair comparisons among hospitals, some adjustment has to be made for differences in the types and severity of illness in the people being treated. Otherwise, the hospitals that care for the sickest people would be at an unfair disadvantage in such a comparison.

Standardization of Death Rates

Standardized rates, which are also called **adjusted rates,** are crude rates that have been modified (adjusted) to control for the effects of age or other characteristics and thereby allow for valid comparisons of rates. Standardization is usually applied to death rates but may be used to adjust any type of rate.

In the case of death rates, the comparison of many age-specific death rates (ASDRs) can become unwieldy. Therefore, to obtain a summary death rate that is free from age bias, investigators can age-standardize (age-adjust) the crude death rates by a direct or an indirect method.

Direct Standardization. Direct standardization is the most commonly used method to remove the biasing effect of the differing age structure of different populations. In the direct method of standardization, the ASDRs of the two (or more) populations to be compared are applied to a single standard population. This is done by multiplying each ASDR from a population to be compared by the number of persons in the corresponding age group in the **standard population.** Because the age structure of the standard population is the same for all of the death rates applied to it, the distorting effect of having different age distributions in the different real populations is eliminated. Overall death rates can then be compared without age bias.

BOX 2–1. Direct Standardization of Crude Death Rates of Two Populations, Using the Averaged Weights as the Standard Population (Fictitious Data)

Part 1. Calculation of the crude death rates:

	Population A			Population B		
Age Group	Population Size	Age-Specific Death Rate	Expected Number of Deaths	Population Size	Age-Specific Death Rate	Expected Number of Deaths
Young	1,000 ×	0.001 =	1	4,000 ×	0.002 =	8
Middle-aged	5,000 ×	0.010 =	50	5,000 ×	0.020 =	100
Older	4,000 ×	0.100 =	400	1,000 ×	0.200 =	200
Total	10,000		451	10,000		308
Crude death rate	451/10,000 = 4.51%			308/10,000 = 3.08%		

Part 2. Direct standardization of the above crude death rates, with the two populations combined to form the standard weights:

	Population A			Population B		
Age Group	Population Size	Age-Specific Death Rate	Expected Number of Deaths	Population Size	Age-Specific Death Rate	Expected Number of Deaths
Young	5,000 ×	0.001 =	5	5,000 ×	0.002 =	10
Middle-aged	10,000 ×	0.010 =	100	10,000 ×	0.020 =	200
Older	5,000 ×	0.100 =	500	5,000 ×	0.200 =	1,000
Total	20,000		605	20,000		1,210
Standardized death rate	605/20,000 = 3.03%			1,210/20,000 = 6.05%		

The standard population may be any real (or any realistic) population, and it is often a larger population of which the populations to be compared are a part. Thus, the death rates of two cities in a state can be compared using the state's population as the standard population. Likewise, the death rates of states may be standardized using the population of the USA.

The direct method shows the total number of deaths that *would have occurred* in the standard population *if* the ASDRs of the individual populations had occurred there. The total expected number of deaths from each of the comparison populations is then divided by the standard population to give a standardized "crude" death rate, which may be compared with any other death rate standardized using the same standard population. The direct method may be applied to compare incidence rates of disease or injury as well as deaths.

Standardized rates are *fictitious*. They are only "what if" rates, but they do allow investigators to make fairer comparisons of death rates than would be possible with crude rates. A simplified example is shown in Box 2–1, where two populations, A and B, are divided into "young," "middle-aged," and "older" people, and the ASDR for each age group in population B is twice as high as that for each age group in population A. Population A has a higher overall crude death rate (4.51%) than population B (3.08%), despite the fact that the ASDRs in B are twice those in A. After the death rates are standardized (here the standard population is simply the sum of the two individual populations), the adjusted death rate for population B correctly reflects the fact that its ASDRs are twice as high as those of population A.

Indirect Standardization. Indirect standardization is used if ASDRs are not available in the population whose crude death rate is to be adjusted. It is also used if the population to be standardized is small, which makes the ASDRs statistically unstable. The indirect method uses **standard rates** and applies them to the known age (or other stratum) groups in the population to be standardized.

Suppose, for example, that an investigator wanted to see if the death rates for male workers in a particular company were similar to or greater than the death rates for males in the US population. To start, the investigator would need the observed crude death rate and the ASDRs for US males for a similar year. These would serve as the **standard death rates.** Next, the investigator would determine the number of workers in each of the same age categories that were used in the US male population. Then the investigator would determine the observed total deaths for 1 year for all of the male workers in the company.

The first step in calculation is to multiply the standard death rates from each age group in the standard population times the number of workers in the corresponding age groups in the company. This gives the number of deaths that would be expected in

each age group of workers if they had the death rates of the standard population. The expected numbers of worker deaths for the various age groups are then added to obtain the total number of deaths that would be expected if the ASDRs in the company were the same as those in the standard population. Next, the *observed* total deaths among the workers is divided by the *expected* total deaths among the workers to obtain a ratio called the **standardized mortality ratio** (SMR). Finally, the SMR is multiplied by 100 to get rid of fractions, so that the expected mortality rate among the standard population equals 100. If the employees in this example had an SMR of 140, it means that their mortality was 40% greater than was expected on the basis of the ASDRs of the standard population. (For further discussion, see Chan et al. 1988.) An illustration of indirect standardization is presented in Box 2–2.

Cause-Specific Rates

Whereas creating age-specific or sex-specific death rates makes the denominators of the rates homogeneous, cause-specific death rates make the numerators homogeneous according to diagnosis. Comparing cause-specific death rates over time or between countries is often risky, because there may be differences in diagnostic styles or efficiency between countries. For example, in countries with inadequate medical care, 10–20% of deaths may be signed out as "symptoms, signs, and ill-defined conditions." This also happens among people who die without adequate medical care in the USA (Becker et al. 1990).

Cause-specific death rates have the following general form:

$$\text{Cause-specific death rate} = \frac{\begin{array}{c}\text{Number of deaths due to}\\ \text{a particular cause}\\ \text{(defined place and}\\ \text{time period)}\end{array}}{\begin{array}{c}\text{Midperiod population}\\ \text{(same place and time period)}\end{array}} \times 1000$$

Table 2–3 provides data on the leading causes of death in the USA for 1950 and 1991, as reported by the National Center for Health Statistics (NCHS) based on the underlying cause of death indicated on death certificates. These data are rarely accurate enough for epidemiologic studies of causal factors (Burnand and Feinstein 1992), but they are useful for understanding how important the different disease groups are relative to each other. They are also useful for studying trends in causes of death over time. For example, it appears that the rates for deaths due to diseases of the heart and deaths due to cerebrovascular disease have been dropping steadily for approximately two decades, whereas the rate for deaths due to malignant neoplasms has remained approximately constant and the rate for deaths due to AIDS has been rising rapidly.

BOX 2–2. Indirect Standardization of the Crude Death Rate for Males in a Company, Using the Age-Specific Death Rates for Males in a Standard Population (Fictitious Data)

Part 1. Beginning data:

	Males in the Standard Population				Males in the Company		
Age Group	Proportion of Standard Population	Age-Specific Death Rate	Observed Death Rate		Number of Workers	Age-Specific Death Rate	Observed Number of Deaths
Young	0.40	× 0.0001 =	0.00004		2,000	× ? =	?
Middle-aged	0.30	× 0.0010 =	0.00030		3,000	× ? =	?
Older	0.30	× 0.0100 =	0.00300		5,000	× ? =	?
Total	1.00		0.00334		10,000		48

Observed death rate 0.00334, or 334/100,000 48/10,000, or 480/100,000

Part 2. Calculation of the expected death rate, using indirect standardization of the above rates and applying the age-specific death rates from the standard population to the numbers of workers in the company:

	Males in the Standard Population				Males in the Company		
Age Group	Proportion of Standard Population	Age-Specific Death Rate	Observed Death Rate		Number of Workers	Standard Death Rate	Expected Number of Deaths
Young	0.40	× 0.0001 =	0.00004		2,000	× 0.0001 =	0.2
Middle-aged	0.30	× 0.0010 =	0.00030		3,000	× 0.0010 =	3.0
Older	0.30	× 0.0100 =	0.00300		5,000	× 0.0100 =	50.0
Total	1.00		0.00334		10,000		53.2

Expected death rate 53.2/10,000, or 532/100,000

Part 3. Calculation of the standardized mortality ratio (SMR):

$$SMR = \frac{\text{Observed death rate for males in the company}}{\text{Expected death rate for males in the company}} \times 100$$

$$= \frac{0.00480}{0.00532} \times 100$$

$$= (0.90)(100) = 90$$

= Males in the company actually had a death rate that was only 90% of the value that would be expected, based on the death rates in the standard population

Commonly Used Rates That Reflect Maternal and Infant Health

Many of the rates commonly used in public health, especially the infant mortality rate, reflect the health of mothers and infants. The definitions used for terms relating to the reproductive process are especially important to have clearly in mind.

Definitions of Terms

The official international definition of a **live birth** is the delivery of a product of conception that shows any sign of life after complete removal from the mother. A **sign of life** may consist of a breath or a cry, any spontaneous movement, a pulse or a heartbeat, or pulsation of the umbilical cord.

Fetal deaths are categorized as early, intermediate, or late fetal deaths. An **early fetal death,** which is better known as a **miscarriage,** occurs when a dead fetus is delivered within the first 20 weeks of gestation. According to international agreements, an **intermediate fetal death** is one in which a dead fetus is delivered between 20 and 28 weeks of gestation. A fetus born dead at 28 weeks of gestation or greater is a **late fetal death,** better known as a **stillbirth.** Because it is easier just to fill out a fetal death certificate than both a birth certificate and a death certificate for an infant, if there is any doubt about the presence of signs of life, an infant barely alive at birth might be treated as a late fetal death. It is not known how often this happens, nor is it known how many fetuses delivered by induced abortion have any sign of life after birth.

An **infant death** is the death of a live-born child before that child's first birthday.

Definitions of Specific Types of Rates

Crude Birth Rate. The crude birth rate is the number of live births divided by the midperiod population:

$$\text{Crude birth rate} = \frac{\substack{\text{Number of live births} \\ \text{(defined place and time period)}}}{\substack{\text{Midperiod population} \\ \text{(same place and time period)}}} \times 1000$$

Crude Death Rate and Age-Specific Death Rate. These are discussed earlier in this chapter (see Use of Crude Rates versus Specific Rates, above).

Infant Mortality Rate. Because the health of infants is unusually sensitive to maternal health practices (especially maternal use of tobacco, alcohol, and illegal drugs), environmental and nutritional factors, and the quality of health services, the infant

mortality rate (IMR) is often used as an overall index of the health status of a nation. The IMR has the added advantages of being available for most countries and of being age-specific. Moreover, both the numerator and the denominator of the IMR are obtained from the same kind of data collection system (vital statistics reporting), so that in areas where infant deaths are reported, births are also likely to be reported, and in areas where reporting is poor, this should affect births and deaths almost equally. The formula for the IMR is as follows:

$$\text{Infant mortality rate} = \frac{\substack{\text{Number of deaths to infants} \\ \text{under 1 year of age} \\ \text{(defined place and time period)}}}{\substack{\text{Number of live births} \\ \text{(same place and time period)}}} \times 1000$$

Most infant deaths occur in the first month (in fact, in the first week) of life and are due to prematurity and the resulting immaturity, which often lead to respiratory failure. Some infant deaths in the first month are due to congenital anomalies.

A subtle point, which is seldom of concern in large populations, is that for any given year—for example, 1991—there is not an exact correspondence between the numerator and denominator of the IMR. This is because some of the infants born in 1991 will not die until 1992, and some of the infants dying in 1991 were born in 1990. Although this does not ordinarily influence the rate of a large population, it could do so in a small population. For studies of small populations, taking the average of 3 or 5 years is better. For detailed epidemiologic studies of causation, it is necessary to link each infant death with the corresponding birth.

Neonatal and Postneonatal Mortality Rates. Epidemiologists distinguish between neonatal and postneonatal mortality. Neonatal deaths are those occurring in infants under 28 days of age, whereas postneonatal deaths are those occurring in infants from the 28th day of life to the first birthday. The formulas for the rates are as follows:

$$\text{Neonatal mortality rate} = \frac{\substack{\text{Number of deaths to infants} \\ \text{under 28 days of age} \\ \text{(defined place and time period)}}}{\substack{\text{Number of live births} \\ \text{(same place and time period)}}} \times 1000$$

$$\text{Postneonatal mortality rate} = \frac{\substack{\text{Number of deaths to infants} \\ \text{between 28 and 365 days of age} \\ \text{(defined place and time period)}}}{\substack{\text{Number of} \\ \text{live births} \\ \text{(same place and} \\ \text{time period)}} - \substack{\text{Number of} \\ \text{neonatal deaths} \\ \text{(same place and} \\ \text{time period)}}} \times 1000$$

The formula for the neonatal mortality rate is fairly obvious, because it is so close to that for the infant mortality rate. For the postneonatal mortality rate,

TABLE 2–3.   Age-Adjusted Death Rates for Selected Causes of Death in the USA, 1950 and 1991

Cause of Death	Age-Adjusted Death Rate per 100,000 per Year	
	1950	1991
Diseases of the heart	307.2	148.2
Malignant neoplasms	125.3	134.5
Unintentional injuries	57.5	31.0
Cerebrovascular disease	88.6	26.8
Chronic obstructive pulmonary disease	4.4	20.1
Influenza and pneumonia	26.2	13.4
Diabetes	14.3	11.8
Suicide	11.0	11.4
Acquired immunodeficiency syndrome (AIDS)	—	11.3
Homicide	5.4	10.9
Chronic liver disease and cirrhosis	8.5	8.3
Other causes	192.1	86.0
All causes	840.5	513.7

Source: National Center for Health Statistics. Health, United States, 1993. Washington, D. C., US Government Printing Office, 1994.

however, investigators must keep in mind the criteria for a valid rate, especially the criterion that all those in the denominator must be at risk for the numerator. Infants born alive are not at risk for dying in the postneonatal period if they die during the neonatal period. Therefore, the correct denominator for the postneonatal mortality rate is the number of live births *minus* the number of neonatal deaths. When the number of neonatal deaths is small, however, as is true in the USA at this time (fewer than 7 per 1000 live births), there is little difference between the two formulas, and the following approximate formula is perfectly adequate for almost all purposes:

$$\text{Approximate postneonatal mortality rate} = \text{Infant mortality rate} - \text{Neonatal mortality rate}$$

As a rough general rule, the neonatal mortality rate provides a better reflection of the quality of medical services and of maternal prenatal behavior (smoking, alcohol, drugs, etc.), whereas the postneonatal mortality rate offers a better reflection of the quality of the home environment.

Perinatal Mortality Rate and Ratio. The use of the infant mortality rate has its limitations, not only because the probable causes of death change rapidly as the time from birth progresses but also because the number of infants born alive is influenced by the effectiveness of prenatal and perinatal care. It is conceivable that an improvement in care could actually increase the infant mortality rate; this would occur, for example, if the improvement keeps very sick fetuses alive long enough to be born, so that they die after being born and are counted as infant deaths rather than as stillbirths. In order to avoid this problem, the **perinatal mortality rate** was developed. This rate is defined slightly differently from country to country. In the USA, it is defined as follows:

Perinatal mortality rate =

$$\frac{\text{Number of stillbirths (defined place and time period)} + \text{Number of deaths to infants under 7 days of age (same place and time period)}}{\text{Number of stillbirths (same place and time period)} + \text{Number of live births (same place and time period)}} \times 1000$$

Perinatal means "around the time of birth." In the formula shown here, stillbirths are included in the numerator to capture the deaths around the time of birth. The stillbirths are included in the denominator because of the criteria for a valid rate and, more specifically, because all of those fetuses who reach the 28th week of gestation are at risk for being late fetal deaths, and their number is equal to those who die before birth (the stillbirths) and those who are born alive (the live births).

An approximation of the perinatal mortality rate is the **perinatal mortality ratio,** in which the denominator does not include the stillbirths. In another

variation, the numerator uses neonatal deaths instead of deaths under 7 days of life (hebdomadal deaths). The primary use of the perinatal mortality rate is to evaluate progress in prenatal and perinatal care of pregnant women and their infants.

Maternal Mortality Rate. Although pregnancy is generally considered a "normal" biologic process, there is no question that it puts considerable strain on the pregnant woman and places her at risk for a number of hazards that she would not usually face otherwise, such as hemorrhage, infection, and toxemia of pregnancy. Pregnancy complicates the course of other conditions, such as heart disease, diabetes, and tuberculosis. Therefore, a useful measure of the progress of a nation in providing adequate nutrition and medical care for pregnant women is the maternal mortality rate (MMR), calculated as follows:

Maternal mortality rate =

$$\frac{\text{Number of pregnancy-related deaths (defined place and time period)}}{\text{Number of live births (same place and time period)}} \times 100,000$$

Note that the equation is based on the number of **pregnancy-related (puerperal) deaths.** The death of a pregnant woman or of a woman who was recently delivered is not pregnancy-related in the case of an automobile injury, homicide, and so forth, but care must be taken here. For example, was a suicide pregnancy-related, or was a cancer made worse by the pregnancy?

Technically, the denominator of the equation should be the number of pregnancies rather than live births, but this number is not easy to obtain in any country, and therefore the number of live births is used instead. The constant multiplier used is usually 100,000, because in recent decades the MMR in many countries has dropped below 1 per 10,000 live births. For example, the MMR for the USA in 1987 was 6.6 per 100,000 live births, although the rates were higher for Hispanics (8.0) and blacks (14.2) than for whites (5.1) (see National Center for Health Statistics 1990).

SUMMARY

Many of the data for epidemiologic studies are collected routinely by various levels of government and are made available to local, state, federal, and international groups. The USA and most other countries undertake a complete population census on a periodic basis. The census in the USA, for example, is taken every 10 years, effective April 1 of every year ending in 0.

Community-wide epidemiologic measurement depends on accurate determination and reporting of (1) numerator data, especially events such as births, deaths, becoming ill (incident cases), and recovery from illness; and (2) denominator data, especially the census. Prevalence data are determined by surveys. These types of data then are used to create community rates and ratios for planning and evaluating

---

BOX 2–3.   Definitions of Basic Epidemiologic Concepts and Measurements

Incidence (incident cases): The frequency (number) of new occurrences of disease, injury, or death—that is, the number of transitions from well to ill, from uninjured to injured, or from alive to dead—in the study population during the time period being examined.

Point prevalence (prevalent cases): The number of persons in a defined population who had a specified disease or condition at a particular point in time, usually the time a survey was done.

Period prevalence: The number of persons who had a specified disease at any time during a specified time interval. Period prevalence is the sum of the point prevalence at the beginning of the interval plus the incidence during the interval. Because period prevalence combines incidence and prevalence, it must be used with extreme care.

Incidence density: The frequency (density) of new events per **person-time** (such as person-months or person-years). Incidence density is especially useful when the event of interest (such as colds, otitis media, or myocardial infarction) can occur in a person more than once during the period of study.

Cohort: A clearly defined group of persons who are studied over a period of time to determine the incidence of death, disease, or injury.

Risk: The proportion of persons who are unaffected at the beginning of a study period but who undergo the **risk event** (death, disease, or injury) during the study period.

Rate: The frequency (number) of new events that occur in a defined time period, divided by the average population at risk. Often, the midperiod population is used as the average number of persons at risk (see Incidence rate, below). Because a rate is almost always less than 1.0 (unless everybody dies or has the risk event), a **constant multiplier** is used to increase both the numerator and the denominator to make the rate easier to think about and discuss.

Incidence rate: A rate calculated as the number of incident cases (see above) over a defined study period, divided by the population at risk at the midpoint of that study period. Rates of the occurrence of births, deaths, and new diseases are all forms of an incidence rate.

Prevalence rate: The proportion (usually the percentage) of a population that has a defined disease or condition at a particular point in time.

Crude rates: Rates that apply to an entire population, without reference to any characteristics of the individuals in it. Crude rates are generally not useful for comparisons, because populations may differ greatly in composition, particularly with respect to age.

Specific rates: Rates that are calculated after a population has been categorized into groups with a particular characteristic. Examples include age-specific rates and sex-specific rates. Specific rates are generally needed for valid comparisons.

Standardized (adjusted) rates: Crude rates that have been modified (adjusted) to control for the effects of age or other characteristics and thereby allow for valid comparisons of rates.

Direct standardization: The preferred method of standardization if the specific rates come from large populations and the needed data are available. The direct method of standardizing death rates, for example, applies the age distribution of a population—the **standard population**—to the actual age-specific death rates of the different populations to be compared. This removes the bias that would occur if an old population was compared to a young population.

Indirect standardization: The method of standardization used either when the populations to be compared are small (so that age-specific death rates are unstable) or when age-specific death rates are not available from one or more populations but data concerning the age distribution and the crude death rate are available. Here **standard death rates** (from the standard population) are applied to the corresponding age groups in the different population or populations to be studied. The result is an "expected" (standardized crude) death rate for each population under study. These "expected" values are those which would have been expected if the standard death rates had been valid for the populations under study.

Standardized mortality ratio (SMR): The **observed crude death rate** divided by the **expected crude death rate.** The SMR is generally multiplied by 100, with the standard population having a value of 100. If the SMR is greater than 100, the **force of mortality** is higher in the study population than in the standard population. If the SMR is less than 100, the force of mortality is lower in the study population than in the standard population.

---

health progress. The collection of such health data is the responsibility of individual countries, and most countries report their data to the United Nations, which then publishes large compendia such as the *Demographic Yearbook* and the *World Health Statistics Annual.*

In large-scale population studies, as much use as possible is made of existing data bases. Some of the most important ongoing health data bases in the USA are the US Vital Statistics System, the US Disease Reporting System, the studies of the National Center for Health Statistics (NCHS), and disease registries, such as the Connecticut Tumor Registry.

In contrast to the types of data above, the data in clinical epidemiologic studies usually come from examination of patients; laboratory, x-ray, and special studies; clinical records; or special questionnaires.

Box 2–3 offers definitions of the basic epidemiologic concepts and measurements discussed in this chapter, while Box 2–4 lists the equations for the most commonly used population rates.

To be valid, a rate must meet certain criteria with respect to the denominator and numerator. First, all of the people counted in the denominator must have been at risk for the events counted in the numerator. Second, all of the events counted in the numerator must have happened to people included in the denominator. Moreover, before comparisons of rates can be made, the following must be true: the numerators for all groups being compared must be defined or diagnosed in the same way; the constant multipliers being used must be the same; and the time intervals being studied must be the same.

BOX 2–4. Equations for the Most Commonly Used Population Data

(1) Crude birth rate $= \dfrac{\text{Number of live births (defined place and time period)}}{\text{Midperiod population (same place and time period)}} \times 1000$

(2) Crude death rate $= \dfrac{\text{Number of deaths (defined place and time period)}}{\text{Midperiod population (same place and time period)}} \times 1000$

(3) Age-specific death rate $= \dfrac{\text{Number of deaths to people in a particular age group (defined place and time period)}}{\text{Midperiod population (same age group, place, and time period)}} \times 1000$

(4) Cause-specific death rate $= \dfrac{\text{Number of deaths due to a particular cause (defined place and time period)}}{\text{Midperiod population (same place and time period)}} \times 1000$

(5) Infant mortality rate $= \dfrac{\text{Number of deaths to infants under 1 year of age (defined place and time period)}}{\text{Number of live births (same place and time period)}} \times 1000$

(6) Neonatal mortality rate $= \dfrac{\text{Number of deaths to infants under 28 days of age (defined place and time period)}}{\text{Number of live births (same place and time period)}} \times 1000$

(7) Postneonatal mortality rate $= \dfrac{\text{Number of deaths to infants between 28 and 365 days of age (defined place and time period)}}{\text{Number of live births (same place and time period)} - \text{Number of neonatal deaths (same place and time period)}} \times 1000$

(8) Approximate postneonatal mortality rate $= \text{Infant mortality rate} - \text{Neonatal mortality rate}$

(9) Perinatal mortality rate $= \dfrac{\text{Number of stillbirths (defined place and time period)} + \text{Number of deaths to Infants under 7 days of age (same place and time period)}}{\text{Number of stillbirths (same place and time period)} + \text{Number of live births (same place and time period)}} \times 1000$

(10) Maternal mortality rate $= \dfrac{\text{Number of pregnancy-related deaths (defined place and time period)}}{\text{Number of live births (same place and time period)}} \times 100{,}000$

References Cited

Becker, T. M., et al. Symptoms, signs, and ill-defined conditions: a leading cause of death among minorities. American Journal of Epidemiology 131:664–668, 1990.

Burnand, B., and A. R. Feinstein. The role of diagnostic inconsistency in changing rates of occurrence for coronary heart disease. Journal of Clinical Epidemiology 45:929–940, 1992.

Centers for Disease Control. Behavioral risk factor surveillance, 1986–1990. Morbidity and Mortality Weekly Report 40(SS-4): 1–47, 1991.

Centers for Disease Control and Prevention. The second 100,000 cases of acquired immunodeficiency syndrome: United States, June 1981 to December 1991. Morbidity and Mortality Weekly Report 41:28–29, 1992.

Chan, C. K., et al. The value and hazards of standardization in clinical epidemiologic research. Journal of Clinical Epidemiology 41:1125–1134, 1988.

Conway, G. A., et al. Underreporting of AIDS cases in South Carolina, 1986 and 1987. Journal of the American Medical Association 262:2859–2863, 1989.

Dorn, H. F. A classification system for morbidity concepts. Public Health Reports 72:1043–1048, 1957.

Jekel, J. F. Publications of the National Center for Health Statistics and their relevance for chronic disease. Journal of Chronic Disease 37:681–688, 1984.

Jekel, J. F., D. H. Freeman, and J. W. Meigs. A study of trends in upper arm soft tissue sarcomas in Connecticut following the introduction of alum-adsorbed allergenic extracts. Annals of Allergy 40:28–31, 1978.

Moriyama, I. M. Inquiring into the diagnostic evidence supporting medical certifications of death. *In* Lilienfeld, A. M., and A. J. Gifford, eds. Chronic Diseases and Public Health. Baltimore, Johns Hopkins University Press, 1966.

National Center for Health Statistics. Health, United States, 1989. Publication No. (PHS)90-1232. Washington, D. C., US Government Printing Office, 1990.

Rubin, D. H., et al. The relationship between infant feeding and infectious illness: a prospective evaluation of infants during the first year of life. Pediatrics 85:464–471, 1990.

US Department of Health and Human Services, Public Health Service. Healthy People 2000: National Health Promotion and Disease Prevention Objectives. Washington, D. C., US Government Printing Office, 1990.

Selected Readings

Centers for Disease Control and Prevention. International Health Data Reference Guide, 1993. Publication No. (PHS)94-1007. Hyattsville, Md., US Department of Health and Human Services, 1994. [International data.]

Chan, C. K., et al. The value and hazards of standardization in clinical epidemiologic research. Journal of Clinical Epidemiology 41:1125–1134, 1988. [Standardization of rates.]

Elandt-Johnson, R. C. Definition of rates: some remarks on their use and misuse. American Journal of Epidemiology 102:267–271, 1975. [Risks, rates, and ratios.]

Gable, C. B. A compendium of public health data sources. American Journal of Epidemiology 131:381–394, 1990. [General information.]

CHAPTER THREE

EPIDEMIOLOGIC

SURVEILLANCE AND

OUTBREAK INVESTIGATION

THE SURVEILLANCE OF DISEASE

Responsibility for Surveillance in the USA

In the USA, the Centers for Disease Control and Prevention (CDC) in Atlanta, Georgia, is the federal agency responsible for the surveillance of most types of acute diseases and, if deemed necessary, the investigation of outbreaks. Data for disease surveillance are passed from local and state governments to the CDC, which then evaluates the data and works with the state and local agencies regarding further investigation and control of problems discovered.

According to the US Constitution, the federal government has jurisdiction over matters concerning interstate commerce, including disease outbreaks with **interstate implications** (outbreaks from a source in one state that have spread to other states or have the potential to do so). Each state government has jurisdiction over disease outbreaks with **intrastate implications** (that is, an outbreak confined within one state's borders). If a disease outbreak has interstate implications, the CDC is a first responder and takes immediate action, rather than waiting for a request for assistance from a state government.

Purposes and Methods for the Surveillance of Disease

Surveillance, generally considered the foundation of public health disease control efforts, has various interrelated functions. A distinction must be made between passive surveillance and active surveillance. Most of the surveillance done on a routine basis is **passive surveillance,** in which those who are required to report disease, such as physicians, laboratories, and hospitals, are given the appropriate mailing forms and instructions, with the expectation that they will report all of the cases of reportable disease that come to their attention. **Active surveillance** requires periodic (usually weekly) telephone calls or personal visits to the reporting individuals to obtain the required data. Active surveillance is obviously more labor-intensive and costly, and it is seldom done on a routine basis.

The percentage of reportable disease cases that are actually reported to public health authorities varies considerably. Harkess et al. (1988) estimated that the percentage reported to state-based passive reporting systems varied from 30% to 62% of cases. These same authors, however, found that 81% of the culture-confirmed cases of shigellosis that occurred in Oklahoma over a 6-month period were reported to the passive surveillance system in that state.

Sometimes a change in medical care practice will uncover a problem that was previously invisible. This occurred, for example, when one hospital in Connecticut began reporting many cases of pharyngeal gonorrhea in young children. This apparent localized outbreak was investigated by a student-faculty rapid response team from Yale University School of Public Health, which discovered that the cases began to appear only after the hospital started examining all throat cultures in children for gonococci as well as for beta-hemolytic streptococci (Helgerson, Jekel, and Hadler 1988).

Establishment of Baseline Data

Usual (baseline) rates and patterns of diseases can only be known if there is a regular reporting and surveillance system. Epidemiologists study the patterns of diseases by the time of occurrence of cases, the geographic location of cases, and the characteristics of the persons involved. Continued surveillance allows epidemiologists to detect deviations from the usual pattern of data, which prompts them to explore whether an epidemic (i.e., an unusual incidence of

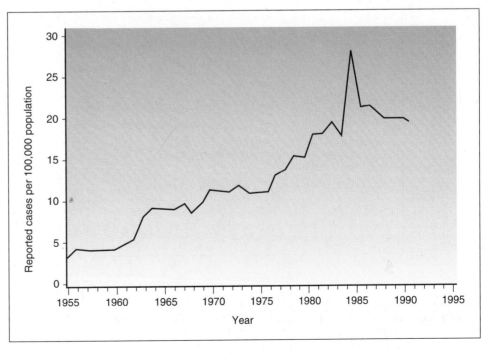

FIGURE 3–1. Incidence rates of salmonellosis (excluding typhoid fever) in the USA, by year of report, 1955–1991. (Source: Centers for Disease Control and Prevention. Summary of notifiable diseases, United States, 1992. Morbidity and Mortality Weekly Report 41: 41, 1992.)

disease) is occurring or whether other factors (such as an alteration in reporting practices) are responsible for the observed changes.

Evaluation of Time Trends

Long-Term Secular Trends. The implications of long-term secular (time) trends of disease are usually different from those of outbreaks or epidemics, and they are often of greater significance. For example, the graph in Fig. 3–1, taken from a CDC surveillance report about salmonellosis, shows that a rise in the number of reported cases of salmonellosis in the USA has been seen over time. The first question to be asked is whether the trend could be explained by changes over time in disease detection, disease reporting, or both, which often happens when an apparent outbreak of a particular disease is reported. When a real or suspected outbreak is announced, this may increase the index of suspicion of physicians, leading to increased diagnosis and to increased reporting of cases that are diagnosed.

Because there have been increasing numbers of outbreaks and because the trend has continued over an extended time period, epidemiologists consider that most of the observed increase in salmonellosis in Fig. 3–1 is real. This is especially true for New England and the East Coast, where a sharp increase in outbreaks due to *Salmonella enteritidis* has been noted since about 1977. A long-term increase in a disease in one region of the country, particularly when it is related to one serotype, is usually of greater public health significance than is a localized outbreak, because it suggests the existence of a more widespread problem.

Fig. 3–2 shows the decline in the reported incidence and mortality from diphtheria in the USA. The data in this figure are presented in the form of a **semilogarithmic graph,** with a **logarithmic scale** used for the y-axis and an **arithmetic scale** for the x-axis. Fig. 3–2 illustrates one advantage of using a logarithmic scale: the lines showing incidence and mortality demonstrate an approximately parallel decline. On a logarithmic scale, this means that the

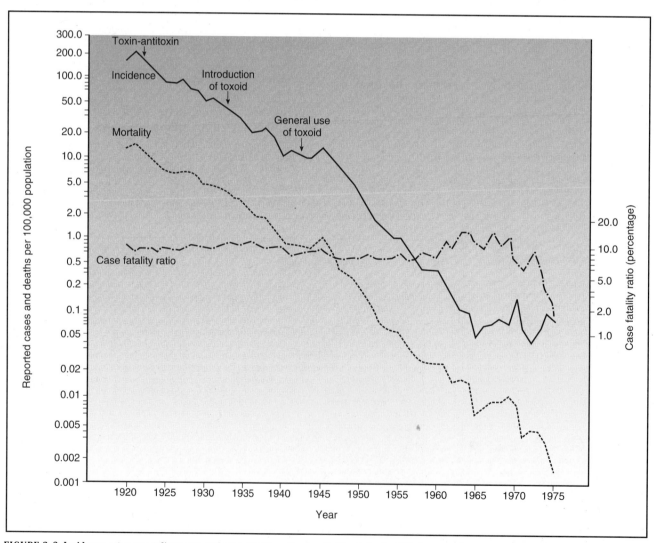

FIGURE 3–2. Incidence rates, mortality rates, and case fatality ratios for diphtheria in the USA, by year of report, 1920–1975. (Source: Centers for Disease Control. Diphtheria Surveillance Summary. Publication No. (CDC)78-8087. Atlanta, Centers for Disease Control, 1978.)

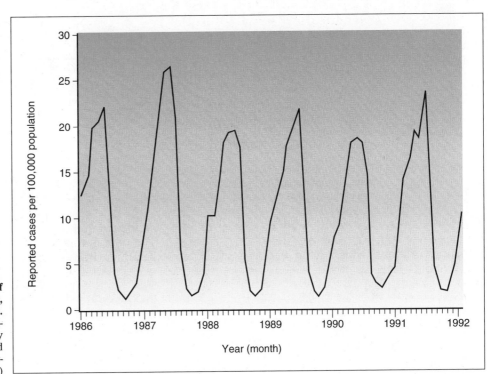

FIGURE 3–3. Incidence rates of varicella (chickenpox) in the USA, by month of report, 1986–1992. (Source: Centers for Disease Control and Prevention. Summary of notifiable diseases, United States, 1992. Morbidity and Mortality Weekly Report 41:53, 1992.)

decline in rates was proportional, so that the percentage of cases that result in death—i.e., the **case fatality ratio**—has remained relatively constant at about 10% over the years. This, in turn, suggests that prevention of disease, rather than treatment of those who are ill, is responsible for the improvement in diphtheria in the USA.

Seasonal Variation. When determining the usual number of cases or rate of disease, epidemiologists must incorporate the expected seasonal variation into their calculations. Many infectious diseases show a strong seasonal variation, with periods of highest incidence usually depending on the **route of spread.**

Infectious diseases that are spread by the **respiratory route,** such as influenza, colds, measles, and varicella (chickenpox), have a much higher incidence in the winter and early spring months in the northern hemisphere. For example, Fig. 3–3 shows the seasonal variation for varicella in the USA by month during the period 1986–1992. Notice the peaks after January and before summer of each year. This pattern is thought to be due to the fact that people spend most of their time close together in indoor environments where the air changes slowly. The drying of mucous membranes, which also occurs in the wintertime because of low humidity and indoor heating, may play a role in promoting respiratory infections. However, diphtheria, when it was common, tended to strike especially in the early autumn, perhaps related to the return of children to school.

Diseases that are spread by **insect or arthropod vectors** (such as viral encephalitis from mosquitoes) have a strong predilection for the summer or early autumn. Lyme disease, spread by *Ixodes* ticks, is usually acquired in the late spring or summer, a pattern explained by the seasonally related life cycle of the ticks and the outdoor activity of people with less protective clothing at that time of the year.

Infectious diseases that are spread by the **fecal-oral route** are most common in the summer, partly because of the ability of the organisms to multiply more rapidly in food and water during warm weather. Fig. 3–4 shows the summer seasonal pattern of waterborne outbreaks of gastrointestinal disease. The peak frequency of outbreaks from drinking water sources occurs from May to August, whereas that for recreational water sources (such as lakes, rivers, and swimming pools) is from June to October. The presence of flies during the summer also contributes to the spread of enteric diseases during this season.

Fig. 3–5 shows a late summer peak for aseptic meningitis, which is usually due to viral infections spread by the fecal-oral route or by insects. Fig. 3–6, which shows a pattern that is similar but has sharper and narrower peaks in late summer and early autumn, describes known arthropod-borne viral infections—in this case due to California-serogroup viruses of the central nervous system.

For reasons that usually are obscure, some noninfectious diseases have a higher incidence during certain seasons. For example, peptic ulcer has classically had a higher incidence in the spring and autumn, but the reasons for this are unknown (Harrison et al. 1958). Although peptic ulcer used to be considered a noninfectious disease, the newest hypothesis is that it is frequently caused by the bacterium *Helicobacter pylori*, which would make some peptic ulcers an infectious disease. The reasons for the seasonal pattern still are unknown.

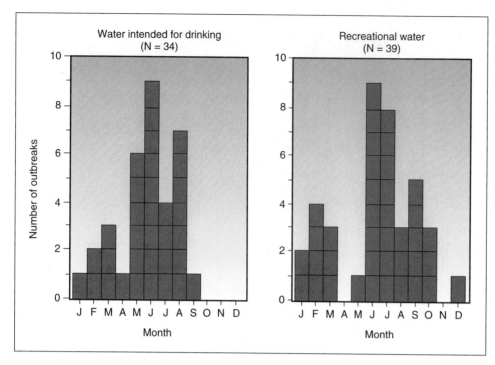

FIGURE 3–4. Incidence of water-borne outbreaks of gastrointestinal disease in the USA, by month of report, 1991–1992. (Source: Centers for Disease Control and Prevention. Surveillance for waterborne disease outbreaks, United States, 1991–1992. Morbidity and Mortality Weekly Report 42(SS-5):1–22, 1993.)

Because the peaks of different patterns occur at different times, the CDC sometimes shows the incidence of diseases by what it calls an epidemiologic year. Unlike the **calendar year,** which runs from January of one year to January of the next year, the **epidemiologic year** for a given disease runs from the month of lowest incidence in one year to the same month in the next year. The advantage of using the epidemiologic year when plotting the incidence of a disease is that it puts the high incidence months near the center of a graph and avoids having the high incidence peak split between the two ends of the graph, as would occur with many respiratory diseases if they were graphed for a calendar year.

Other Types of Variation. Health problems can vary by the day of the week, as is illustrated in Fig. 3–7, which shows that recreational drownings are much more frequent on weekends than during the week.

Identification and Documentation of Outbreaks

An **epidemic,** or **disease outbreak,** is the occurrence of disease at an unusual (unexpected)

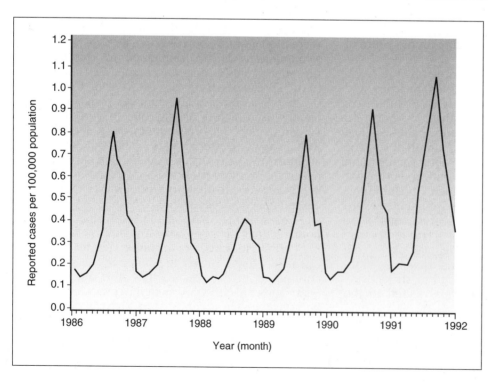

FIGURE 3–5. Incidence rates of aseptic meningitis in the USA, by month of report, 1986–1992. (Source: Centers for Disease Control and Prevention. Summary of notifiable diseases, United States, 1992. Morbidity and Mortality Weekly Report 41:20, 1992.)

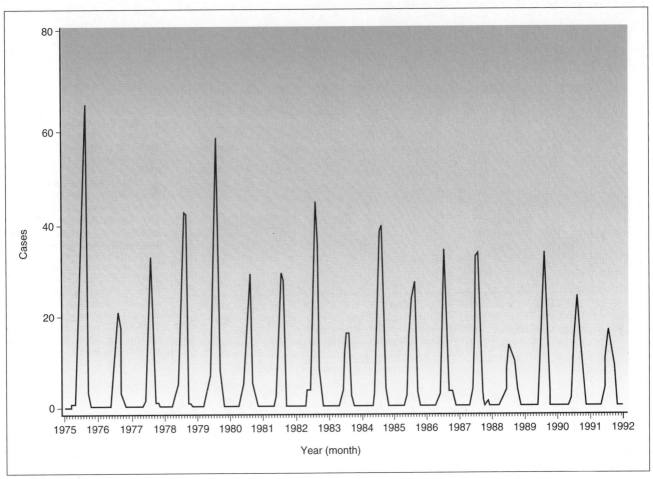

FIGURE 3–6. Incidence of central nervous system infections due to California-serogroup viruses in the USA, by month of report, 1975–1992. (Source: Centers for Disease Control and Prevention. Summary of notifiable diseases, United States, 1992. Morbidity and Mortality Weekly Report 41:18, 1992.)

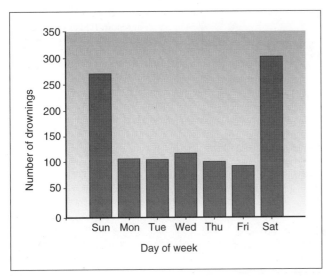

FIGURE 3–7. Number of drownings at the recreation facilities of the US Army Corps of Engineers, by day of week of report, 1986–1990. (Source: Centers for Disease Control and Prevention. Drownings at U.S. Army Corps of Engineers recreation facilities, 1986–1990. Morbidity and Mortality Weekly Report 41:331–333, 1992.)

frequency. Because the word *epidemic* tends to create fear in a population, that term is usually reserved for a problem of wider than local implications, and the term *outbreak* is usually used for a localized epidemic. Nevertheless, the two terms are often used interchangeably.

Whether the level of disease is unusual can only be determined if the usual rates of the disease are known and if reliable surveillance shows that the current rates are in considerable excess of those ordinarily expected. For example, in order to determine when and where influenza and pneumonia outbreaks occur, the CDC uses a seasonally adjusted *expected* number of influenza and pneumonia deaths in the USA—a number called the **epidemic threshold**—to compare with the reported number of cases. (Pneumonias are included because influenza-induced pneumonias often are signed out on the death certificate just as pneumonia, with no mention of influenza.)

Fig. 3–8 provides data concerning the expected number of pneumonia and influenza deaths in 121 US cities for 1988–1993. The lower line is the seasonal baseline, which is the expected number of pneumonia and influenza deaths per week in these cities. The

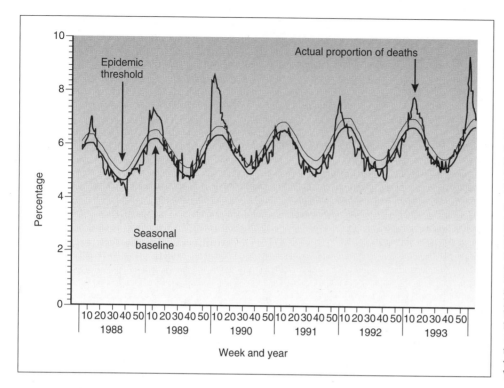

FIGURE 3–8. Epidemic threshold, seasonal baseline, and actual proportion of deaths due to pneumonia and influenza in 121 US cities, 1988–1993. The epidemic threshold is 1.645 standard deviations above the seasonal baseline. The expected seasonal baseline is projected using a robust regression procedure in which a periodic regression model is applied to observed percentages of deaths from pneumonia and influenza since 1983. (Source: Centers for Disease Control and Prevention. Update: influenza activity—United States and worldwide, 1993–1994 season, and composition of the 1994–1995 influenza vaccine. Morbidity and Mortality Weekly Report 43:179–183, 1994.)

upper line is the epidemic threshold, as discussed above. There were major influenza outbreaks in early 1990 and late 1993; moderate outbreaks in early 1988, 1989, 1992, and 1993; and no outbreak at all in the winter of 1990–1991. No other disease has this sophisticated a prediction model, but the basic principles apply to determining whether or not an outbreak is occurring.

Evaluation of Disease Interventions

The introduction of major interventions, especially vaccines, is monitored by looking for changes in long-term disease patterns. Fig. 3–9 shows the impact that the two types of polio vaccine—the inactivated (Salk) vaccine and the oral (Sabin) vaccine—had on the reported incident cases of poliomyelitis. Note that the large graph in this figure

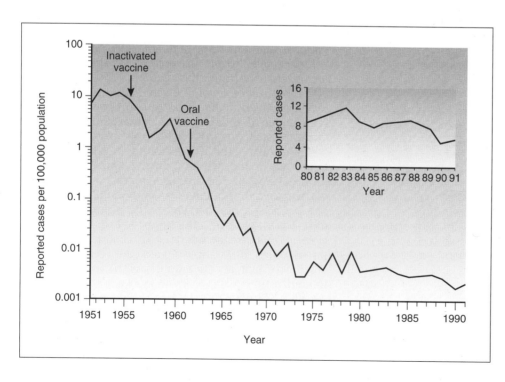

FIGURE 3–9. Incidence rates of paralytic poliomyelitis in the USA, by year of report, 1951–1991. (Source: Centers for Disease Control. Summary of notifiable diseases, United States, 1991. Morbidity and Mortality Weekly Report 40: 37, 1991.)

has a logarithmic scale on the *y*-axis. It is used here because the drop in the poliomyelitis incidence rate was so steep that on an arithmetic scale, no detail would be visible at the bottom after the early 1960s. A logarithmic scale compresses the high rates on a graph compared to lower rates, so that the detail of the latter can be seen.

Fig. 3–9 shows that after the inactivated vaccine was introduced in 1955, the rates of paralytic disease dropped quickly. Unfortunately, the public tended to think the problem had gone away, and many parents became less concerned about immunizing newborn children. However, because the inactivated vaccine did not provide herd immunity, the unimmunized newborns were very much at risk. Fig. 3–9 shows a recurrent poliomyelitis spike in 1958 and 1959. At this time, most of the new cases of paralytic poliomyelitis were among young children who had not been immunized. The rates dropped again in 1960 and thereafter, both because the public was shaken out of its complacency to obtain vaccine and because a newer vaccine was introduced. This live, attenuated oral vaccine provided herd immunity as well as individual immunity. (For a discussion of herd immunity, see Chapter 1 and Fig. 1–3.)

The failure of a vaccine to produce immunity or the failure of people to use the vaccine can be detected by one of the following: (1) a lack of change in disease rates; (2) an increase in disease rates following an initial fall, as occurred in the example of the polio vaccine just discussed; or (3) an increase in disease rates in a recently vaccinated group, as occurred following the use of bad lots of inactivated polio vaccine manufactured by Cutter Laboratories in the 1950s (see Chapter 1).

The importance of surveillance was underscored recently through continued evaluation and close surveillance of measles rates in the USA. Investigators were able to detect the failure of the initial measles vaccines and vaccination schedules to provide long-lasting protection (see Chapter 1). Research into this problem led to a new set of recommendations for immunization against measles. According to the 1994 recommendations (see Centers for Disease Control and Prevention 1994), two doses of measles vaccine should be administered to young children. The first dose should be given when the child is between 12 and 15 months of age (to avoid the greater failure rate if given earlier), and a second dose should be given when the child is between 4 and 6 years old, before school entry.

Setting of Disease Control Priorities

The patterns of diseases for the current time and recent past help governmental and voluntary agencies establish priorities for disease control efforts. This is not a simple counting procedure. A disease will be of more concern if its rates are rising rapidly—as is the case with acquired immunodeficiency syndrome (AIDS) and tuberculosis—than if its rates are steady or declining. Moreover, the severity of the disease is a critical feature, and this usually can be established by good surveillance. AIDS gets high priority because of its severity and its potential for epidemic spread.

Study of the Natural History of Diseases

By studying the patterns of occurrence of a particular disease over time in populations and in subpopulations, epidemiologists can better understand the natural history of the disease. A new pattern of occurrence may be more ominous than a mere increase in the incidence of a disease. In the case of tuberculosis, for example, the incidence is now increasing after falling for decades. More than the increase in numbers, the new patterns of the disease—the association with AIDS and the increase in multiple drug–resistant tuberculosis (MDRTB)—are causes for concern.

Changes in the virulence of infectious organisms are also of concern. For example, beta-hemolytic streptococci are causing more severe infections again after almost a century of behaving as less virulent organisms. This phenomenon is poorly understood and raises the question of whether these organisms have a regular long-term cycle of virulence.

There was a resurgence in the reported number of cases of primary and secondary syphilis among women in the 1980s, with a concomitant sharp increase in the number of cases of congenital syphilis. Fig. 3–10 shows the close relationship between these types of syphilis in New York City.

THE INVESTIGATION OF EPIDEMICS
The Nature of Epidemics

The common definition of an **epidemic** is an unusual or unexpected occurrence of disease. The term comes from the Greek language and means "upon the population."

Although people usually think of an epidemic as something that involves large numbers of people, it is possible to name circumstances under which just *one* case of a disease could be considered an epidemic. For example, because smallpox has been eradicated from the world, a single case would represent a smallpox epidemic. Similarly, if a disease has been eradicated from a particular region (for example, paralytic poliomyelitis in the western hemisphere) or if a disease is approaching elimination from an area and has the potential for spread (as is the case with measles in the USA), the report of even one case in the geographic region is "unexpected" and is cause for concern. Under these circumstances, any occurrence of the disease can be considered an epidemic.

When a disease in a population is occurring regularly and at about its usual level, it is said to be **endemic.** This term, also from the Greek language, means "within the population."

Epidemiologists also distinguish between usual and unusual patterns of diseases in animals. If there is a disease outbreak in an animal population, it is

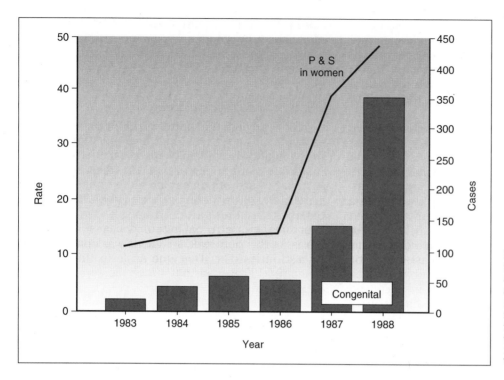

FIGURE 3–10. Incidence of congenital syphilis in infants under 1 year of age (bars) and incidence of primary and secondary syphilis in women (line) in New York City, by year of report, 1983–1988. (Source: Centers for Disease Control. Congenital syphilis, New York City, 1983–1988. Morbidity and Mortality Weekly Report 38:825–829, 1989.)

said to be **epizootic** ("upon the animals"), or if a disease is deeply entrenched in a wild animal population but not changing much, it is said to be **enzootic** ("within the animals").

Investigators of acute disease outbreaks ordinarily use a measure of disease frequency called the **attack rate,** particularly when the period of exposure is short (i.e., considerably less than a year). Rather than being a true rate, the attack rate is really the proportion of exposed persons that becomes ill. It is calculated as follows:

Attack rate =

$$\frac{\text{Number of new cases of a disease}}{\text{Number of persons exposed in a particular outbreak}} \times 100$$

In this equation, 100 is used as the constant multiplier so that the rate can be expressed as a percentage. (For a discussion of other measures of disease frequency, see Chapter 2.)

Procedures for Investigating an Epidemic

If an epidemic occurs, it suggests that something in the equilibrium of factors for and against the occurrence of a particular disease has been disrupted, rather suddenly and probably rather recently. The goal is to discover and correct the recent changes so the balance can be restored and the epidemic controlled. The epidemically oriented physician will not only be concerned to give the correct treatment to individual patients prospectively (i.e., from the time of disease onset forward) but will also ask the following retrospective question: Why did *this* patient become sick with *this* disease at *this* time and place?

Outbreak investigation is somewhat like crime investigation in that both require a lot of "shoe leather" (for good descriptions of epidemic investigation, see Roueché 1991). Although there is no simple way to teach imagination and creativity in the investigation of disease outbreaks, there is an organized way of approaching and interpreting the data that assists in the solution of problems. This section outlines a series of steps to follow in investigating a disease outbreak.

Establish the Diagnosis

This may seem obvious, but it is surprising how many people start investigating an outbreak without taking the first step of establishing the diagnosis. Many cases are "solved" just by making the correct diagnosis and thereby demonstrating that the disease occurrence was not unusual after all. For example, a health department in North Carolina received panic calls from numerous people who lived in a small town and were concerned about the occurrence of smallpox in their county. A physician working in local public health was assigned to investigate the matter and quickly discovered that the reported case of smallpox was actually a typical case of chickenpox in a young child. The child's mother did not speak English well, and the neighbors heard the word "pox" and panicked. The "outbreak" was stopped by a correct diagnosis.

Establish the Case Definition

The case definition is the list of specific criteria used to decide whether or not a person has the disease of concern. Establishing a case definition is especially important if the disease is unknown, as was the case in the early investigations of legionnaires' disease, AIDS, hantavirus respiratory syndrome, and eosinophilia-myalgia syndrome, among others. For example, the CDC case definition for eosinophilia-myalgia syndrome includes (1) a total eosinophil count greater than 1000/μL; (2) generalized myalgia at some point during the course of the illness of sufficient severity to limit the ability to pursue normal activities; and (3) exclusion of other neoplastic or infectious conditions that could account for the syndrome (Slutsker et al. 1990).

No case definition will be perfect, because there will always be some **false positives** (i.e., individuals wrongly included in the affected group) and **false negatives** (i.e., individuals wrongly included in the unaffected group). Nevertheless, the case definition should be developed carefully and adhered to in the collection and analysis of data. Using a generally established case definition also permits epidemiologists to make more accurate comparisons among the findings from many different outbreak investigations (see Centers for Disease Control 1990).

Determine Whether an Epidemic Exists

Even if there are proven cases, are they sufficient in number to constitute an epidemic? As emphasized above, it is difficult to answer this question unless the "usual" number of cases is known by ongoing surveillance.

Characterize the Epidemic by Time, Place, and Person

The epidemic should be characterized using the criteria in the case definition. It is unwise to plan the data collection until the case definition has been established, because the case definition determines the data needed in order to classify persons as affected or unaffected.

Time.   The time dimension of the outbreak is best described by an **epidemic time curve.** This is a graph with time on the x-axis and the number of new cases on the y-axis. The epidemic time curve should be created so that the units of time on the x-axis are considerably smaller than the expected incubation period, and the y-axis is simply the *number* of cases that became symptomatic during the time interval. Rates are not used in creating the epidemic time curve.

The epidemic time curve provides several important clues about what is happening in an outbreak and helps the epidemiologist answer the following questions: What was the **type of exposure** (i.e., common source or propagated)? What was the **route of spread** (respiratory, fecal-oral, skin-to-skin contact, exchange of blood or body fluids, or via insect or animal vectors)? When were the affected persons exposed? What was the incubation period? In addition to **primary cases** (persons infected initially by a common source), were there **secondary cases** (which represent person-to-person transmission of disease

from primary cases to other persons, often members of the same household)?

In a **common source exposure,** many people come into contact with the same source, such as contaminated water or food, usually over a short period of time. If an outbreak is due to this type of exposure, the epidemic curve usually has a sudden onset, a peak, and a rather rapid decline. If the outbreak is due to **person-to-person spread,** however, the epidemic curve usually has a prolonged, irregular pattern. The latter kind of outbreak is often referred to as a **propagated outbreak.**

Fig. 3–11 shows the epidemic time curve from an outbreak of gastrointestinal disease due to a common source exposure to *Shigella boydii* at Fort Bliss in Texas. In this outbreak, spaghetti was contaminated by a food handler. The time scale in this figure is shown in 12-hour periods. Note the rapid increase and rapid disappearance of the outbreak.

Fig. 3–12 shows the epidemic time curve from a propagated outbreak of bacillary dysentery due to *Shigella sonnei,* which was transmitted from person to person at a school for mentally retarded people in Vermont. In this outbreak, the spread of disease was

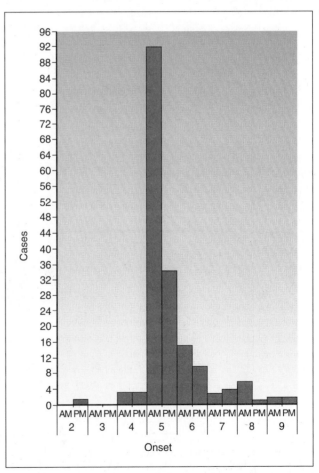

FIGURE 3–11. Epidemic time curve showing the onset of cases of gastrointestinal disease due to *Shigella boydii* in Fort Bliss, Texas, in November 1976. Note that the onset is shown in 12-hour periods for dates in November. (Source: Centers for Disease Control. Food and Waterborne Disease Outbreaks: Annual Summary, 1976. Atlanta, Centers for Disease Control, 1977.)

through contamination of persons, clothing, and the school environment with feces. The time scale here is shown in 5-day periods. Note the ongoing, "dragged-out" appearance of the outbreak.

If conditions are right, a respiratory disease spread by the person-to-person route may produce an epidemic time curve that looks almost like that of a common source epidemic. Fig. 3–13 shows the spread of measles in an elementary school. A widespread initial exposure apparently occurred in the school assembly, so that the air in that assembly can almost be thought of as a common source. The initial case in this situation is called the **index case**—i.e., the case that introduced the organism into the population. However, sporadic cases can be seen during the prior 2 months. The first of these measles cases should have warned school and public health officials to immunize all of the school children immediately. If that had been done, the outbreak would probably have been avoided.

Sometimes an epidemic will have more than one peak, either because of multiple common source exposures or because of secondary cases. This is illustrated in Fig. 3–14, which shows the epidemic time curve for an outbreak of shigellosis among students who attended a camp in the eastern USA.

The campers who drank contaminated water on a trip were infected with *Shigella* organisms. After they returned home, they infected others with shigellosis.

Epidemiologists occasionally encounter situations in which there are two different common source outbreaks that had the same time and place of exposure but had different incubation periods. Say, for example, that a group of people is exposed to contaminated shellfish in a restaurant. The exposure might cause an outbreak of shigellosis in 24–72 hours and also cause an outbreak of hepatitis A about 2–4 weeks after the exposure.

Not only is the epidemic time curve useful in ascertaining the type of exposure, but it is also useful in determining when the affected persons were exposed. If the causative organism is known and the exposure appears to be a common source, the epidemiologist can use knowledge about that organism's usual incubation period to determine the probable time of exposure. Two methods are commonly used. The data in Fig. 3–14, which pertain to *Shigella* infection among campers, will serve as the basis for illustrating each of these methods of determining the probable time of exposure.

Method 1 involves taking the shortest and longest known incubation period for the causative

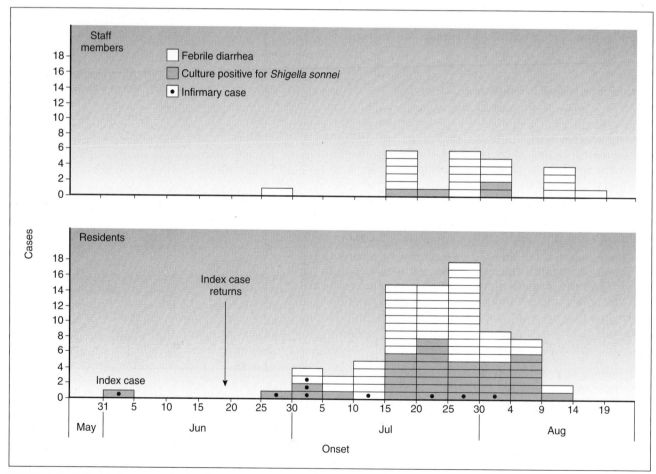

FIGURE 3–12. Epidemic time curve showing the onset of cases of bacillary dysentery due to *Shigella sonnei* at a training school in Brandon, Vermont, from May to August 1974. Note that the onset is shown in 5-day periods for dates in May, June, July, and August. (Source: Centers for Disease Control. Shigella Surveillance. Report No. 37. Atlanta, Centers for Disease Control, 1976.)

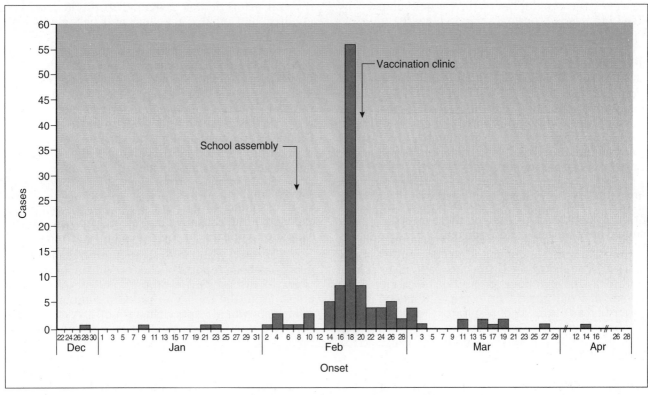

FIGURE 3–13. Epidemic time curve showing the onset of cases of measles at an elementary school from December 1975 to April 1976. Note that the onset is shown in 2-day periods for dates in December 1975 and in January, February, March, and April 1976. (Source: Centers for Disease Control. Measles Surveillance, 1973–1976. Report No. 10. Atlanta, Centers for Disease Control, 1977.)

organism and calculating backward in time from the first and last cases. If these estimates are reasonably close together, they bracket the probable time of exposure. For example, the incubation period for *Shigella* organisms is usually from 1 to 3 days (from 24 to 72 hours), but it may be as short as 12 hours or as long as 96 hours (Benenson 1990). Fig. 3–14 shows

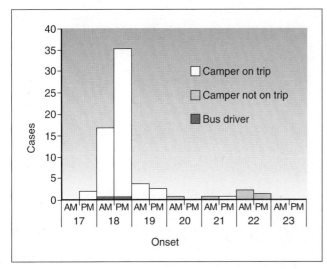

FIGURE 3–14. Epidemic time curve showing the onset of cases of shigellosis in campers from New Jersey and New York in August 1971. Note that the onset is shown in 12-hour periods for dates in August. (Source: Centers for Disease Control. Shigella Surveillance: Annual Summary, 1971. Atlanta, Centers for Disease Control, 1972.)

that the first two cases of shigellosis occurred after noon on August 17. If these cases had a 12-hour incubation period, the exposure was sometime before noon on August 17 (without knowing the exact hours, it is not possible to be more specific). The longest known incubation period for *Shigella* is 96 hours, and the last camper case was August 21 after noon. Ninety-six hours before that would be August 17 after noon. The most probable exposure time, therefore, was either before noon or after noon on August 17. If the same procedure is used but applied to the *most common* incubation period (from 24 to 72 hours), the result is an estimate of after noon on August 16 from the early cases and an estimate of after noon on August 18 from the last case. These two estimates still center on August 17, so it is reasonable to assume that the campers were exposed sometime during August 17.

Method 2 is closely related to the above method but involves taking the average incubation period and measuring backward from the epidemic peak, if that were clear. In Fig. 3–14, the peak is after noon on August 18. An average of 48 hours (2 days) earlier would be after noon on August 16, slightly earlier than the previous estimates. Therefore, the most probable time of exposure was either after noon on August 16 or any time during August 17.

Place.   The accurate characterization of an epidemic involves defining the geographic location of cases. A geographic clustering of cases may give important clues as to what is going on. Usually, however, the geographic picture is not sufficient by itself but needs other data to complete the interpretation.

Sometimes a **spot map** showing where each affected person lives or works will be helpful to the solution of an epidemic puzzle. One of the best examples came from a study done in the 1850s in London by John Snow, who showed that most of the persons affected by an outbreak of cholera lived in the blocks immediately surrounding the Broad Street water pump. Based on this information, Snow had the pump removed from service.

Spot maps are not used very much in outbreak investigations nowadays, because they only show the numerator (the number of cases) and do not provide information on the denominator. Epidemiologists prefer to show **incidence rates by location,** such as by hospital ward (in a hospital infection outbreak), by work area or classroom (in an occupational or school outbreak), or by block or section of a city (in a community outbreak). For example, Roueché (1991) described an outbreak of respiratory fungal infection in an Arkansas school and showed how classroom incidence rates provided a clue to the cause of the outbreak. All of the classrooms except one had 3 or fewer cases each. The exception, a room named the Liberace Room after a pet parakeet, had 14 cases. This room was located directly over the coal chute, and coal had been dumped on the ground and then shoveled into the chute over several windy days. The Liberace Room had become very dusty from the coal, which had come from a strip mine and apparently had been contaminated with *Histoplasma capsulatum* in the soil before it was delivered to the school. The children had inhaled the dust and become ill with histoplasmosis.

When epidemiologists wish to determine the general location of a disease and how it is spreading, they may compare trends in incidence rates in different regions. For example, Fig. 3–15 shows the rates of reported *Salmonella enteritidis* infections by region in the USA, 1976–1989. According to this figure, there was an unusually high rate for the New England region from 1978 to 1989. Beginning in about 1984, the mid-Atlantic states also began to show an excessive rate of salmonellosis from the same serotype, suggesting that the problem was spreading down the East Coast. Fig. 3–16 uses a map to demonstrate the spread of epidemic cholera in South and Central America from January 1991 through July 1992.

A special type of investigation problem in recent years has been reports of clusters of cancer or other types of disease in neighborhoods or other small areas. From the theory of random sampling, epidemiologists would expect clusters of disease to happen by chance alone, but that does not comfort the people involved. Distinguishing **"chance" clusters** from **"real" clusters** is often difficult, but the types of cancer in a cluster may help epidemiologists decide fairly quickly whether or not the cluster might be an environmental problem.

If the types of cancer in the cluster vary considerably and are of the more common cell types (e.g., lung, breast, colon, prostate, etc.), the cluster probably is not due to a hazardous local exposure (see Brooks-Robinson, Helgerson, and Jekel 1987; Jacquez

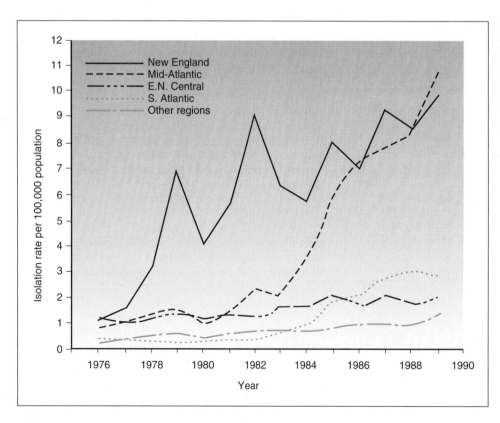

FIGURE 3–15. Isolation rate of *Salmonella enteritidis* infections per 100,000 population in various regions of the USA, by year of report, 1976–1989. (Source: Centers for Disease Control. Update: *Salmonella enteritidis* infections and shell eggs, United States, 1990. Morbidity and Mortality Weekly Report 39:909–912, 1990.)

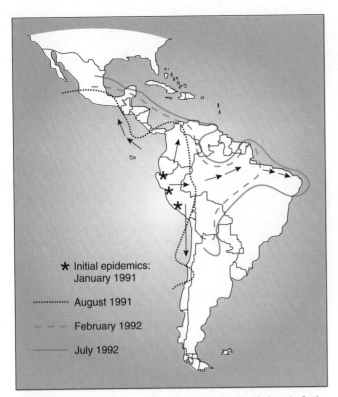

FIGURE 3-16. **Map showing the spread of epidemic cholera in Latin America from January 1991 to July 1992.** (Source: Centers for Disease Control and Prevention. Update: cholera, western hemisphere. Morbidity and Mortality Weekly Report 41:667–668, 1992.)

★ Initial epidemics:
January 1991

·········· August 1991

– – – February 1992

——— July 1992

1993; and National Conference on Clustering of Health Events 1990). If, however, most of the cases are of only one type or are of a limited number of related types of cancer (especially leukemia or brain cancer), a more intensive investigation is indicated.

The next step is to begin at the time the "cluster" is reported and observe the situation prospectively. The hypothesis is that the unusual number of cases will not continue. Because this is a prospective hypothesis, as will be explained in Chapter 10, an appropriate statistical test can be used to decide whether the number of cases continues to be excessive. If the answer is "yes," there may be a true environmental problem in the area.

Person.   Knowing the characteristics of persons affected by an outbreak may help clarify the problem and its cause. Among the important characteristics are age; sex; race; religion; source of water, milk, and food; immunization status; type of work or schooling; and contacts with other affected persons.

Figs. 3–17 and 3–18 illustrate the value of analyzing the personal characteristics of affected individuals for clues regarding the cause of the outbreak. Fig. 3–17 shows the age distribution of measles cases among children in the Navajo nation, while Fig. 3–18 shows the age distribution of measles cases among residents of Cuyahoga County, Ohio. The fact that measles in the Navajo nation tended to occur in very young children is consistent with the hypothesis that the outbreak in this instance was due to lack of initial immunization of newborns.

In contrast, the fact that very young children in Cuyahoga County were almost exempt from measles and that school-aged children tended to be the ones infected suggests that the outbreak in this instance was due to failure of measles vaccine to produce long-lasting immunity. If they were not immunized early, the children of Cuyahoga County probably would have had measles earlier in life and would therefore have been immune by the time they entered school.

Develop Hypotheses Regarding Source, Type, and Route of Spread

The **source of infection** is the vehicle (e.g., food, water) or person (the index case) that brought the infection into the affected community in the first place. For example, the source of infection in the outbreak of gastrointestinal illness at Fort Bliss (see Fig. 3–11) was an infected food handler, who contaminated spaghetti that was eaten by many persons more or less simultaneously.

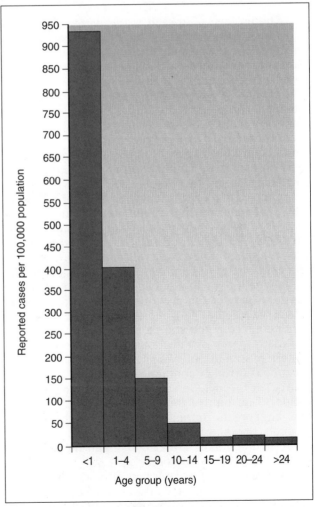

FIGURE 3–17. **Incidence rates of measles in members of the Navajo nation, by age group, 1972–1975.** (Source: Centers for Disease Control. Measles Surveillance, 1973–1976. Report No. 10. Atlanta, Centers for Disease Control, 1977.)

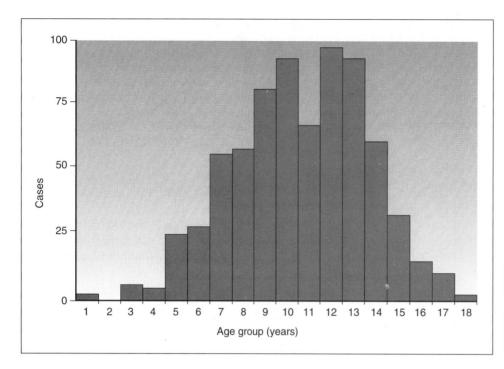

FIGURE 3–18. Incidence of measles in residents of Cuyahoga County, Ohio, by age group, from October 1973 to February 1974. (Source: Centers for Disease Control. Measles Surveillance, 1973–1976. Report No. 10. Atlanta, Centers for Disease Control, 1977.)

The **pattern of spread** is the pattern by which infection can be spread from the source to those infected. The primary distinction is between a **common source pattern,** such as occurs when contaminated water is drunk by many people in the same time period, and a **propagated pattern,** in which the infection "propagates itself" by spreading directly from person to person over an extended period of time. There is also a **mixed pattern,** in which persons who acquired a disease through a common source then spread it to family members or others (the secondary cases) by personal contact.

Affected persons in common source outbreaks may have just one short **point source exposure,** or they may have a **continuous common source exposure.** In the Fort Bliss outbreak, the infected spaghetti was the point source. In Milwaukee in 1993, an epidemic of *Cryptosporidium* infection was caused by contamination of the public water supply for the southern part of the city over a several-day period (MacKenzie et al. 1994), and this was an example of a continuous common source exposure.

Many types of infections have more than one pattern of spread. *Shigella* infection, for example, can be spread through contaminated water (a common source) or through person-to-person contact (propagation). The human immunodeficiency virus (HIV) can be spread to many intravenous drug users through the sharing of one infected needle and syringe (a common source), or it can be passed to others through sexual contact.

The **mode of transmission** of epidemic disease may be respiratory, fecal-oral, vector-borne, skin-to-skin, or via exchange of serum or other body fluids. In some cases, transmission is via contact with fomites—that is, objects that can passively carry organisms from one person to another, such as

unclean sheets or bedside water containers in hospitals.

Test the Hypotheses

Laboratory studies are important in testing the hypotheses and may include one or more of the following: (1) cultures from patients and, if appropriate, from possible vehicles such as food or water; (2) stool examinations for ova and parasites; (3) serum tests for antibodies to the organism suspected of causing the disease (e.g., tests of "acute" and "convalescent" serum samples to determine if there has been a rise in antibodies to the organism over time); and (4) tests for nonmicrobiologic agents, such as toxins or drugs.

A common, efficient way of testing hypotheses is to do **case-control studies** (see Chapter 5). For example, if there has been a food-borne outbreak of disease, the investigator assembles the persons who have the disease (the cases) and a sample of the persons who ate at the same place at the suspected time of exposure but did not have the disease (the controls). Then the investigator looks for what exposures (e.g., food items eaten) were considerably more common in the cases than in the controls. Both groups are questioned regarding the specific foods they did or did not eat prior to the outbreak. For each item of food and drink, the percentage of controls who consumed it is subtracted from the percentage of cases who consumed it. The food or drink showing the greatest difference in percentage is the most likely suspect. The case-control study can be used in an epidemic of noninfectious disease as well. Herbst, Ulfelder, and Poskanzer (1971) noted that 8 young women with adenocarcinoma of the vagina were treated at one hospital between 1966 and 1969.

Because of the rarity of this type of cancer, the number of cases would qualify as an outbreak. When the investigators did a case-control study, they used 32 controls (4 matched controls for every case). They were able to demonstrate that the only significant difference between the 8 cases and 32 controls was that 7 of the 8 cancer patients had been exposed to diethylstilbestrol (DES) in utero. Their mothers had been given DES, a synthetic estrogen, during the first semester of pregnancy in an effort to prevent miscarriage or premature labor. In contrast, none of the 32 controls were the offspring of mothers given DES during pregnancy. The probability of finding this distribution by chance alone was infinitesimal.

Initiate Control Measures

When an outbreak occurs, there is usually a general outcry that something be done immediately. It may be necessary to begin control measures before the source of the outbreak and other pertinent details are known for certain. If at all possible, the measures should be initiated in such a way as not to interfere with the investigation of the outbreak.

There are four common types of intervention. The first is **sanitation,** which often involves modification of the environment. Sanitation efforts may consist of removing the pathogenic agent from the sources of infection (water, food, etc.); removing the human source of infection from where he or she can spread it to others; or removing susceptible people from the environment. The second type is **prophylaxis,** which implies putting a barrier to the infection within the susceptible hosts. While a variety of immunizations are recommended for the entire population and are usually begun during infancy, other measures that offer short-term protection are also available for people who plan to travel to other countries. These include antimalarial drugs and hyperimmune globulin against hepatitis A. The third type of intervention consists of **diagnosis and treatment** of those who are infected (such as in outbreaks of tuberculosis, syphilis, and meningococcal meningitis) so that the infected persons cannot spread the disease to others. The fourth type of intervention involves **control of the disease vector,** such as mosquitoes in malaria, dengue, or yellow fever.

Although an outbreak may require one or more of the above interventions, sometimes an outbreak may simply fade away if enough people have been infected and there is a lack of susceptible individuals.

One important aspect of the control effort is the written and oral communication of findings to the appropriate authorities, the appropriate health professionals, and the public. This enables local and state authorities to assist in disease control, contributes to the professional fund of knowledge about the causes and control of outbreaks, and also adds to the information regarding prevention that the public has at its disposal.

Initiate Specific Follow-Up Surveillance to Evaluate the Control Measures

No medical or public health intervention is adequate without follow-up surveillance of the disease or problem that initially caused the outbreak. The importance of a sound surveillance program is not only to detect subsequent outbreaks but also to evaluate the effect of the control measures. If possible, the surveillance following an outbreak should be active surveillance (defined at the beginning of this chapter).

A Brief Example of the Investigation of an Outbreak

In January 1991, a liberal arts college with a population of about 400 students reported 82 cases of acute gastrointestinal illness, mostly among students, over a period of 102 hours. The president of this small college in New England sought help from local and state health authorities to determine whether the college cafeteria should be closed or even whether the entire college should be closed and the students sent home, which would have been terribly disruptive to their academic year.

Initial investigation focused on making a diagnosis. Clinical data suggested that the illness was of short duration, with most students found to be essentially well in 24 hours. The data also suggested that the illness was relatively mild. Only one student was hospitalized, and the need for hospitalization in this case was uncertain. In most cases, the symptoms consisted of nausea and vomiting, with little or no diarrhea and only mild systemic symptoms such as headache and malaise. Examination revealed only a low-grade fever. Initial food and stool cultures for pathogenic bacteria yielded negative results.

BOX 3–1. Disease Surveillance and Outbreak Investigation

Functions of disease surveillance
(1) Establishment of baseline data
(2) Evaluation of time trends
(3) Identification and documentation of outbreaks
(4) Evaluation of disease interventions
(5) Setting of disease control priorities
(6) Study of the natural history of diseases

Procedures for outbreak investigation
(1) Establish the diagnosis
(2) Establish the case definition
(3) Determine whether an epidemic exists
(4) Characterize the epidemic by time, place, and person
(5) Develop hypotheses regarding source, type, and route of spread
(6) Test the hypotheses
(7) Initiate control measures
(8) Initiate specific follow-up surveillance to evaluate the control measures

Based on this information, the investigating team developed a case definition. A case was defined as any person in the college who complained of either diarrhea or vomiting between Monday, January 28, and Thursday, January 31, 1991. The large percentage of cases over this short time made it clear that the situation was unusual and that the problem could be considered a disease outbreak.

The people meeting the criteria of the case definition included resident students, commuter students, and employees. When the investigating team interviewed samples of these groups of affected people, they found that most, but not all, of the resident students had eaten only at the campus cafeteria. The epidemic time curve (Fig. 3–19) suggested that if cafeteria food were the source, one or more meals on 2 days in January could have been responsible, although a few cases had occurred before and after the peak of the outbreak. Near the beginning of the outbreak, two food handlers had worked while feeling ill with typical symptoms. Health department records, however, revealed that the school cafeteria had always received high scores for sanitation, and officials who conducted an emergency reinspection of the facilities and equipment during the outbreak found no change. They detected no problem with sanitary procedures, except for the food handlers working while not feeling well.

Most of the commuter students with symptoms had brought food from home during the time of question. Almost none of them had eaten at the college cafeteria, although a few had eaten at an independently run snack bar in the student center. Further questioning revealed that the family members of several of the affected commuter students had also had a similar illness during the weeks preceding the outbreak or concurrent with it. One public school in a nearby town had closed briefly because of a similar illness in the majority of the children and staff members.

Although a college-wide questionnaire was distributed and analyzed, this took several days, and the president wanted some answers as soon as possible. Within 2 days of being summoned, the investigation team was able to make the following recommendations: the college, including the cafeteria, should remain open; college-wide assemblies and indoor sports events should be canceled for 2 weeks; and no person should be allowed to work as a food handler while ill. To demonstrate their confidence in the cafeteria, the members of the investigation team ate lunch there and sat in a prominent place. The outbreak quickly faded away, and the college schedule was able to proceed more or less normally.

Why was the investigation team able to make these recommendations so quickly? While the epidemic time curve and information gathered from interviews offered numerous clues, past knowledge gained from similar outbreaks, from disease surveillance, and from research concerning the natural history of diseases all helped the investigators make their recommendations with confidence. The self-limiting, mild course of disease, the lack of diarrhea, and the fact that no bacterial pathogens could be cultured from the food and stool samples that had been collected all made the diagnosis of bacterial infection unlikely. A staphylococcal toxin was considered initially, but the consistent story of a low-grade fever made a toxin unlikely; fever is a sign of infections but not external (ingested) toxins.

The clinical and epidemiologic pattern was most consistent with an outbreak due to a Norwalk-like viral agent, the laboratory demonstration of which is exceedingly difficult and costly. For Norwalk-like agents, the fecal-oral route of spread has been demonstrated for both food and water, but many outbreaks show a pattern also suggesting a respiratory route of spread, although that has not been confirmed. The latter was the reason for suggesting cancellation of assemblies and indoor sports events.

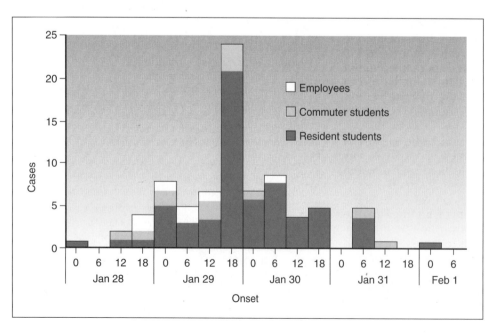

FIGURE 3–19. Epidemic time curve showing the onset of cases of gastroenteritis in a small college in New England from January 28 to February 1, 1991. Note that the onset is shown in 6-hour periods for dates in January and February.

The team was comfortable in recommending that the cafeteria remain open, because the commuters who had become ill had not eaten at the cafeteria and because a similar illness was reported in the surrounding community. These factors made it unlikely that the cafeteria was the only source of infection, although there was a possibility that the ill food handlers had spread their disease to some. The short duration and mild nature of the illness meant that there was no need to close the college, even though there probably would be a certain amount of disruption and class absenteeism for a few more days.

Continued surveillance was established at the college, and this confirmed that the outbreak was dying out. Cultures continued to yield negative results for bacterial pathogens, and the analysis of the major questionnaire survey did not change any conclusions. This outbreak illustrates, among other things, that even without a definitive diagnosis, epidemiologic evidence enabled the investigators to rule out the biggest concern, bacterial food contamination, with a high degree of probability. In contrast to viral gastroenteritis, bacterial gastroenteritis is often quite serious, requiring hospitalization. In outbreaks, negative evidence (i.e., evidence that shows what the problem is not) often can permit epidemiologists to calm a nervous population.

SUMMARY

Surveillance is the foundation of public disease control. It may be active or passive. Its functions are varied and include determining the baseline rates of disease, detecting outbreaks, and evaluating control measures. Surveillance data are used for setting disease control policy.

The investigation of disease outbreaks is one of the primary functions of public health agencies, but the practicing physician has an important role of detecting and reporting disease and assisting in the investigation. The approach to the investigation of disease outbreaks has been developed and standardized during this century. The procedure involves making a diagnosis, establishing a case definition, and determining whether or not there is a definite outbreak.

If an outbreak is occurring, the cases of disease are characterized by time (especially using an epidemic time curve), place (usually determining rates in people who live and work in different locations), and person (determining the personal characteristics and patterns of the persons involved in the outbreak and ascertaining how they differ from those of persons not involved). Following this, hypotheses are developed and tested regarding the source of the infection, the pattern of spread, and the mode of transmission. These hypotheses are tested with cultures, paired sera, analysis for toxins, or case-control studies, depending on the hypotheses. Control measures are initiated as soon as practicable, and follow-up surveillance is initiated to evaluate the control measures.

References Cited

Benenson, A. S. Control of Communicable Diseases in Man, 15th ed. Washington, D. C., American Public Health Association, 1990.

Brooks-Robinson, S., S. D. Helgerson, and J. F. Jekel. An epidemiologic investigation of putative cancer clusters in two Connecticut towns. Journal of Environmental Health 50:161–164, 1987.

Centers for Disease Control. Case definitions for public health surveillance. Morbidity and Mortality Weekly Report 39(RR-13):1–43, 1990.

Centers for Disease Control and Prevention. Recommendations of the Advisory Committee on Immunization Practices. Morbidity and Mortality Weekly Report 43(RR-1):1–38, 1994.

Harkess, J. F., et al. Is passive surveillance always insensitive? American Journal of Epidemiology 128:878–881, 1988.

Harrison, T. R., et al. Principles of Internal Medicine, 3rd ed. New York, McGraw-Hill Book Company, 1958.

Helgerson, S. D., J. F. Jekel, and J. L. Hadler. Training public health students to investigate disease outbreaks: examples of community service. Public Health Reports 103:72–76, 1988.

Herbst, A. L., H. Ulfelder, and D. C. Poskanzer. Adenocarcinoma of the vagina: association of maternal stilbestrol therapy with tumor appearance in young women. New England Journal of Medicine 284:878–881, 1971.

Jacquez, G. M., ed. Workshop on Statistics and Computing in Disease Clustering. Statistics in Medicine 12:1751–1968, 1993.

MacKenzie, W. R., et al. A massive outbreak in Milwaukee of *Cryptosporidium* infection transmitted through the public water supply. New England Journal of Medicine 331:161–167, 1994.

National Conference on Clustering of Health Events. American Journal of Epidemiology 132:S1–202, 1990.

Roueché, B. The Medical Detectives. New York, Truman Talley Books, 1991.

Slutsker, L., et al. Eosinophilia-myalgia syndrome associated with exposure to tryptophan from a single manufacturer. Journal of the American Medical Association 264:213–217, 1990.

Selected Readings

Centers for Disease Control. Case definitions for public health surveillance. Morbidity and Mortality Weekly Report 39(RR-13):1–43, 1990. [Surveillance.]

Centers for Disease Control. Guidelines for evaluating surveillance systems. Morbidity and Mortality Weekly Report 37(S-5):1–19, 1988. [Surveillance.]

Epidemiology Program Office, Centers for Disease Control and Prevention. Principles of Epidemiology: Self-Study Course 3030-G, 2nd ed. Atlanta, Centers for Disease Control and Prevention, 1992. [Outbreak investigation.]

Goodman, R. A., J. W. Buehler, and J. P. Koplan. The epidemiologic field investigation: science and judgment in public health practice. American Journal of Epidemiology 132:9–16, 1990. [Outbreak investigation.]

Gregg, M. B., and J. Parsonnet. The principles of an epidemic field investigation. *In* Holland, W. W., et al., eds. Oxford Textbook of Public Health, 2nd ed. Oxford, Oxford University Press, 1991. [Outbreak investigation.]

Kelsey, J. L., W. D. Thompson, and A. S. Evans. Methods in Observational Epidemiology. New York, Oxford University Press, 1986. [Outbreak investigation; see especially Chapter 9, entitled Epidemic Investigation.]

Langmuir, A. D. The surveillance of communicable diseases of national importance. New England Journal of Medicine 268:182–192, 1963. [Surveillance.]

Rhot, L. H., et al. Principles of Epidemiology: A Self-Teaching Guide. New York, Academic Press, 1982. [Outbreak investigation.]

CHAPTER FOUR

THE STUDY OF CAUSATION

IN EPIDEMIOLOGIC

INVESTIGATION AND

RESEARCH

Epidemiologists are frequently involved in studies to determine causation—that is, to find the specific cause or causes of a disease. This is a more difficult and elusive task than might be supposed, and it leaves considerable room for obfuscation, as was demonstrated in an article in *The New York Times* (September 24, 1991) that focused on cigarette smoking. In this article, Thomas Lauria, a spokesman for the Tobacco Institute (a trade association for cigarette manufacturers) was quoted as saying that he did "not deny that smoking was a risk factor, though not a cause, of a variety of diseases."

Is a risk factor, then, a cause, or is it not? To answer this question, this chapter begins with a review of basic concepts concerning causation.

TYPES OF CAUSAL RELATIONSHIPS

Most scientific research seeks to identify causal relationships. The three fundamental types of causation, which are discussed below in the order of decreasing strength or sufficiency as a cause, are (1) a sufficient cause, (2) a necessary cause, and (3) a risk factor. The three types of association, discussed in the order of decreasing directness in bringing about an effect, are (1) a directly causal association, (2) an indirectly causal association, and (3) a noncausal association.

Sufficient Cause

A sufficient cause precedes a disease and has the following relationship with it: if the cause is present, the disease will always occur. Examples in which this proposition holds true are rare, apart from certain genetic abnormalities which, if homozygous, inevitably lead to a fatal disease (e.g., Tay-Sachs disease).

Smoking is not a sufficient cause of bronchogenic lung cancer, because many people who smoke do not acquire lung cancer before they die of something else. It is not known whether all smokers would get lung cancer if they lived and smoked long enough, but within the human life span, smoking cannot be considered a sufficient cause of lung cancer.

Necessary Cause

A necessary cause precedes a disease and has the following relationship with it: if the cause is absent, the disease cannot occur. For example, in the absence of the organism *Mycobacterium tuberculosis,* the disease of tuberculosis cannot occur. Therefore, *M. tuberculosis* can be called a necessary cause, or prerequisite, of tuberculosis. It cannot be called a sufficient cause of tuberculosis, however, because it is possible for people to carry the organism in their bodies and yet have no symptoms of the disease.

The initial exposure to *M. tuberculosis* usually leads to a primary infection with few or no symptoms. Primary tuberculosis commonly leaves a healed lesion filled with dormant mycobacteria at the initial infection site in the lungs, in the hilar lymph nodes, or in both locations. The mycobacteria remain alive for the rest of the infected person's life, as demonstrated by the results of skin testing with purified protein derivative (PPD). The mycobacteria usually remain dormant, held in check by the cell-mediated immunity that developed during the first infection. If there is a decline in cell-mediated immunity against the mycobacteria, however, the organisms may reactivate and cause a recurrence of clinical disease.

Cigarette smoking is not a necessary cause of bronchogenic lung cancer, because lung cancer can and does occur in the absence of both active and passive cigarette smoking. Furthermore, exposure to other agents, such as radon gas, radiation, arsenic, asbestos, chromium, nickel, coal tar, and some organic chemicals, has been shown to be associated with lung cancer, even in the absence of cigarette smoking (Doll and Peto 1981).

Risk Factor

A risk factor is a characteristic which, if present and active, clearly increases the probability of a particular disease in a group of persons who have the factor compared to an otherwise similar group of persons who do not. A risk factor, however, is neither a necessary cause nor a sufficient cause of the disease. Even though smoking is the most important risk factor for bronchogenic carcinoma, producing up to 20 times as high a risk of lung cancer in males who are heavy smokers as in males who are nonsmokers, smoking is neither a sufficient cause nor a necessary cause of lung cancer.

What about the quotation cited above, in which the spokesman from the Tobacco Institute did "not deny that smoking was a risk factor, though not a cause, of a variety of diseases"? If by "cause" the speaker includes only necessary and sufficient causes, he is correct. If, however, the concept of causation includes those situations in which possession of the risk factor clearly increases the probability of the disease, he is wrong. The overwhelming proportion of scientists who have studied the question of smoking and lung cancer (98% of them, according to the article in *The New York Times*) believe that cigarette smoking is a cause of lung cancer and, in fact, is the most important cause, despite the fact that it is neither a necessary nor a sufficient cause of the disease.

Directly or Indirectly Causal Association

If an association is causal, the causal pathway may be direct or indirect. The classification here depends on the absence or presence of **intermediary factors,** which are called **intervening variables.**

A **directly causal association** occurs when the factor under consideration exerts its effect without intermediary factors. For example, a severe blow to the head will cause brain damage and death without other external causes being required.

BOX 4–1. Types of Causal Relationship

Sufficient cause: If the factor (cause) is present, the effect (disease) will always occur.

Necessary cause: If the factor (cause) is absent, the effect (disease) cannot occur.

Risk factor: If the factor is present and active, the probability that the effect (disease) will occur is increased.

Directly causal association: The factor exerts its effect in the absence of intermediary factors (intervening variables).

Indirectly causal association: The factor exerts its effect via intermediary factors.

Noncausal association: The relationship between two variables is statistically significant, but no causal relationship exists, either because the temporal relationship is incorrect (the presumed cause comes after, rather than before, the presumed effect) or because another factor is responsible for both the presumed cause and the presumed effect.

An **indirectly causal association** occurs when one factor influences one or more other factors which are, in turn, directly causal. For example, poverty per se may not cause disease and death, but by preventing adequate nutrition, housing, and medical care, it may lead to ill health and a higher risk of premature death. Education appears to lead to better health indirectly, presumably because it increases the amount of knowledge about health, the level of motivation to maintain health, and the extent of financial resources.

Noncausal Association

A statistical association may be strong and yet not be causal. One of the most important principles of data analysis is that association does *not* prove causation. If a statistically significant association is found between two variables but the presumed cause occurs after the effect, rather than before it, the association is noncausal. Likewise, if a statistically significant association is found between two variables but some other factor causes both the presumed cause and the effect, the association is noncausal. For example, baldness may be associated with the risk of coronary artery disease, but it is probably a noncausal association, because both baldness and coronary artery disease are functions of age and gender.

STEPS IN THE DETERMINATION OF CAUSE AND EFFECT

Investigators must have a model of causation to guide their thinking. The scientific method for determining causation can be summarized as having three steps, which should be considered in the following order: (1) investigation of the statistical association, (2) investigation of the temporal relationship, and (3) elimination of all known alternative explanations (Bauman 1980). These steps in epidemiologic studies are similar in many ways to the steps followed in murder investigations, as discussed below.

Investigation of the Statistical Association

Investigations may focus on risk factors or may involve the study of protective factors. For causation to be identified, the presumed **risk factor** must be present significantly more often in persons with the particular disease of interest than in persons without the disease. Conversely, the presumed **protective factor** must be present significantly less often in those with the disease than in those without it. When the presumed factor (either a risk factor or a protective factor) is not associated with a different frequency of disease, the factor cannot be considered causal. It might be argued that something else could be obscuring a real association between the factor and the disease. If that occurs, however, this principle is not violated, because proper research design and statistical analysis would demonstrate the real association.

While the first step in an epidemiologic study is to demonstrate statistical association between the presumed risk or protective factor and the disease, the equivalent first step in a murder investigation is to demonstrate a geographic association between the accused murderer and the victim—that is, to show that both were in the same place or that the murderer was in a place from which he or she could have caused the murder.

The relationship between smoking and lung cancer provides an example of how an association can lead to the understanding of causation. The earliest epidemiologic studies showed that smokers had an average overall death rate approximately 2 times that for nonsmokers, and the studies also indicated that the death rate for lung cancer among smokers was approximately 10 times that among nonsmokers (see US Surgeon General 1964). These studies led to other research efforts, which clarified the role of cigarette smoking as a risk factor for lung cancer and for many other diseases as well.

In epidemiologic studies, the research design must allow a statistical association to be shown, if it exists. This usually means comparing the rate of disease before and after an intervention or comparing groups with and without the exposure or the treatment. Statistical analysis is needed both to demonstrate that the difference associated with the intervention or exposure is greater than would be expected by chance alone and to estimate how large this difference is. Research design and statistical analysis, therefore, work closely together. (For a detailed discussion of the types of research design, see Chapter 5).

If a statistically significant difference in risk of disease or rate of recovery is seen, the investigator must first consider the direction and extent of the difference: Did the therapy make the patients better or worse, on the average? Was the difference large enough to be etiologically or clinically important? Even if the difference observed is real and large, statistical association does not prove causation. It may initially appear that an association is causal, when in fact it is not. For example, in the era before antibiotics were developed, syphilis was treated with arsenic compounds (e.g., salvarsan), despite their toxicity. An outbreak of fever and jaundice occurred in many of the patients treated with arsenicals (see Anderson, Arnstein, and Lester 1962). At the time, it seemed obvious to those concerned that the outbreak was due to the arsenic. Many years later, however, medical experts realized that the outbreak of fever and jaundice was most likely due to an infectious agent—probably hepatitis B or C virus—spread via the use of inadequately sterilized needles during the administration of the arsenic compounds.

There are several criteria which, if met, increase the probability that a statistical association is causal (Susser 1973). Many of the criteria can be traced back to the philosopher John Stuart Mill (1856) and are often called **Mill's canons.** In general, an association is more likely to be causal if the following are true: (1) The association shows **strength**—i.e., the differ-

ence is large. (2) The association demonstrates **consistency**—i.e., the difference is always observed if the risk factor is present. (3) The association shows **specificity**—i.e., the difference does not appear if the risk factor is not present. (4) The association has **biologic plausibility**—i.e., it makes sense, based on what is known about the natural history of the disease. (5) The association exhibits a **dose-response relationship**—i.e., the risk of disease is greater with stronger exposures to the risk factor.

An example of a dose-response relationship is shown in Fig. 4–1 and is based on an early study of cigarette smoking and lung cancer. In this study, Doll and Hill (1956) found the following rates of lung cancer deaths, expressed as the number of deaths per 100,000 population per year: 7 deaths in men who did not smoke; 47 deaths in men who smoked about one-half pack of cigarettes a day; 86 deaths in men who smoked about one pack a day; and 166 deaths in men who smoked two or more packs a day.

Even if all of the above-mentioned criteria for an association hold true, the proof of a causal relationship will also depend on the demonstration of the necessary temporal relationship and the elimination of alternative explanations, which are the next two steps discussed below.

FIGURE 4–1. An example of a dose-response relationship in epidemiology. The x-axis is the approximate "dose" of cigarettes per day, and the y-axis is the rate of deaths due to lung cancer. (Source of data: Doll, R., and A. B. Hill. Lung cancer and other causes of death in relation to smoking. British Medical Journal 2:1071, 1956.)

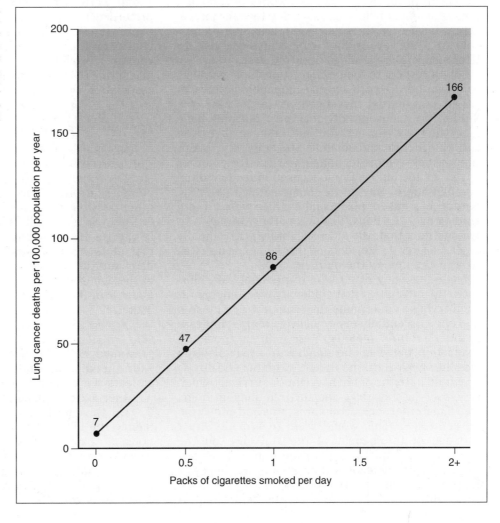

Investigation of the Temporal Relationship

Although some philosophical traditions consider time as circular, Western science assumes that time runs only one way. To demonstrate causation, the suspected causal factor must have occurred or been present before the effect (e.g., the disease) developed. This is more complex than it might seem unless **experimental control**—i.e., randomization followed by measurement of the risk factor and disease in both groups before and after the experimental intervention—is possible.

With chronic diseases, the onset of the "effect" is often unclear: When did atherosclerosis begin? When did the first bronchial cell become cancerous? Likewise, the onset of the risk factor may be unclear: When did the blood pressure begin to rise? When did the diet first become unhealthy? Because of long but varying latent periods between the onset of risk factors and the onset of the diseases they cause, the temporal relationships may be obscured.

Research design has an important role in determining the temporal sequence of cause and effect. If information on both the cause and the effect is obtained simultaneously, as in a survey, it is difficult to decide whether the presumed cause or the effect began first. On the one hand, basic demographic variables such as gender and race—factors that are present from birth—presumably would have begun to have an effect before diseases due to external risk factors began. On the other hand, it is often impossible in a survey or in a single medical visit to determine which variables occurred first.

With respect to temporal relationships, parallels can again be drawn between epidemiologic investigations and murder investigations. In the case of a murder, the accused individual must not only have been with the victim at some time but must have been with the victim immediately preceding the death (unless some remote technique was used). In murder mysteries, the innocent but accused individual often stumbles onto the scene immediately after the murder has taken place and is discovered there bending over the body. The task of the attorney is to demonstrate that the accused individual actually appeared after the murder and that someone else was there at the time of the murder.

The following discussion of prenatal care illustrates the difficulties that epidemiologists encounter when trying to determine the temporal relationship of events. Essentially every analysis of prenatal care in the literature demonstrates a direct (positive) association between the number of prenatal visits and the health of the infant, whether health is measured in terms of birth weight or survival (which are closely associated), and this relationship holds even if maternal socioeconomic status and education are controlled. This would seem to provide direct evidence of the benefit of prenatal care on the pregnancy and infant, but a major problem arises. Prenatal visits are made with increasing frequency as the pregnancy nears term, often weekly in the last 4 weeks and biweekly in the 2 months before that. A

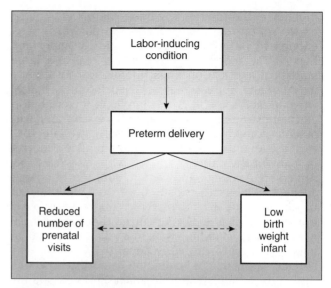

FIGURE 4–2. An illustration of causal association (arrows with solid lines) and possible noncausal association (arrow with dotted lines) in studies of infant birth weights and prenatal care.

pregnancy that terminates at 36 weeks of gestation will, on the average, have had 4 fewer prenatal visits than a pregnancy that terminates at 40 weeks of gestation, regardless of the reason that the pregnancy ended early. Therefore, any cause that induces preterm delivery will also produce a reduced number of prenatal visits (Fig. 4–2). Studies that attempted to control for this problem have suggested that prenatal care does provide some benefits to the child, but the magnitude of these benefits is smaller than the crude association would suggest.

Elimination of All Known Alternative Explanations

In a murder case, the verdict of "not guilty"—i.e., "not proved beyond a reasonable doubt"—can usually be obtained for the accused person if that person's attorney can demonstrate that there are other possible scenarios for what happened and that one of them is at least as likely as the scenario which implicates his or her client. For example, evidence that another person was at the scene of the crime and had a murder motive as great as or greater than that of the accused person would usually cast sufficient doubt on the guilt of the latter to result in an acquittal.

In the case of an epidemiologic investigation concerning the causation of disease, even if the presumed causal factor is associated statistically with the disease and occurs before the disease appears, it is necessary to demonstrate that there are no other likely explanations for the association.

On the one hand, proper research design can reduce the likelihood of competing causal explanations. For example, randomization, if done correctly, ensures that neither self-selection nor investigator bias will influence the allocation of subjects into experimental and control groups. Randomization also means that the treatment and control groups should be reasonably comparable with regard to disease susceptibility and disease severity. Hard work by the investigator can reduce measurement bias (discussed in detail below) and other potential problems, such as a difference between the number of subjects lost to follow-up in each group.

On the other hand, the criterion that all alternative explanations be eliminated can never be fully met for all time, because it is violated as soon as someone proposes a new explanation that fits the data and cannot be ruled out. For example, the classic theory of the origin of peptic ulcers (stress and hypersecretion) has been challenged recently by the theory that an infection by *Helicobacter pylori* is the primary cause of these ulcers. The fact that scientific explanations are always tentative—even when they seem perfectly satisfactory and meet the criteria concerning statistical association, timing, and elimination of known alternatives—is demonstrated in the following additional examples concerning the causation of cholera, cardiovascular disease, and eosinophilia-myalgia syndrome.

Explanations for Cholera

In 1849, there was an almost exact correspondence between the predicted cholera rates and the observed cholera rates in London, England, at various levels of elevation above the Thames River, as shown in Fig. 4–3. The accuracy of the prediction of cholera rates in London was hailed as an impressive confirmation of miasma theory, on which the rates had been based (Langmuir 1961). According to this theory, cholera was due to noxious vapors, which have their highest and most dangerous concentrations at low elevations. Subsequently, the germ theory of cholera became popular, and this theory is held to the present. Although nobody accepts the miasma theory today, it would be difficult to improve on the prediction of the cholera rates that were based on that theory in 1849.

Explanations for Cardiovascular Disease

Several recent studies of cardiovascular diseases, including atherosclerosis and myocardial infarction (MI), have focused on the levels of iron stored in the body (the iron burden). These studies have challenged the previously accepted idea that the most important risk factors for MI are related to smoking and to levels of various lipid fractions in the blood, which, in turn, are influenced by diet, exercise, and estrogen levels.

In 1981, Sullivan published a study concerning iron and the differences in risk of MI for men and women. He suggested that the lower risk of MI in premenopausal women was attributable to the loss of iron in menstrual flow, rather than to a direct effect of estrogen levels on atherosclerosis. Prior to Sullivan's hypothesis (the iron hypothesis), it had been widely

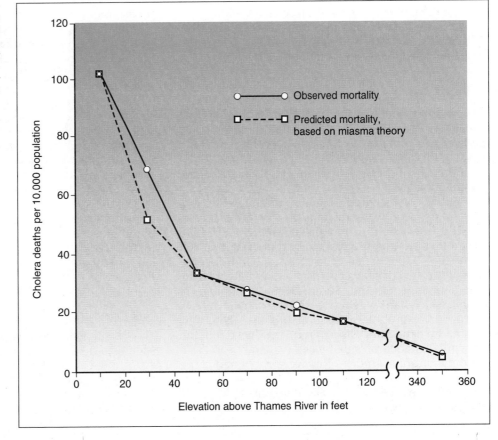

FIGURE 4–3. Predicted and observed cholera rates at various levels of elevation above the Thames River in London, England, in 1849. (Reproduced with permission from Langmuir, A. D. Epidemiology of airborne infection. Bacteriological Reviews 24: 173–181, 1961.)

assumed that hormonal factors, particularly estrogen levels, were directly protective against MI.

The iron hypothesis holds that the association between estrogen levels and MI is indirectly causal, because the hormonal effects are mediated through the loss of blood in the menstrual flow, keeping the iron burden in women's bodies lower than that in men's bodies. After menopause, women begin building up iron stores, and this leads to the increase in rates of MI. The level of iron in the body, therefore, is an intervening variable between hormones and atherosclerosis.

In 1992, Salonen et al. reported that a high level of stored iron was associated with an excess risk of MI in Eastern Finnish men. This finding in men added support to the iron hypothesis.

The iron hypothesis has the advantage of possibly explaining other associations, such as that between a high level of red meat intake and an increased risk of MI, because red meat provides, in addition to saturated fat, considerable iron. The iron hypothesis, then, also partly challenges the direct role of dietary saturated fats in the etiology of MI.

From the public health viewpoint, the iron hypothesis is an important hypothesis to test because, if established, it could suggest new methods of intervention, such as removing iron supplements from daily vitamins and from foods (e.g., cereals); altering the daily diet to avoid foods that are rich in iron, in addition to avoiding foods that are high in saturated fats; and pursuing treatments for elevated iron levels, perhaps including the removal and donation of blood.

The iron question is far from settled and may well prove to be false or of minor importance. Nevertheless, it demonstrates that any hypothesis is open to challenges from alternative hypotheses.

Explanations for Eosinophilia-Myalgia Syndrome

Another example of an explanation that met the causal criteria of association and temporal sequence and yet was replaced by a better hypothesis was the association of eosinophilia-myalgia syndrome (EMS) with the use of dietary supplements of L-tryptophan, an amino acid.

Initially, investigators thought that high doses of the amino acid were responsible for EMS. Subsequently, however, this hypothesis was replaced by a new one, based on the discovery that essentially all of the EMS patients had used L-tryptophan from only one of the two primary chemical companies making the supplements, the Showa-Denka Company in Japan, which had switched to a new strain of bacteria in the company's fermentation process. This new strain, investigators discovered, produced an unknown substance or substances (called "peak E" in chromatographic studies) that were contained in the L-tryptophan pills and were probably responsible for the EMS (Slutsker et al. 1990; Belongia et al. 1990; Philen et al. 1993).

COMMON PITFALLS IN CAUSAL RESEARCH

Among the most frequently encountered pitfalls in causal research are bias, random error, confounding, synergism, and effect modification, each of which is defined below.

Bias

Bias, also known as **differential error,** is a dangerous source of error in epidemiologic research. Bias usually produces deviations or distortions that are consistently in one direction. It may occur when there is unequal allocation of subjects, unequal detection of the outcome (as occurs, for example, with measurement bias or recall bias), or unequal loss to follow-up of subjects in the various groups being studied. Bias becomes a problem when it weakens a true association, produces a spurious association, or distorts the apparent direction of association between variables.

Measurement Bias

Bias may occur in collecting baseline data or follow-up data. Bias could result, for example, from measuring the patients' height with their shoes on, in which case all the heights would be too great, or measuring the patients' weight with their clothes on, in which case all the weights would be too large. Even this is complicated, because the heels of men's shoes may differ in height from those of women's shoes and also because there will be variation in heel size within each group. Nevertheless, all people measured with their shoes on will be overmeasured to some extent.

In the case of blood pressure values, bias can occur if some investigators or some study sites have blood pressure cuffs that measure incorrectly and cause the measurements they take to be higher or lower than the true values.

Chemistry data from various medical laboratories are subject to bias. Some laboratories consistently report higher or lower values than other laboratories. Clinical investigators who collect laboratory data over time in the same institution or who compare laboratory data from different institutions must obtain the normal standards for each laboratory at the appropriate times and adjust their findings accordingly. For example, differences in reported blood glucose levels are meaningful only if adjusted to the same level of "normal." The differences in laboratory standards are a potential source of bias that can be corrected by the investigator.

Recall Bias

People who have experienced an adverse event, such as a disease, may cogitate more about why the event might have happened and therefore be more likely to recall previous risk factors than the people who have never experienced the event. Recall bias is a major problem in research into causes of congenital anomalies. For example, mothers who give birth to abnormal infants tend to think more about their pregnancy and are more likely to remember infections, medications, or injuries. This may produce a spurious (falsely positive) association between a risk factor (such as respiratory infections) and the outcome (congenital abnormality).

Selection Bias

Bias in allocation of subjects to groups is often called selection bias or assembly bias. If subjects are allowed to choose whether they are in the intervention group or the placebo group in a study, those who are more educated, more adventuresome, or more health-conscious may want to try a new therapy or preventive measure. Differences subsequently found may be due partly or entirely to differences between the subjects rather than to an effect of the intervention.

A good illustration of selection bias occurred in the 1954 polio vaccine trials, which involved one intervention group and two control groups (Francis et al. 1955). Earlier studies of paralytic poliomyelitis had shown that the rates of this disease were greater in upper socioeconomic groups than in lower socioeconomic groups. When a polio vaccine was first developed, some parents (usually those with more education) wanted their children to have a chance to receive the vaccine, so they agreed to let their children be randomly assigned to either the intervention group (the group to be immunized) or the primary control group (control group I). Other parents (usually those with less education) stated that they did not want their children to act as "guinea pigs" and receive the vaccine; their children were followed as a secondary control group (control group II). The investigators correctly predicted that the rate of poliomyelitis would be greater in control group I, whose parents were of a higher socioeconomic level, than in control group II, whose socioeconomic status was lower. During the study period, the rate of paralytic poliomyelitis was 0.057% in control group I but only 0.035% in control group II.

Another example of selection bias is found in studies of treatment methods for terminal diseases. In these studies, the most severely ill patients are often the ones who are the most willing to try a new treatment, despite its known or unknown dangers. This is presumably because these patients believe that they have little to lose. Because of self-selection, a new treatment might be given to the patients who are sickest, with relatively poor results. These results could not be fairly applied to those patients who were not as sick.

Bias in the selection of subjects creates a frequent problem for randomized trials. On the one hand, the results presumably are valid for participants, which means that the study has **internal validity.** On the other hand, it is not clear to whom the results can be generalized, because the study group is not fully representative of any easily defined population. In other words, the study may lack **external validity.**

Questions of external validity have arisen in regard to the Physicians' Health Study, a costly and well-performed study consisting of a field trial of aspirin to reduce cardiovascular events and a field trial of beta-carotene to prevent cancer (see Physicians' Health Study Steering Committee 1989). The approximately 22,000 participants in the study were US physicians who were between 40 and 75 years of age and met the exclusion criteria (baseline criteria) of never having had heart disease, cancer, gastrointestinal disease, a bleeding tendency, or an allergy to aspirin. The participants had to agree to take part in the study, and after a trial period, those with poor compliance were dropped. To what group of people in the population can investigators generalize the results obtained from a study of predominantly white, exclusively male, middle-aged or older physicians? Certainly not women and young men, probably not blacks, and probably not members of the lower socioeconomic groups.

Random Error

Random error, also known as **nondifferential error,** produces findings that are too high and too low in approximately equal amounts, owing to random factors. Even though it is a serious problem, random error is ordinarily less serious than bias because it is less likely to distort (i.e., reverse the direction of) findings. It does, however, decrease the probability of finding a real association by reducing the statistical power of a study (Kelsey, Thompson, and Evans 1986).

Confounding

Confounding (from the Latin meaning "to pour together") is the confusion of two supposedly causal variables, so that part or all of the purported effect of one variable is actually due to the other. For example, the percentage of gray hairs on the heads of adults is associated with the risk of myocardial infarction, but presumably that is not a causal association. Age increases both the proportion of gray hairs and the risk of myocardial infarction.

The next example is similar but concerns the risks of breast cancer. Women who had high parity (had given birth to many children) were found to have lower rates of breast cancer, and investigators assumed that childbearing was protective against subsequent breast cancer. Later, it was discovered that the best predictor was childbearing at an early age. When the woman's age at the time of her first delivery was entered into statistical analyses, the number of offspring no longer predicted the rate of breast cancer. As Fig. 4–4 shows, because childbearing at a young age was associated with high parity, there was an association between parity and breast

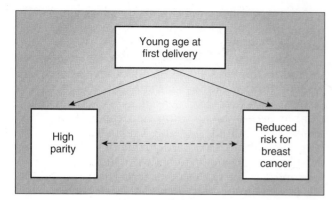

FIGURE 4–4. An illustration of causal association (arrows with solid lines) and noncausal association (arrow with dotted lines) in studies of childbearing and breast cancer.

cancer, but apparently it was not causal (Kelsey, Thompson, and Evans 1986).

Confounding can also obscure a true causal relationship, as this final example illustrates. In the early 1970s, the author (JFJ) and a colleague were involved in a study of the predictors for educational success among teenage mothers. An analysis of the data concerning these young women revealed that both their age and their grade level were positively associated with their ultimate educational success: the older a young mother was and the higher her grade level in school, the more likely she was to stay in school and graduate. But age was strongly associated with grade level in school (the older she was, the more likely she was to be in a high grade). When the effect of age was studied *within* each grade level, age was shown to be negatively associated with educational success. That is, the older a teenage mother was for a given grade level, the less successful she was (Klerman and Jekel 1973). This was apparently due to the fact that a woman who was old for a given grade level had been kept back because of academic or social difficulties, which were negative predictors of success. Thus, one important aspect of the association of age and educational success was obscured by its confounding with grade level.

Synergism

Synergism (from the Greek meaning "to work together") is the interaction of two or more presumably causal variables, so that the combined effect is clearly greater than the sum of the individual effects. For example, the risk of lung cancer is greater when a person has exposure to both asbestos and smoking than would be expected on the basis of the observed risks from each factor acting alone (Hammond, Selikoff, and Seidman 1979).

Fig. 4–5 shows the relationship between the percentage of infants with a low birth weight and the number of adverse factors present during the pregnancy. Low birth weight in this study was defined as 2500 g or less, and examples of adverse factors were teenage pregnancy and maternal smoking. For infants

with white mothers, the risk was 1.7% (12/708) if no adverse factor was present; 4.5% (32/715) if one adverse factor was present; 15.4% (35/228) if two adverse factors were present; and 29.7% (19/64) if three or more adverse factors were present (Miller and Jekel 1987). Similarly, for infants with black mothers, the figure shows how adverse factors interacted synergistically to produce low birth weight infants.

Effect Modification (Interaction)

Sometimes the direction or strength of association between two variables will differ depending on the value of a third variable. This is usually called **effect modification** by epidemiologists and **interaction** by biostatisticians.

In addition to providing an example of synergism, Fig. 4–5 provides an example of effect modification. The number of adverse factors during pregnancy has a similar *pattern* of impact on the birth weights of infants born to white mothers and those born to black mothers. However, the *size* of the impact is modified at each level by the reported race of the mother. A greater impact is consistently seen in infants born to black mothers, and this is an example of effect modification. Notice that this is not confounding; the adverse impact of the risk factors in pregnancy is not being questioned (based on the available data, it is the risk factors themselves that produce the effect).

A more biologic example of effect modification is seen in the ways in which Epstein-Barr virus infection is manifested in different geographic areas (Kelsey, Thompson, and Evans 1986). While the virus usually results in infectious mononucleosis in the USA, it often produces Burkitt's lymphoma in African regions where malaria is endemic. To test whether malaria modifies the effects of Epstein-Barr virus, investigators instituted a malaria suppression program in an African region where Burkitt's lymphoma was usually found and followed the number of new cases. They reported that the incidence of Burkitt's lymphoma fell after malaria was suppressed, although other factors appeared to be involved as well (Geser, Brubaker, and Draper 1989).

IMPORTANT REMINDERS ABOUT RISK FACTORS AND DISEASE

While it is essential to avoid the specific types of pitfalls described above, it is also necessary to keep two important concepts in mind.

First, one causal factor may increase the risk for several different diseases. For example, cigarette smoking is a risk factor for cancer of the lungs, larynx, mouth, and esophagus, as well as for chronic bronchitis and chronic obstructive pulmonary disease.

Second, one disease may have several different risk factors. Even though smoking is a strong risk factor for chronic obstructive pulmonary disease, it may be only one of several contributing factors in a

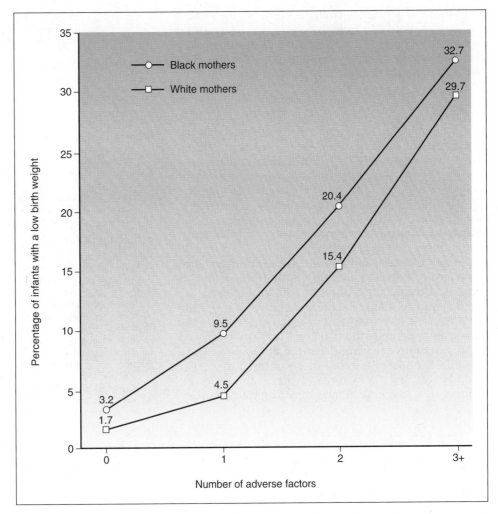

FIGURE 4–5. Relationship between the percentage of infants with a low birth weight and the number of adverse factors present during the pregnancy. Low birth weight was defined as 2500 g or less, and examples of adverse factors were teenage pregnancy and maternal smoking. (Source of data: Miller, H. C., and J. F. Jekel. Incidence of low birth weight infants born to mothers with multiple risk factors. Yale Journal of Biology and Medicine 60:397–404, 1987.)

given case. Other factors may include occupational exposure to dusts (e.g., coal dust or silicon) and genetic factors (e.g., alpha₁-antitrypsin deficiency). Similarly, the risk of myocardial infarction is influenced not only by a patient's genes, diet, exercise, and smoking but also by other conditions such as high blood pressure and diabetes. One of the tasks of epidemiologists, therefore, is to determine the relative amount that each risk factor contributes to a disease. This contribution, called the attributable risk, is discussed in Chapter 6.

The possibility of confounding and effect modification makes the interpretation of epidemiologic studies more difficult. Age may be a confounder because it has a direct effect on the risk of death and of many diseases, so that its impact must be removed before the causal impact of other variables can be known. But advancing age also can be an effect modifier, when it changes the magnitude of the risk of other variables (Jacobsen et al. 1992). For example, the risk of myocardial infarction increases both with age and with increasing levels of cholesterol and blood pressure. But both cholesterol levels and blood pressure also increase with age. To determine whether there is an association between cholesterol levels and myocardial infarction, the effects of both

age and blood pressure must be controlled. Likewise, to determine the association of blood pressure and myocardial infarction, the effects of age and choles-

---

BOX 4–2.   Problems That Obscure True Causal Relationships

Bias: A differential error that usually produces findings which are consistently distorted in one direction, owing to nonrandom factors.

Random error: A nondifferential error that produces findings which are too high and too low in approximately equal amounts, owing to random factors.

Confounding: The confusion of two supposedly causal variables, so that part or all of the purported effect of one variable is actually due to the other.

Synergism: The interaction of two or more presumably causal variables, so that the total effect is clearly greater than the sum of the individual effects.

Effect modification (interaction): A phenomenon in which a third variable alters the direction or strength of association between two other variables.

terol levels must be controlled. Although controlling sometimes can be done by research design and sample selection (e.g., by selecting study subjects in a narrow range of age and blood pressure), usually this is accomplished in the statistical analysis.

SUMMARY

Epidemiologists are concerned with discovering the causes of disease in the environment, nutrition, life-style, and genes of individuals and populations—that is, the causes or factors that when removed or modified will be followed by a reduction in the disease burden. Research to determine causation is complicated, particularly because epidemiologists usually do not have experimental control and must rely on observational methods.

Several criteria must be met to establish a causal relationship between a factor and a disease. First, a statistical association must be shown between the factor and the disease. The association is more impressive if it is strong and consistent. Second, the factor must precede the disease. Third, there should be no alternative explanations that fit the data equally well. Demonstrating that these criteria are met is complicated by the hazards of bias, random error, confounding, synergism, and effect modification.

References Cited

Anderson, G., M. Arnstein, and M. R. Lester. Chapter 17 in Communicable Disease Control, 4th ed. New York, Macmillan Company, 1962.

Bauman, K. E. Research Methods for Community Health and Welfare. New York, Oxford University Press, 1980.

Belongia, E. A., et al. An investigation of the cause of the eosinophilia-myalgia syndrome associated with tryptophan use. New England Journal of Medicine 323:357–365, 1990.

Doll, R., and A. B. Hill. Lung cancer and other causes of death in relation to smoking. British Medical Journal 2:1071, 1956.

Doll, R., and R. Peto. The Causes of Cancer. Oxford, Oxford University Press, 1981.

Francis, T., Jr., et al. An evaluation of the 1954 poliomyelitis vaccine trials. American Journal of Public Health, April supplement, 1955.

Geser, A., G. Brubaker, and C. C. Draper. Effect of a malaria suppression program on the incidence of African Burkitt's lymphoma. American Journal of Epidemiology 129:740–752, 1989.

Hammond, E. C., I. J. Selikoff, and H. Seidman. Asbestos exposure, cigarette smoking and death rates. Annals of the New York Academy of Sciences 330:473–490, 1979.

Jacobsen, S. J., et al. Cholesterol and coronary artery disease: age as an effect modifier. Journal of Clinical Epidemiology 45:1053–1059, 1992.

Kelsey, J. L., W. D. Thompson, and A. S. Evans. Chapter 9 in Methods in Observational Epidemiology. New York, Oxford University Press, 1986.

Klerman, L. V., and J. F. Jekel. School-Age Mothers: Problems, Programs, and Policy. Hamden, Conn., Linnet Books, 1973.

Langmuir, A. D. Epidemiology of airborne infection. Bacteriological Reviews 24:173–181, 1961.

Mill, J. S. A System of Logic (1856). Summarized in J. M. Last. A Dictionary of Epidemiology, 2nd ed. New York, Oxford University Press, 1988.

Miller, H. C., and J. F. Jekel. Incidence of low birth weight infants born to mothers with multiple risk factors. Yale Journal of Biology and Medicine 60:397–404, 1987.

Philen, R. M., et al. Tryptophan contaminants associated with eosinophilia-myalgia syndrome. American Journal of Epidemiology 138:154–159, 1993.

Physicians' Health Study Steering Committee. Final report on the aspirin component of the ongoing Physicians' Health Study. New England Journal of Medicine 321:129–135, 1989.

Salonen, J. T., et al. High stored iron levels are associated with excess risk of myocardial infarction in Eastern Finnish men. Circulation 86:803–811, 1992.

Slutsker, L., et al. Eosinophilia-myalgia syndrome associated with exposure to tryptophan from a single manufacturer. Journal of the American Medical Association 264:213–217, 1990.

Sullivan, J. L. Iron and the sex difference in heart disease risk. Lancet 1:1293–1294, 1981.

Susser, M. Causal Thinking in the Health Sciences. New York, Oxford University Press, 1973.

US Surgeon General. Smoking and Health. Public Health Service publication No. 1103. Washington, D. C., US Government Printing Office, 1964.

Selected Readings

Greenland, S., ed. Issues in causal inference. Part I in Evolution of Epidemiologic Ideas. Chestnut Hill, Mass., Epidemiology Resources, 1987.

Susser, M. Causal Thinking in the Health Sciences. New York, Oxford University Press, 1973.

CHAPTER FIVE

COMMON RESEARCH

DESIGNS USED IN

EPIDEMIOLOGY

FUNCTIONS OF RESEARCH DESIGN

The basic function of most epidemiologic research designs is to permit a fair, unbiased contrast to be made between a group with and a group without a risk factor or intervention. In a case-control study, the contrast is between the frequency of the risk factor among the cases and the frequency of the risk factor among the controls.

A good research design must perform the following functions: (1) enable a comparison of a variable (such as disease frequency) between two or more groups at one point in time or, in some cases, between one group before and after receiving an intervention or being exposed to a risk factor; (2) allow the contrast to be quantified either in absolute terms (as with a risk difference or rate difference) or in relative terms (as with a relative risk or odds ratio), as discussed in detail in Chapter 6; (3) permit the investigators to determine when the risk factor and the disease occurred, in order to determine the temporal sequence; and (4) minimize biases, confounding, and other problems that would complicate interpretation of the data.

The research designs discussed in this chapter are the primary ones used in epidemiologic research. Cross-sectional surveys and ecologic studies are useful for developing hypotheses; cohort studies and case-control studies can be used both to develop hypotheses and to test them, although the hypothesis development and hypothesis testing must always be done on different data sets; and randomized clinical trials or field trials are usually the best for testing new treatments or preventive measures.

Hypothesis development is a critical step in the scientific process. Hypotheses are used to make predictions, which are then tested by further research. If the test results are consistent with the hypothesis, the likelihood of the hypothesis being true is strengthened. If the results are not consistent with the hypothesis, it needs modification.

TYPES OF RESEARCH DESIGN

Because some research questions can be answered by more than one type of research design, the choice of design depends on a variety of considerations, including speed, cost, and availability of data. Each type of research design has advantages and disadvantages, as discussed below and summarized in Table 5–1.

Observational Designs for Generating Hypotheses
Cross-Sectional Surveys

A cross-sectional survey is a survey of a population at a single point in time. Among the examples are an **interview survey** and a **mass screening program.**

Cross-sectional surveys have the advantages of being fairly quick and easy to perform. They are useful for determining the prevalence of risk factors and the frequency of prevalent cases of disease for a defined population. They are also useful for measuring current health status and planning for some health services, including setting priorities for disease control. For example, many surveys have been undertaken to determine the knowledge, attitudes, and health practices of various populations regarding the human immunodeficiency virus (HIV) and acquired immunodeficiency syndrome (AIDS).

A major disadvantage of using a cross-sectional survey is that data about both the exposure to risk factors and the presence or absence of disease are collected simultaneously. This creates problems in determining the temporal relationship of a presumed cause and effect. Another disadvantage is that a cross-sectional survey selects for longer-lasting and more indolent diseases. Such diseases are more likely to be found by a survey because people live longer with them, enabling the affected individuals to be interviewed, whereas severe diseases that tend to be rapidly fatal are less likely to be found by a survey. This phenomenon is called **Neyman bias**. It is called

TABLE 5–1. Advantages and Disadvantages of Common Types of Studies Used in Epidemiology

Studies	Advantages	Disadvantages
Cross-sectional surveys	Are fairly quick and easy to perform; are useful for hypothesis generation.	Do not offer evidence of a temporal relationship between risk factors and disease; are subject to late look bias; are not good for hypothesis testing.
Ecologic studies	Are fairly quick and easy to perform; are useful for hypothesis generation.	Do not allow for causal conclusions to be drawn, since the data are not associated with individual persons; are subject to ecologic fallacy; are not good for hypothesis testing.
Cohort studies	Can be performed retrospectively or prospectively; can be used to obtain a true (absolute) measure of risk; can study many disease outcomes; are good for studying rare risk factors.	Are time-consuming and costly (especially prospective studies); can study only those risk factors measured at the beginning; can be used only for common diseases; may have losses to follow-up.
Case-control studies	Are fairly quick and easy to perform; can study many risk factors; are good for studying rare diseases.	Can obtain only a relative measure of risk; are subject to recall bias; selection of controls may be dfficult; temporal relationships may be unclear; can study only one disease outcome at a time.
Randomized controlled trials	Are the "gold standard" for evaluating treatment interventions (clinical trials) or preventive interventions (field trials); allow investigator to have extensive control over research process.	Are time-consuming and usually costly; can study only interventions or exposures that are controlled by investigator; may have problems related to therapy changes and dropouts; may be limited in generalizability; are often unethical to perform at all.

late look bias if it results in selecting fewer individuals with severe disease because they died before detection. It is called **length bias** in screening programs, which tend to select less aggressive cases for treatment.

Repeated cross-sectional surveys may be used to determine changes in risk factors and changes in disease frequency in populations over time (but not the nature of their association). The data derived from these surveys also can be examined for associations in order to generate hypotheses, but they are not good for testing the effectiveness of interventions. For example, in a cross-sectional survey, investigators might find that subjects who indicated that they had been immunized against a disease had fewer cases of the disease. However, the investigators would not know whether this finding was due to the fact that those who sought immunization were more concerned about their health and less likely to expose themselves to the disease. If they randomized the subjects into two groups and immunized only one of the groups, this would exclude self-selection as a possible explanation for the association.

Cross-sectional surveys are of particular value in infectious disease epidemiology, where the prevalence of antibodies against infectious agents, when analyzed by age or other variables, may provide evidence about when and in whom infection has occurred. Proof of a recent acute infection can be obtained by two serum surveys separated by a short interval. The first serum samples, called the **acute sera,** are collected soon after symptoms of an infectious disease appear. The second serum samples, called the **convalescent sera,** are collected 10–28 days later. A significant increase in the serum titer of antibody to a particular infectious agent is taken as proof of recent infection.

Even if two serum samples are not taken, important inferences can be drawn on the basis of findings concerning IgG and IgM, two immunoglobulin classes, in a single serum sample. A high IgG titer without an IgM titer of antibody to a particular infectious agent suggests that the infection occurred in the distant past. A high IgM titer with a low IgG titer suggests a current or very recent infection. A high IgM titer in the presence of a high IgG titer suggests that the infection occurred in the fairly recent past.

Cross-Sectional Ecologic Studies

Cross-sectional ecologic studies relate the frequency with which some characteristic (e.g., smoking) and some outcome of interest (e.g., lung cancer) occur in the same geographic area. These studies are often useful for suggesting hypotheses, but they cannot be used to draw causal conclusions, because there is no information as to whether the people who smoked are the same people who got the lung cancer. This problem with ecologic studies is often referred to as the **ecologic fallacy.**

Concerned citizens sometimes are unaware of the problem of ecologic fallacy and use the findings in surveys to make statements such as the following: "There are high levels of both toxic pollution and cancer in northern New Jersey, so the toxins are causing the cancer." This conclusion may or may not be correct. Remember that statistical association does not prove causation (see Chapter 4). Are the data adjusted for age? Has it been established that the cause came before the effect? And have all other explanations for the association been eliminated?

There are, of course, cases in which important hypotheses initially suggested by cross-sectional ecologic studies were later proved correct by other types of studies. For example, the rate of dental caries in children was found to be much higher in areas with low levels of natural fluoridation in the water than in areas with high levels of natural fluoridation (Arnim, Aberle, and Pitney 1937). Subsequent research established that this association was causal, and the introduction of water fluoridation and fluoride treatment of teeth has been followed by striking reductions in the rate of dental caries (Ast 1962).

Longitudinal Ecologic Studies

Longitudinal ecologic studies use ongoing surveillance or frequent cross-sectional studies to measure trends in disease rates over many years in a defined population. By comparing the trends in disease rates with other changes in the society (such as wars, immigration, or the introduction of a vaccine or antibiotics), epidemiologists attempt to determine the impact of these changes on the disease rates.

For example, as discussed in Chapter 3 and illustrated in Fig. 3–9, the introduction of the inactivated (Salk) polio vaccine and, subsequently, of the oral (Sabin) polio vaccine resulted in a precipitous drop in the rate of paralytic poliomyelitis in the US population. In this case, because of the large number of people involved in the immunization program and the relatively slow rate of change of other factors in the population, longitudinal ecologic studies were useful for determining the impact of the public health intervention. Nevertheless, confounding with other factors can distort the conclusions drawn from ecologic studies in circumstances like this, so if time is available (i.e., it is not an epidemic situation), investigators should perform field studies, such as randomized controlled field trials, before pursuing a large-scale, new public health intervention.

Another example of longitudinal ecologic research is the study of the rates of malaria in the US population since 1930. As shown in Fig. 5–1, the peaks in malaria rates can be readily related to social events such as wars and immigration. (The use of a logarithmic scale in the figure visually minimizes the relative drop in disease frequency, making it less impressive to the eye, but enables the reader to see in detail the changes occurring when the rates are low.)

Important causal associations have been suggested by longitudinal ecologic studies. For example,

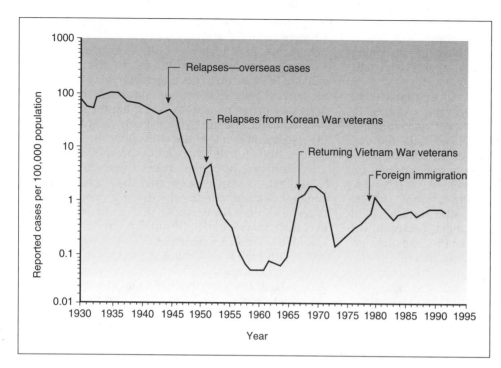

FIGURE 5–1. Incidence rates of malaria in the USA, by year of report, 1930–1992. (Source: Centers for Disease Control and Prevention. Summary of notifiable diseases, United States, 1992. Morbidity and Mortality Weekly Report 41: 38, 1992.)

about 20 years after there was an increase in the smoking rates in men, the lung cancer rate in the male population began rising rapidly. Similarly, about 20 years after women began to smoke in large numbers, the lung cancer rate in the female population began to rise. The studies in this case were ecologic studies in the sense that they used only national data, which did not relate the cases of lung cancer to individual smokers; the task of establishing a causal relationship was left to cohort and case-control studies.

Observational Designs for Generating or Testing Hypotheses

Cohort Studies

A cohort is a clearly identified group to be studied. In cohort studies, investigators begin by assembling one or more cohorts, either by choosing persons specifically because they were and were not exposed to one or more risk factors to be studied or else by taking a random sample of a population. A form of random sampling was used, for example, in the Framingham Study of heart disease, in which about 5000 people were studied (Dawber, Meadors, and Moore 1951). After the cohort of study subjects is selected, the subjects are followed over time to determine whether or not they develop the diseases of interest and whether the risk factors that were measured at the beginning of the study predict the diseases that occur.

There are two general types of cohort study, the prospective type and the retrospective type. The time relationships of the two are shown in Fig. 5–2.

Prospective Cohort Studies.   In a prospective cohort study, the investigator assembles the study groups in the present time, collects baseline data on them, and continues to collect data over time.

There are several advantages of performing prospective studies. The first is that the investigator is able to control the data collection as the study progresses and can check the outcome events carefully when they occur, thereby making sure that they are correctly classified. The second advantage is that the estimates of risk obtained from prospective cohort studies are true (absolute) risks for the groups studied. The third advantage is that many different disease outcomes can be studied, including some that were not anticipated at the beginning of the study.

Cohort studies have disadvantages, however. In a cohort study, only those risk factors defined and measured at the beginning of the study can be used. Other disadvantages of cohort studies are their high costs and the long wait until their results are obtained.

The classic cohort study is the Framingham Heart Study, which was begun in 1950 (see Dawber, Meadors, and Moore 1951) and still continues today. Table 5–2 shows the 8-year risk of heart disease as calculated from the Framingham Study's equations (Breslow 1978). Although the risk ratios are not based on the most recent findings from the Framingham Study, the length of follow-up and clarity of the message make them useful for sharing with patients.

Retrospective Cohort Studies.   Some of the time and cost limitations of the cohort study can be mitigated by doing a retrospective cohort study. In this approach, the investigator goes back into history to define a risk group (e.g., those exposed to the Hiroshima atomic bomb in August 1945) and follows the group members up to the present to see what outcomes (e.g., cancer and death) have occurred.

A retrospective cohort study was done by Mac-Mahon (1962), who was interested in investigating

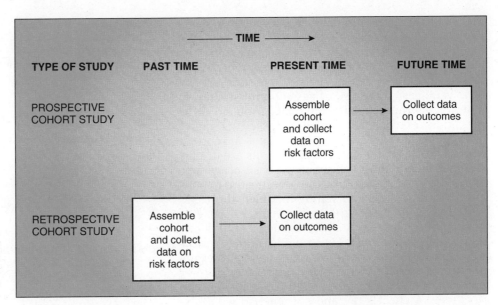

FIGURE 5–2. Illustration of the relationship between the time of assembling the study subjects and the time of data collection in a prospective cohort study and a retrospective cohort study.

the effects of prenatal x-ray exposure. In the past, radiographs were often used to measure the pelvic size of pregnant women, and this exposed their offspring to x-rays in utero. MacMahon identified one group of subjects who had been exposed in utero and another group who had not. He followed these subjects to see how many from each group had gotten cancer during childhood or early adulthood (up to the time he did the study). He found that those who had been exposed to x-rays in utero had a 40% increase in the risk of childhood cancers (i.e., a risk ratio of 1.4) after adjustments had been made for other factors.

Case-Control Studies

The investigator in a case-control study selects the case group and the control group on the basis of the outcome (i.e., having the disease of interest versus not having the disease of interest) and compares the groups in terms of their frequency of past exposure to possible risk factors. This can be thought of as comparing the "risk of having the risk factor" in the two groups. The actual risk of the outcome cannot be determined from case-control studies, because the underlying population is not known. However, an estimate of the relative risk of the outcome, called the odds ratio, can be determined in case-control studies.

In this kind of study, the cases and controls are assembled and then they are questioned (or their relatives or medical records are consulted) regarding past exposure to risk factors. In past decades, case-control studies were often called retrospective studies for this reason. The time relationships in a case-control study are similar to those in a cross-sectional study in that the investigator learns simultaneously about the current disease state and any risk factors that may have existed in the past. In terms of assembling the subjects, however, a case-control study differs from a cross-sectional study in that the

sample for the case-control study is chosen specifically from groups with and without the disease of interest.

Case-control studies are especially useful when a study must be done quickly and inexpensively or when the disease being studied is rare. In a cohort study, a huge number of study subjects would have to be followed to find even a few cases of a rare disease, and the search might take a long time even if the funds were available. Although in case-control studies only one outcome (one disease) can be considered per study, many risk factors may be considered, and this makes case-control studies useful for generating hypotheses concerning the causes of a disease. Methodologic standards have been developed so that

TABLE 5–2. The Risk That a 45-Year-Old Man Will Have Cardiovascular Disease Within 8 Years

Risk Group	Characteristics of Risk Group	Risk	Risk Ratio
Lowest	All of the following factors: - Nonsmoker - No glucose intolerance - No hypertrophy of left ventricle - Low systolic blood pressure ($\leq$ 105 mm Hg) - Low cholesterol level ($\leq$ 185 mg/dL)	2.2%	—
Highest	All of the factors listed below	77.8%	35.4
Intermediate	One of the following factors: - Smoker - Glucose intolerance - Hypertrophy of left ventricle - Severe hypertension (systolic blood pressure $\geq$ 195 mm Hg) - High cholesterol level ($\geq$ 335 mg/dL)	 3.8% 3.9% 6.0% 8.4% 8.5%	 1.7 1.8 2.7 3.8 3.8

Sources of data: (1) Pearson, T., and D. Becker. Cardiovascular risk. Computer program for IBM-compatible systems, using the Framingham Study 8-year risk equations. Developed at Johns Hopkins University on a Parke-Davis Educational Grant. (2) Breslow, L. Risk factor intervention for health maintenance. Science 200:908–912, 1978.

the quality of information obtained from case-control studies can approximate that obtained from the much more difficult, costly, and time-consuming randomized clinical trials (Imperiale and Horwitz 1989).

Despite these advantages, there are several disadvantages to the use of case-control studies. In determining the risk factors, a major problem is the potential for recall bias, a pitfall discussed in Chapter 4. Moreover, it is not easy to know what is the correct control group for the cases. The controls are usually matched individually to cases on the basis of age, sex, and often race. If possible, the investigator obtains controls from the same setting in which the cases were found, in order to avoid potential bias (e.g., having the disease more likely to be detected in one group than in another). For example, if the controls were taken from the same hospital and were examined for a disease of the same organ system (e.g., pulmonary disease), presumably a similar workup (including a chest x-ray and spirometry) would be done, so that cases of the disease would be less likely to be missed and classified as controls. Similarly, if a study concerns birth defects, the control subject for each case might be the next infant who was born at the same hospital, was of the same sex and race, and had a mother of similar age and from the same town. This would control for season, location, sex, race, and age of mother and infant. Often, the investigator assembles two or more control groups, one of which is from the general population.

Case-control studies were used to clarify the etiology of the 1989 epidemic of eosinophilia-myalgia syndrome (EMS), which was associated with dietary supplements of L-tryptophan (see Chapter 4). Investigators initially thought that the L-tryptophan itself was responsible for EMS, but additional investigation suggested that the problem was linked with pills produced by a particular manufacturer, the Showa-Denka Company. Two case-control studies were done to test this hypothesis and determine the odds that the source of the pills made a difference. If the source made no difference, the expected odds ratio would be 1. When Slutsker et al. (1990) compared the use of pills from Showa-Denka Company versus the use of

TABLE 5–3. Data from a Case-Control Study Showing the Source of L-Tryptophan Used by Subjects with Eosinophilia-Myalgia Syndrome (Cases) and the Source of L-Tryptophan Used by Subjects without Eosinophilia-Myalgia Syndrome (Controls)

Source of L-Tryptophan	Cases	Controls	Calculation of Odds Ratio
Showa-Denka Company	45	18	$\dfrac{45 \times 23}{18 \times 1} = 57.5$
Other manufacturers	1	23	
Total	46	41	

Source of data: Slutsker, L., et al. Eosinophilia-myalgia syndrome associated with exposure to tryptophan from a single manufacturer. Journal of the American Medical Association 264:213–217, 1990.

pills from all other manufacturers, their data permitted calculation of an odds ratio of 57.5, as shown in Table 5–3. When Belongia et al. (1990) undertook a similar case-control study, they found an odds ratio of 19.3. Thus, in both studies, the odds ratio for association of EMS with the Showa-Denka Company's L-tryptophan was strongly elevated.

Experimental Designs for Testing Hypotheses

Two types of randomized controlled trials are discussed below: randomized controlled clinical trials (RCCTs) and randomized controlled field trials (RCFTs). While both types follow the same series of steps shown in Fig. 5–3 and have many of the same advantages and disadvantages, the major difference between the two is that clinical trials are usually used to test therapeutic interventions in ill persons, while field trials test preventive interventions in well persons.

Randomized Controlled Clinical Trials

In a randomized controlled clinical trial (RCCT), patients are enrolled in a study and then randomly assigned to one of the following groups: (1) the intervention group, which will receive the experimental treatment, or (2) the control group, which will receive the nonexperimental treatment, consisting

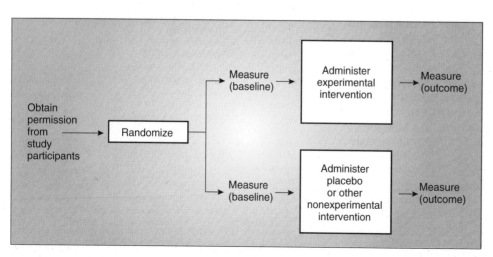

FIGURE 5–3. Illustration of the relationship between the time of assembling the study subjects and the time of data collection in a randomized controlled clinical trial (RCCT) or a randomized controlled field trial (RCFT).

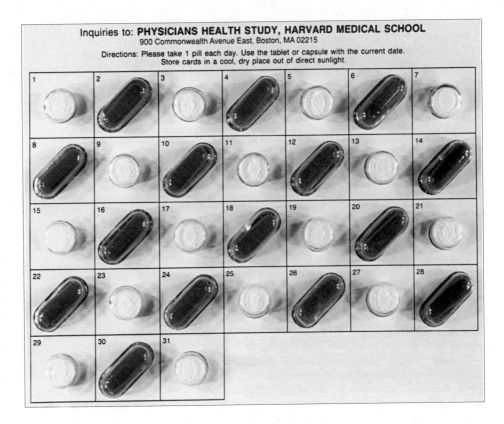

FIGURE 5–4. Photograph of the "bubble" pill packet provided monthly to the 22,000 physicians in the Physicians' Health Study, which consists of a simultaneous trial of aspirin to reduce cardiovascular disease and of beta-carotene to prevent cancer. The round white tablets contain either aspirin or a placebo, and the elongated capsules contain either beta-carotene or a placebo. The participants do not know which substances they are taking. (Courtesy of Dr. Charles Hennekens, Director, Physicians' Health Study, Boston.)

either of a placebo (inert substance) or a standard method of treatment.

RCCTs are considered the "gold standard" for studying interventions, because of their ability to minimize bias in the information obtained from the study subjects. Nevertheless, they do not entirely eliminate bias, and they pose some challenges and ethical dilemmas for investigators.

To be enrolled in an RCCT, the patients must agree to participate without knowing whether they will be given the experimental or nonexperimental treatment. If possible, the observers who collect the data are also prevented from knowing which type of treatment each patient is given. When this is done, the trial is said to be a **double-blind study.** To have true blinding, the nonexperimental treatment must appear identical to the experimental treatment. Fig. 5–4 shows the pill packet from a trial of two preventive measures from the Physicians' Health Study (see Chapter 4). The round tablets are either aspirin or a placebo, but the study subjects cannot tell which. The elongated capsules are either beta-carotene or a placebo, but the study subjects cannot tell which.

It is usually impossible as well as unethical to have patients participate blindly in a study involving a surgical intervention, because blinding would require a sham operation. But in studies involving nonsurgical interventions, investigators can usually develop an effective placebo. For example, when Rubin et al. (1986) designed a computer game to teach asthmatic children how to care for themselves with the goal of reducing hospitalizations, they distributed similar-looking computer games to the children in both the intervention group and the control group, but the games for the control group were without asthma content.

Undertaking an RCCT would be unethical if the intervention is strongly believed to be the best available, whether or not that has been established scientifically by carefully designed and controlled studies. There have been no RCCTs to compare prenatal care versus no prenatal care, so there is no conclusive proof that prenatal care is valuable, and questions about this are raised from time to time. However, because prenatal care is strongly thought to be of value, it would be unethical to undertake an RCCT in which some pregnant women were deprived of prenatal care.

In RCCTs, many biases still are possible, even though some biases have been minimized by the randomized, prospective design and by double-blinding. For example, in the two groups being compared, there may be different rates at which patients drop out of the study or become lost to follow-up, and this could produce a greater change in the characteristics of the remaining study subjects in one group than in the other.

Therapy changes and dropouts are special problems in RCCTs involving severe diseases, such as advanced cancer. The patients receiving the new treatment may continue to fail to respond, and either they or their physicians may decide to try a different treatment, which they must be allowed to do. Patients may also leave a study if the new treatment has unpleasant side effects, even though the treatment may be effective. For example, some medications for hypertension reduce male potency, and many men will discontinue their medication when this happens, regardless of its beneficial effect on their hypertension.

Randomized Controlled Field Trials

A randomized controlled field trial (RCFT) is similar to a randomized controlled clinical trial (RCCT) (see Fig. 5–3), except that ordinarily the intervention in an RCFT is preventive rather than therapeutic. Appropriate subjects are randomly allocated to receive the preventive measure (e.g., a vaccine or oral drug) or to receive the placebo (e.g., an injection of sterile saline or an inert pill). They are then followed over time to determine the rate of disease in each group.

Examples of RCFTs include trials involving vaccines to prevent paralytic poliomyelitis (Francis et al. 1955); trials involving the administration of a 6-month course of isoniazid (INH) to tuberculin skin test converters to prevent the reactivation of dormant infections with *Mycobacterium tuberculosis* (Ferebee 1963); trials of aspirin to reduce cardiovascular disease (see Physicians' Health Study Steering Committee 1989); and trials of beta-carotene to prevent cancer (see Physicians' Health Study Steering Committee 1989).

RCFTs and RCCTs have similar advantages and disadvantages. One disadvantage is that results may take a long time to obtain. The Physicians' Health Study (see above and Chapter 4) illustrates this problem. This trial of the preventive benefits of aspirin and beta-carotene was begun in 1982. The final report on the aspirin component of the trial was released 7 years later, and the final report on the beta-carotene component had not been released by 1995, which was 13 years after the trial began.

Another disadvantage of RCFTs and RCCTs has to do with **external validity,** which is the ability to generalize the findings to other groups in the population (as opposed to **internal validity,** which concerns the validity of results for the persons in the study). After the study subjects for a randomized trial have been assembled and various potential subjects have been excluded according to the study's exclusion criteria, it may not be clear whom the remaining people in the trial actually represent. Moreover, even if it is clear whom they represent, the people studied may be a limited subgroup of the population who might benefit from the intervention tested.

For example, the very carefully performed Physicians' Health Study of the preventive effects of aspirin on cardiovascular disease and of beta-carotene on cancers has been criticized because of questionable generalizability (i.e., external validity). The subjects included in the ongoing study are middle-aged and older male physicians with no history of heart disease, digestive tract disorders, cancer, or bleeding tendencies (Manson et al. 1991). While minorities were not excluded, there were few in

the study. Therefore, the results cannot be generalized to women, young men, and minorities and perhaps not even to nonphysicians who might have less health knowledge and financial resources. The findings probably are valid for healthy male physicians who are 40 years of age and older. The best evidence that the subjects in the study are a selected group was reported recently in the *Physicians' Health Study Newsletter* (see Harvard Medical School 1990): the 22,000 physicians participating in the study had less than 20% of the mortality rate that was expected for their age and sex, based on the general population. Surely they are a highly selected subgroup of the population.

SUMMARY

Observational research designs suitable for generating hypotheses include cross-sectional surveys, cross-sectional ecologic studies, and longitudinal ecologic studies. A cross-sectional study collects data about a population at one point in time, while a longitudinal study is done over a period of time. Cross-sectional surveys are useful in determining the prevalence of risk factors and diseases in the population, but they are weak in determining the temporal relationship between variables. In ecologic studies, both the rate of a disease and the frequency of exposure to a risk factor are obtained for an entire population, but the unit of study is the population and not individuals within it, so the exposure and the disease cannot be linked in individual persons.

Observational research designs suitable for generating or testing hypotheses include prospective cohort studies, retrospective cohort studies, and case-control studies. For cohort studies, one group consists of persons exposed to risk factors, while another group consists of persons not exposed. The groups are studied to determine and compare their rates of disease. Fig. 5–2 illustrates the difference between a prospective and a retrospective cohort study. For case-control studies, the case group consists of persons who have a particular disease, and the control group consists of persons who do not have the disease but are matched individually to the cases (e.g., in terms of age, sex, and type of medical workup). Each group is studied to determine the frequency of past exposure to possible risk factors. Based on this information, the relative odds that a disease is linked with a particular risk factor (the odds ratio) can be calculated.

The experimental designs suitable for testing hypotheses are randomized controlled clinical trials and randomized controlled field trials. Both types of trials follow the steps shown in Fig. 5–3. The major difference between the two types is that clinical trials are used to test therapeutic interventions, while field trials are used to test preventive interventions. A trial is called a double-blind study if neither the subjects who participate in it nor the observers who collect the data know which type of intervention each participant is given.

References Cited

Arnim, S., S. Aberle, and E. Pitney. A study of dental changes in a group of Pueblo Indian children. Journal of the American Dental Association 24:478, 1937.

Ast, D. B. Effectiveness of water fluoridation. Journal of the American Dental Association 65:581, 1962.

Belongia, E. A., et al. An investigation of the cause of the eosinophilia-myalgia syndrome associated with tryptophan use. New England Journal of Medicine 323:357–365, 1990.

Breslow, L. Risk factor intervention for health maintenance. Science 200:908–912, 1978.

Dawber, T. R., G. F. Meadors, and F. E. Moore, Jr. Epidemiologic approaches to heart disease: the Framingham Study. American Journal of Public Health 41:279–286, 1951.

Ferebee, S. United States Public Health Service trials of isoniazid prophylaxis. In Proceedings of the XVIIth International Tuberculosis Conference. International Congress Series No. 69, Rome, 1963.

Francis, T., Jr., et al. An evaluation of the 1954 poliomyelitis vaccine trials. American Journal of Public Health, April supplement, 1955.

Harvard Medical School. Physicians' Health Study Newsletter. Cambridge, Mass., Harvard University, Fall 1990.

Imperiale, T. R., and R. I. Horwitz. Scientific standards and the design of case-control research. Biomedicine and Pharmacotherapy 43:187–196, 1989.

MacMahon, B. Prenatal x-ray exposure and childhood cancer. Journal of the National Cancer Institute 28:1173, 1962.

Manson, J. E., et al. Baseline characteristics of participants in the Physicians' Health Study: a randomized trial of aspirin and beta-carotene in US physicians. American Journal of Preventive Medicine 7:150–154, 1991.

Physicians' Health Study Steering Committee. Final report on the aspirin component of the ongoing Physicians' Health Study. New England Journal of Medicine 321:129–135, 1989.

Rubin, D. H., et al. Educational intervention by computer in childhood asthma. Pediatrics 77:1–10, 1986.

Slutsker, L., et al. Eosinophilia-myalgia syndrome associated with exposure to tryptophan from a single manufacturer. Journal of the American Medical Association 264:213–217, 1990.

Selected Readings

Feinstein, A. R. Clinical Epidemiology. Philadelphia, W. B. Saunders Company, 1985.

Hennekens, C. H., and J. E. Buring. Epidemiology in Medicine. Boston, Little, Brown, and Company, 1987.

Hulley, S. B., and S. R. Cummings. Designing Clinical Research. Baltimore, Williams and Wilkins Company, 1988.

Kelsey, J. L., et al. Methods in Observational Epidemiology. New York, Oxford University Press, 1986.

Morgenstern, H. Uses of ecologic analysis in epidemiologic research. American Journal of Public Health 72:1336–1344, 1982.

Schlesselman, J. J. Case-Control Studies: Design, Conduct, Analysis. New York, Oxford University Press, 1982.

CHAPTER SIX

ASSESSMENT OF RISK IN

EPIDEMIOLOGIC STUDIES

Causal research in epidemiology requires that two fundamental distinctions be made. The first distinction is between those who do have and those who do not have the risk factor being studied (the **independent variable**), while the second distinction is between those who do have and those who do not have the disease being studied (the **dependent variable**). These distinctions are seldom simple, and they are subject to both random errors and biases.

In addition, epidemiologic research may be complicated by other requirements. The first is the need to analyze several independent (possibly causal) variables at the same time, including how they interact. For example, the frequency of hypertension is related to age and gender, and these variables interact in the following manner: before the age of about 50, men are more likely to be hypertensive; but after the age of 50, women are more likely to be hypertensive. The second complication involves the need to measure different degrees of strength of exposure to the risk factor, duration of exposure to the risk factor, or both. Investigators study strength and duration in combination, for example, when they measure exposure to cigarettes in terms of pack-years, which is the average number of packs smoked per day times the number of years of smoking. Depending on the risk factor, it may be difficult to determine the time of onset of exposure to it. This is true, for example, for risk factors such as sedentary life-style and excess intake of fat in the diet. Another complication involves the need to measure different levels of disease severity.

Despite these complexities, much epidemiologic research still relies on the dichotomies first mentioned—dichotomies that in the literature are commonly presented in the form of a **standard 2 × 2 table,** as shown in Table 6–1.

TABLE 6–1. Standard 2 × 2 Table for Demonstrating the Association between a Risk Factor and a Disease

		DISEASE STATUS		
		Present	Absent	Total
RISK FACTOR STATUS	Present	a	b	$a+b$
	Absent	c	d	$c+d$
	Total	$a+c$	$b+d$	$a+b+c+d$

Interpretation of the cells:

a = subjects with both the risk factor and the disease
b = subjects with the risk factor but not the disease
c = subjects with the disease but not the risk factor
d = subjects with neither the risk factor nor the disease

$a+b$ = all subjects with the risk factor
$c+d$ = all subjects without the risk factor
$a+c$ = all subjects with the disease
$b+d$ = all subjects without the disease

$a+b+c+d$ = all study subjects

DEFINITION OF STUDY GROUPS

Causal research depends on the measurement of contrast. In cohort studies, the contrast is between the frequency of disease in **persons exposed** to a risk factor and the frequency of disease in **persons not exposed** to a risk factor. In case-control studies, the contrast is between the frequency of the risk factor in **case subjects** (those with the disease) and the frequency of the risk factor in **control subjects** (those without the disease).

The exposure may be to a nutritional factor (e.g., a high-fat diet), an environmental factor (radiation following the Chernobyl disaster), a behavioral factor (cigarette smoking), a physiologic characteristic (a high total cholesterol level in the blood), a medical intervention (an antibiotic), or a public health intervention (a vaccine). This list is far from exhaustive.

COMPARISON OF RISKS IN DIFFERENT STUDY GROUPS

Although differences in risk can be measured either in absolute terms or in relative terms, the method used will depend on the type of study performed. For reasons discussed in Chapter 5, case-control studies allow investigators to obtain only a relative measure of risk, while cohort studies allow them to obtain both absolute and relative measures of risk. Whenever possible, it is important to examine both absolute and relative risks, because they provide different information.

After the differences in risk are calculated by the methods outlined in detail below, the level of statistical significance must be determined to ensure that the observed difference is probably not due to chance. If the difference is statistically significant but not clinically important, it is trivial. If the difference appears to be clinically important but is not statistically significant, it may be a false-negative (beta) error if the sample size is small (see Chapter 12) or it may be a chance finding.

Absolute Differences in Risk

Absolute differences in risk can be expressed as a risk difference or as a rate difference. The **risk difference** is the risk in the exposed group minus the risk in the unexposed group. Similarly, the **rate difference** is the rate in the exposed group minus the rate in the unexposed group. The discussion here will focus on risks, which are used more often than rates in cohort studies.

When the level of risk in the exposed group is the same as the level of risk in the unexposed group, the risk difference is 0. If an exposure is harmful (as in the case of cigarette smoking), the risk difference is expected to be greater than 0. If an exposure is protective (as in the case of a vaccine), the risk difference will be less than 0. The risk difference is also known as the **attributable risk** because it is an estimate of the amount of risk that is attributable to the risk factor after all other known causes of the disease have been taken into account.

In Table 6–1, the risk of disease in the exposed individuals is $a/(a + b)$, and the risk of disease in the unexposed individuals is $c/(c + d)$. Thus, when these symbols are used, the attributable risk (AR) can be expressed as the difference between the two:

$$AR = Risk_{(exposed)} - Risk_{(unexposed)}$$

$$= [a/(a + b)] - [c/(c + d)]$$

Fig. 6–1 provides data on age-adjusted death rates for lung cancer among adult male smokers and nonsmokers in the US population in 1986 (see Centers for Disease Control 1989 for a report of the 1986 data) and in the UK population (Doll and Hill 1956). For the USA in 1986, the rate in smokers was 191 per 100,000 population per year, while that in nonsmokers was 8.7 per 100,000 per year. Because the death rates for lung cancer in the population were low (under 1% per year) in the year for which data are shown, the rate and the risk for lung cancer death would be essentially the same. Therefore, the attributable risk in the USA can be calculated as follows: 191/100,000 minus 8.7/100,000 equals 182.3/100,000. Similarly, the attributable risk in the UK can be calculated as follows: 166/100,000 minus 7/100,000 equals 159/100,000.

Relative Differences in Risk

Relative risk can be expressed in terms of a risk ratio or in terms of an odds ratio.

The Relative Risk (Risk Ratio)

The relative risk, which is also known as the risk ratio (both being abbreviated as RR), is the ratio of the risk in the exposed group to the risk in the unexposed group. If the risks in the exposed group and unexposed group are the same, the RR will equal 1. If the risks in the two groups are not the same, calculating the RR will provide a straightforward way of showing in relative terms how much different (greater or smaller) the risks for the exposed group are. Remember that the risk for the disease in the exposed group will be greater if an exposure is harmful (as in the case of cigarette smoking) or will be smaller if an exposure is protective (as in the case of a vaccine).

In terms of the groups and symbols defined in Table 6–1, relative risk (RR) would be calculated as follows:

$$RR = Risk_{(exposed)}/Risk_{(unexposed)}$$

$$= [a/(a + b)]/[c/(c + d)]$$

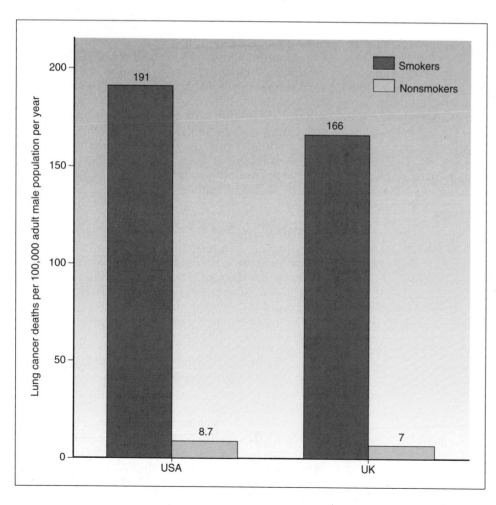

FIGURE 6–1. Comparison of the risks of death from lung cancer per 100,000 adult male population per year for smokers and nonsmokers in the USA and UK. (Source of US data: Centers for Disease Control. Chronic disease reports: deaths from lung cancer—United States, 1986. Morbidity and Mortality Weekly Report 38:501–505, 1989. Source of UK data: Doll, R., and A. B. Hill. Lung cancer and other causes of death in relation to smoking. British Medical Journal 2:1071, 1956.)

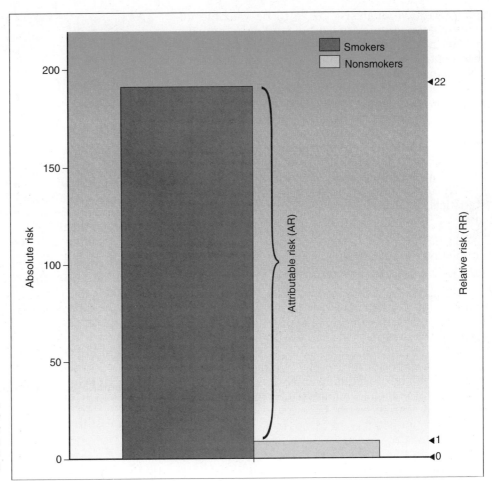

FIGURE 6–2. Diagram showing the risks of death from lung cancer per 100,000 adult male population per year for smokers and nonsmokers in the USA, expressed both in absolute risk terms (left axis) and in relative risks terms (right axis).

Earlier, the data on lung cancer deaths in Fig. 6–1 were used to determine the attributable risk, or AR. This time, the same data can be used to calculate the RR. For adult males in the USA, 191/100,000 divided by 8.7/100,000 gives an RR of 22. The conversion from absolute to relative risks can be seen in Fig. 6–2. Absolute risk is shown on the left axis, and relative risk is on the right axis. Note that in relative risk terms, the value of the risk for lung cancer death in the unexposed group is 1. Compared to that, the risk for lung cancer death in the exposed group is 22 times as great, and the attributable risk is the difference, which is 182.3/100,000 in absolute risk terms and is 21 in relative risk terms.

For the data in the UK study on lung cancer deaths, 166/100,000 divided by 7/100,000 gives an RR of 23.7, indicating that smokers were almost 24 times as likely to die of lung cancer as nonsmokers were. This estimate is very similar to the estimate from the US study, in which the RR was 22.

It is important to remember the number of people to whom the relative risk applies. A large relative risk that applies to a small number of people may actually produce few excess deaths or cases of disease, whereas a small relative risk that applies to a large number of people may produce many excess deaths or cases of disease.

The Odds Ratio

People who do not bet may be unfamiliar with the concept of odds and with the difference between the concepts of risk and odds. Based on the symbols used in Table 6–1, the **risk** of disease in the exposed group is $a/(a + b)$, whereas the **odds** of disease in the exposed group is simply a/b. If a is small compared to b, the odds will be similar to the risk. If the risk of the disease is relatively large (say, more than 5%), the odds ratio is not a very good estimate of the risk ratio.

The odds ratio can be calculated by dividing the odds of exposure in the diseased group by the odds of exposure in the nondiseased group. In the terms used in Table 6–1, the formula for the odds ratio (OR) is as follows:

$$OR = (a/c)/(b/d)$$

$$= ad/bc$$

In mathematical terms, it would make no difference whether the odds ratio were calculated as $(a/c)/(b/d)$ or as $(a/b)/(c/d)$, because cross-multiplication in either case would yield ad/bc. In conceptual terms, it makes no sense to use $(a/b)/(c/d)$, because cells a and b come from different study groups. However, the fact that the odds ratio is the same whether it is developed from a horizontal analysis of the table or from a vertical analysis proves to be valuable for analyzing data from case-control studies. Although a risk or a risk ratio cannot be calculated from a case-control study, an odds ratio can. Moreover, under most real world circumstances, the odds ratio from a case-control study is a good estimate of the risk ratio that would have been obtained from a prospective cohort study, and yet the case-control study is much less costly and time-consuming. Therefore, the odds ratio may be used as an estimate of the risk ratio if the risk of disease in the population is low (say, less than 5%).

The odds ratio also is used in logistic methods of statistical analysis (logistic regression, log-linear models, Cox regression analyses), which are discussed briefly in Chapter 11.

Which Side Is Up in the Risk Ratio and Odds Ratio?

If the risk for a disease is the same in the group exposed to a particular risk factor or protective factor as it is in the group not exposed to the factor, the risk ratio is expressed simply as 1. Hypothetically, the risk ratio could be as low as 0 (i.e., if the individuals exposed to a protective factor have no risk and the unexposed individuals have some risk), or it may be as high as infinity (i.e., if the individuals exposed to a risk factor have some risk and the unexposed individuals have no risk). In practical terms, however, because there usually is some disease in every large group, these extremes of the risk ratio are rare.

When risk factors are discussed, placing the exposed group in the numerator is a convention that makes intuitive sense (because the number gets larger as the risk has a greater impact), and this convention is followed in the literature. However, one of the interesting properties of the risk ratio is that it can also be expressed with the exposed group in the denominator. Consider the case of cigarette smoking and myocardial infarction, where the risk of this disease for smokers is greater than that for nonsmokers. On the one hand, it is acceptable to put the smokers in the numerator and express the risk as 2/1 (i.e., 2), meaning that the risk of myocardial infarction is about twice as high for smokers as for nonsmokers of otherwise similar age, sex, and health status. On the other hand, it is acceptable to put the smokers in the denominator and express the risk as 1/2 (i.e., 0.5), meaning that nonsmokers have half the risk as smokers do.

Another risk factor might produce, say, 4 times the risk of a disease, in which case the ratio could be expressed either as 4 or as 1/4. When the risk ratio is plotted on a logarithmic scale, as shown in Fig. 6–3, it is easy to see that regardless of which way the ratio is expressed, the distance to the risk ratio of 1 is the same. Mathematically, it does not matter whether the risk for the exposed group or the unexposed group is in the numerator: either way the risk ratio is easily interpretable. However, almost always the risk of the exposed group is expressed in the numerator.

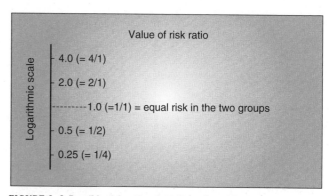

FIGURE 6–3. Possible risk ratios plotted on a logarithmic scale, showing that reciprocal risks are equidistant from the neutral point, where the risk ratio is equal to 1.0.

Although the equation for calculating the odds ratio differs from that for calculating the risk ratio, once the ratio is calculated the same observations apply: the ratio is usually expressed with the exposed group in the numerator, but mathematically it can be interpreted equally well if the exposed group is placed in the denominator.

OTHER MEASURES OF THE IMPACT OF RISK FACTORS

One of the most useful applications of epidemiology is to estimate how much disease burden is caused by certain modifiable risk factors. This is useful for policy development, because the impact of risk factors or interventions can be compared to costs in cost-benefit and cost-effectiveness analyses. In addition, health education is more effective when educators can demonstrate how big an impact a given risk factor has on individual risks.

The most common measures of the impact of exposures are (1) the attributable risk percent in the exposed, (2) the population attributable risk, and (3) the population attributable risk percent. In the discussion of these measures, smoking and lung cancer will be used as the examples of risk factor and disease, and the calculations will be based on 1986 rates for the USA (see Fig. 6–1).

Attributable Risk Percent in the Exposed

If an investigator wanted to answer the question, "Among smokers, what percentage of the total risk for fatal lung cancer is due to smoking?" it would be necessary to calculate the attributable risk percent in the exposed, which is abbreviated as $AR\%_{(exposed)}$. There are two methods of calculation, one based on absolute differences in risk and the other based on relative differences in risk.

The following equation is based on absolute differences:

$$AR\%_{(exposed)} = \frac{Risk_{(exposed)} - Risk_{(unexposed)}}{Risk_{(exposed)}} \times 100$$

If the 1986 US data on the lung cancer death rates in

adult male smokers and nonsmokers is used, the calculation is as follows:

$$AR\%_{(exposed)} = \frac{(191 - 8.7)}{191} \times 100 = \frac{182.3}{191} \times 100 = 95.4\%$$

If the absolute risk is not known, the risk ratio (RR) can be used instead, with the following formula:

$$AR\%_{(exposed)} = \frac{RR - 1}{RR} \times 100$$

Earlier in this chapter, the RR for the US data was calculated as 22, so this figure can be used in the equation:

$$AR\%_{(exposed)} = \frac{(22 - 1)}{22} \times 100 = 95.5\%$$

Note that the percentage based on the formula using relative risk is about the same as the percentage based on the formula using absolute risk. Why does this work? The important thing to remember is that the relative risk for the unexposed group is always 1, because that is the group to which the exposed group is compared. Therefore, the attributable risk, which is the amount of risk in excess of the risk in the unexposed group, is RR minus 1.

Because the odds ratio may be used to estimate the risk ratio if the risk of disease in the population is small, the AR%$_{(exposed)}$ also can be estimated by using odds ratios obtained from case-control studies and substituting them for the RR in the formula above.

Population Attributable Risk

The population attributable risk is defined as the risk in the total population minus the risk in the unexposed group. In the case of smoking and lung cancer, calculation of the population attributable risk allows an investigator to answer the question, "Among the general population, how much of the total risk for fatal lung cancer is due to smoking?" The answer to this question is not as useful to know for counseling patients, but it is of considerable importance to policy makers.

Using the US data for 1986, the investigator would subtract the risk in the adult male nonsmokers (8.7/100,000 per year) from the risk in the total adult male population (72.5/100,000 per year) to find the population attributable risk (63.8/100,000 per year). It can be presumed in this case that if there had never been any smokers or effects of second-hand smoke in the USA, the total US lung cancer death rate in adult males would be only 8.7/100,000 per year. Therefore, the excess over this figure—i.e., 63.8/100,000 per year—could be attributed to smoking.

Population Attributable Risk Percent

The population attributable risk percent (PAR%) answers the question, "Among the general population, what percentage of the total risk for fatal lung cancer is due to smoking?" As with the AR%$_{(exposed)}$,

the PAR% can be calculated using either absolute or relative differences in risk.

The following equation is based on absolute differences:

$$PAR\% = \frac{Risk_{(total)} - Risk_{(unexposed)}}{Risk_{(total)}} \times 100$$

When the US data discussed above for males are used, the calculation is as follows:

$$PAR\% = \frac{(72.5 - 8.7)}{72.5} \times 100 = \frac{63.8}{72.5} \times 100 = 88\%$$

The PAR% could instead be calculated using the risk ratio (or the odds ratio if the data come from a case-control study). But first it is necessary to incorporate another measure into the formula—namely, the proportion exposed, which is abbreviated as *Pe* and is defined as the effective proportion of the population exposed to the risk factor. The equation is then as follows:

$$PAR\% = \frac{(Pe)(RR - 1)}{1 + (Pe)(RR - 1)} \times 100$$

In the case of smoking, the *Pe* would be the *effective* proportion of the adult population who smoked. There are two reasons that this figure must be estimated, rather than being obtained directly. The first is that smoking is not linked with death in the same year. This means, for example, if the deaths occurred in the year 1986, using the proportion of smokers in 1986 would not offer a good estimate of the effective smoking rate that caused the 1986 deaths. The second is that the proportion of smokers has been dropping over time (now down to less than 30% of adults). Here, the *Pe* is assumed to be 0.35, or 35%.

As calculated earlier, the relative risk (RR) for lung cancer in the USA was 22. Thus, if this number is used, the calculation can be completed as follows:

$$PAR\% = \frac{(0.35)(22 - 1)}{1 + (0.35)(22 - 1)} \times 100 = \frac{7.35}{1 + 7.35} \times 100 = 88\%$$

Fig. 6–4 shows diagrammatically how the formula for PAR% works.

USES OF RISK ASSESSMENT DATA

After the various measures of the impact of smoking on lung cancer deaths have been calculated, the results can be used both in policy analysis and in counseling patients. For purposes of the discussion here, the baseline data and risk calculations are summarized in Table 6–2.

Application of Attributable Risk to Policy Analysis

Once the population attributable risk percent (PAR%) is known, the potential costs and benefits of programs that might reduce smoking by a defined percentage—say, by 50%—can be considered. Because the formula for PAR% involves the risk ratio (RR) and the effective proportion of people who

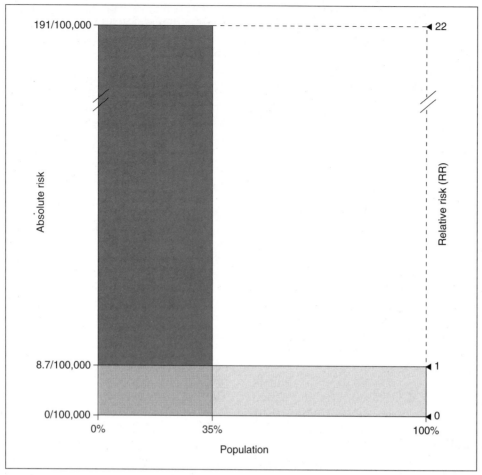

FIGURE 6–4. Diagram showing how the equation for population attributable risk percent (PAR%) works. The x-axis shows the population, divided into two groups: the 35% of the population representing the proportion exposed *(Pe)* to the risk factor (i.e., the effective population of smokers), and the remaining 65% of the population, who are nonsmokers. The right side of the y-axis shows the relative risk (RR) of lung cancer death. For reference, the left side of the y-axis shows the absolute risk of lung cancer death. Orange shading, gray shading, and a combination of the two are used to show the relationship between the risk factor (smoking) and the disease outcome (lung cancer death) in the smokers and nonsmokers. The purely orange part represents outcomes that are not attributable to the risk factor in nonsmokers. The purely gray part represents outcomes that are attributable to the risk factor in smokers. The overlapping gray and orange part represents outcomes that are not attributable to the risk factor in smokers (i.e., lung cancer deaths that are not attributable to smoking, even though they occurred in smokers). The equation is as follows:

$$PAR\% = \frac{(Pe)(RR - 1)}{1 + (Pe)(RR - 1)} \times 100$$

$$= \frac{(0.35)(22 - 1)}{1 + (0.35)(22 - 1)} \times 100$$

$$= \frac{7.35}{1 + 7.35} \times 100 = 88\%$$

smoked *(Pe)*, reduction of either of these measures would reduce the PAR%. If some people continued to smoke but reduced the amount they smoked (and there is evidence that this often happens), this would reduce the RR and thereby reduce the PAR%. If some people stopped smoking, this would reduce the *Pe* and thereby reduce the PAR%. Therefore, the impact of a prevention policy can be predicted from the anticipated reduction in packs per day for smokers and the reduction in the percentage of people who smoke at all.

Earlier, the population attributable risk (PAR) of lung cancer due to smoking was calculated to be 63.8/100,000 per year, while the attributable risk (AR,

or the difference between the risk in the exposed and the risk in the unexposed) was 182.3/100,000 per year. Either of these figures can be used to determine the benefits of a program designed to reduce the risk factor by 50%.

In the first method, the PAR is multiplied by the percentage of reduction of the risk factor to find the rate of lung cancer deaths that would result: 63.8/100,000 per year × 50% = 31.9/100,000 per year.

In the second method, the AR is multiplied by the effective percentage of the population with the risk factor and by the percentage of reduction of the risk factor to find the rate of lung cancer deaths that would result: 182.3/100,000 per year × 35% × 50% =

TABLE 6–2. Measures of Smoking and Lung Cancer Deaths in Adult Males in the USA, 1986

Measure	Amount
*Lung cancer deaths among smokers	191 per 100,000 per year
*Lung cancer deaths among nonsmokers	8.7 per 100,000 per year
†Proportion exposed *(Pe)* to the risk factor (effective population of smokers, averaged over time)	35%, or 0.35
†Population risk of lung cancer death	72.5 per 100,000 per year
†Relative risk, or RR	22 [191/8.7 = 22]
Attributable risk, or AR	182.3 per 100,000 per year [191 − 8.7 = 182.3]
Attributable risk percent in the exposed, or AR%(exposed)	95.4% [182.3/191 × 100 = 95.4]
Population attributable risk, or PAR	63.8 per 100,000 per year [72.5 − 8.7 = 63.8]
†Population attributable risk percent, or PAR%	88% [63.8/72.5 × 100 = 88]

*These rates were calculated from the data marked with a dagger.

†The source of data for measures shown with a dagger is as follows: Centers for Disease Control. Chronic disease reports: deaths from lung cancer—United States, 1986. Morbidity and Mortality Weekly Report 38:501–505, 1989.

31.9/100,000 per year. This result is the same as the result from the first method of calculation.

The risk of death from lung cancer in the total adult male population was 72.5/100,000. Reducing this rate by about 31.9/100,000 would leave a residual death rate from lung cancer in the population of about 40.6/100,000. This represents a 44% reduction from 72.5/100,000. Of the remaining 40.6 deaths per 100,000 adult male population per year, 31.9 would be due to smoking (on the average) and 8.7 would be due to other causes. The PAR% would have been reduced from 88% to 78.6%.

Application of Attributable Risk to the Counseling of Patients

Suppose a physician's patient is resistant to the idea of quitting smoking but is willing to be convinced. Or suppose the physician has been asked to give a short talk summarizing the effect of smoking on the lung cancer death rates, which is roughly equivalent to talking about the incidence of lung cancer, because most lung cancer patients die of their disease. Using the measures of risk discussed here and summarized in Table 6–2, the physician could make the following estimates of the impact of smoking (although the data come from studies in males, they apply reasonably well to females also): (1) Smokers are about 22 times as likely as nonsmokers to die of lung cancer. (2) About 95 out of every 100 lung cancer deaths in people who smoke can be attributed to the fact that they smoke. (3) There are about 133,000 deaths from lung cancer in the USA each year, and because about 88% can be attributed to smoking, this means that smoking is responsible for about 117,000 lung cancer deaths per year.

BOX 6–1. Equations for Comparing Risks in Different Groups and Measuring the Impact of Risk Factors

(1) Risk difference = Attributable risk (AR)

$$= \text{Risk}_{(\text{exposed})} - \text{Risk}_{(\text{unexposed})}$$

$$= [a/(a+b)] - [c/(c+d)]$$

where a represents subjects with both the risk factor and the disease; b represents subjects with the risk factor but not the disease; c represents subjects with the disease but not the risk factor; and d represents subjects with neither the risk factor nor the disease

(2) Relative risk = Risk ratio (RR)

$$= \text{Risk}_{(\text{exposed})}/\text{Risk}_{(\text{unexposed})}$$

$$= [a/(a+b)]/[c/(c+d)]$$

(3) Odds ratio (OR) $= (a/c)/(b/d)$

$$= ad/bc$$

(4) Attributable risk percent in the exposed $= \text{AR\%}_{(\text{exposed})}$

$$= \frac{\text{Risk}_{(\text{exposed})} - \text{Risk}_{(\text{unexposed})}}{\text{Risk}_{(\text{exposed})}} \times 100$$

$$= \frac{RR - 1}{RR} \times 100$$

$$\approx \frac{OR - 1}{OR} \times 100$$

(5) Population attributable risk (PAR) $= \text{Risk}_{(\text{total})} - \text{Risk}_{(\text{unexposed})}$

(6) Population attributable risk percent $= \text{PAR\%}$

$$= \frac{\text{Risk}_{(\text{total})} - \text{Risk}_{(\text{unexposed})}}{\text{Risk}_{(\text{total})}} \times 100$$

$$= \frac{(Pe)(RR - 1)}{1 + (Pe)(RR - 1)} \times 100$$

where Pe stands for the effective proportion of the population exposed to the risk factor

SUMMARY

Epidemiologic research is usually designed to permit one or more primary contrasts in risk, rate, or odds of disease or exposure. The most straightforward of these measures are the risk difference (the attributable risk) and the rate difference, which show in absolute terms how much the risk of one group (usually the group that is exposed to a risk factor or a preventive factor) differs from that of another group. This contrast can also be expressed as a ratio of risks, rates, or odds; the greater this ratio, the more difference the exposure makes.

The impact of the risk factor on the total disease burden can be measured in terms of an attributable risk percent for the exposed group or for the population in general. If it is known by how much a preventive program can reduce the risk ratio and in whom, the total benefit of the program, including its cost-effectiveness, can be calculated.

References Cited

Centers for Disease Control. Chronic disease reports: deaths from lung cancer—United States, 1986. Morbidity and Mortality Weekly Report 38:501–505, 1989.
Doll, R., and A. B. Hill. Lung cancer and other causes of death in relation to smoking. British Medical Journal 2:1071, 1956.

Selected Readings

Kleinbaum, D. G., L. L. Kupper, and H. Morgenstern. Epidemiologic Research: Principles and Quantitative Methods. London, Lifetime Learning Publications, 1982. [Advanced text.]
Rothman, K. J. Modern Epidemiology. Boston, Little, Brown and Company, 1986. [Moderately advanced text.]

SECTION II

BIOSTATISTICS

CHAPTER SEVEN

UNDERSTANDING AND

REDUCING ERRORS IN

CLINICAL MEDICINE

GOALS OF DATA COLLECTION AND ANALYSIS

It may not be comforting to talk about errors in medicine, but they occur and are difficult to eliminate. Statistical methods are used to measure and explain overall variation, some of which is due to errors; to distinguish between random and meaningful variation; and to facilitate interpretations of data needed for medical diagnosis, prognosis, and treatment.

Promoting Accuracy and Precision

Two distinct but related goals of data collection and analysis are accuracy and precision. **Accuracy** refers to the ability of a measurement to be correct on the average. If a measure is not accurate, it is biased. **Precision,** sometimes known as **reproducibility** or **reliability,** is the ability of a measurement to give the same result or a very similar result with repeated measurements of the same thing. Random error alone, if large, will result in lack of precision.

To ask whether accuracy or precision is more important in data collection and analysis would be somewhat like asking which wing of an airplane is more important. As shown in Figs. 7–1 and 7–2, unless both qualities are present, the data would be generally useless. The accuracy of Fig. 7–1A is reflected in the fact that the mean is the true value (correct value), while the precision (reliability) of Fig. 7–1A is evident in the fact that all values are

close to the true value. Fig. 7–1B shows a measure that is accurate but not precise, meaning that it gives the correct answer only on the average. Such a measure might be useful for some kinds of research, but even so it would not be reassuring to the investigator. Moreover, for an individual patient, there is no value in something being correct on the average. To guide diagnosis and treatment, each observation must be accurate. Fig. 7–1C shows data that are precise but are biased, rather than being accurate, and are therefore misleading. Fig. 7–1D shows data that are neither accurate nor precise and are obviously of no value. Finally, Fig. 7–2 uses a target and bullet holes to demonstrate the same concepts.

Reducing Differential and Nondifferential Errors

As discussed in Chapter 4, there are several types of errors to avoid in the collection and analysis of data. **Bias** is a **differential error**—that is, a nonrandom, systematic, or consistent error in which the values tend to be inaccurate in a particular direction. Bias results, for example, from measuring the heights of patients with their shoes on or from measuring blood pressures with an arm cuff that reads too high or too low. Statistical analysis cannot correct for bias unless the amount of bias in each individual measurement is known. In the example of the patients' height measurements, bias could only

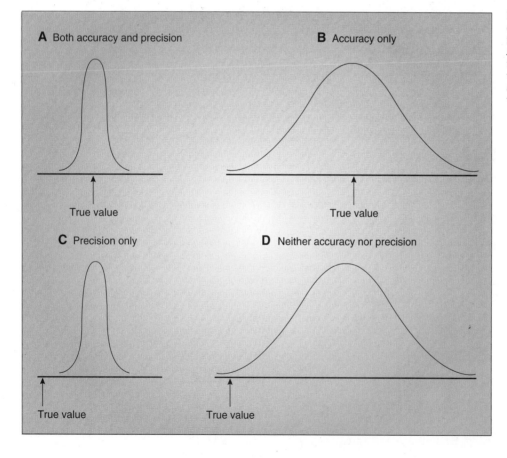

FIGURE 7–1. Possible combinations of accuracy and precision in describing a continuous variable. The x-axis is a range of values, with the arrow indicating the true value. The curves are the probability distributions of observed values.

A Both accuracy and precision

True value

B Accuracy only

True value

C Precision only

True value

D Neither accuracy nor precision

True value

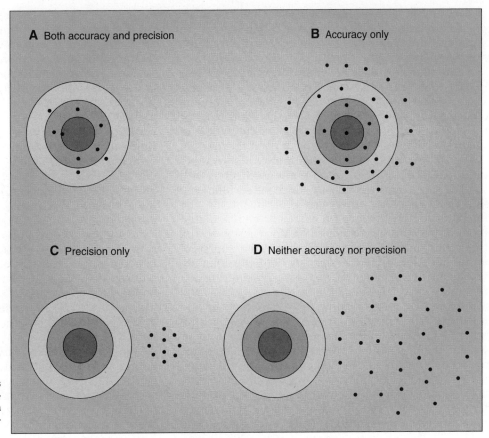

A Both accuracy and precision

B Accuracy only

C Precision only

D Neither accuracy nor precision

FIGURE 7–2. Possible combinations of accuracy and precision in describing a continuous variable, using a target and bullet holes to demonstrate the concepts.

be corrected if the height of each patient's heel was known and subtracted from that patient's reported measurement.

While measuring patients in their bare feet could eliminate bias, it would not necessarily eliminate **random errors,** or **nondifferential errors.** When data have only random errors, some observations will be too high and some will be too low. It is possible for random errors to produce biased results (Dosemeci, Wacholder, and Lubin 1990). However, on the average, at least if there are enough observations, data with random errors can at best produce a correct estimate of the mean.

Reducing Intraobserver and Interobserver Variability

If the same physician takes successive measurements of the blood pressure or height of the same person or if the same physician examines the same x-ray several times without knowing that it is the same x-ray, there will usually be some differences in the measurements or interpretations obtained. This is known as **intraobserver variability.** If two different physicians measure the same blood pressure or examine the same x-ray independently, there will usually be some differences. This is called **interobserver variability.** A goal of data collection and analysis is to reduce the amount of intraobserver (within observer) and interobserver (between observers) variability.

STUDYING THE ACCURACY AND USEFULNESS OF SCREENING AND DIAGNOSTIC TESTS

One way to judge the usefulness of a medical test for a particular disease is to evaluate how often its results are correct in two groups: (1) a group of persons in whom the disease is known to be present and therefore in whom the test results should be positive and (2) a group of persons in whom the disease is known to be absent and therefore in whom the test results should be negative. This kind of research is not as easy as it might initially appear, because several factors influence whether the results for an individual subject will be accurate and whether the test in general will be useful in diagnosing or screening for a particular disease. Among these factors are the stage of the disease and the spectrum of disease in the study population. As emphasized by Ransohoff and Feinstein (1978), the population in which the diagnostic or screening test is evaluated should have characteristics similar to those of the populations in which the test will be used.

False-Positive and False-Negative Results

In science, if something is said to be true when it is not true, that is variously called a **type I error,** a **false-positive error,** or an **alpha error.** If something is said to be false when it is true, that is called a **type II error,** a **false-negative error,** or a **beta error.** Therefore, the finding of a positive result in a patient in whom the disease is absent is called a **false-positive result,** and the finding of a negative result in a patient in whom the disease is present is called a **false-negative result.**

The **stage of disease** often influences the test results. For example, tests for infectious diseases, such as the blood test for the human immunodeficiency virus (HIV) and the tuberculin skin test for tuberculosis, may be more accurate in the middle of the period of infection than in the early or late period. Weeks or months may be required for detectable blood antibodies to appear in persons infected with the HIV virus, and weeks may be required following infection with the tuberculosis organism for the infected person to develop sufficient cell-mediated immunity to produce a positive skin reaction to the tuberculin antigen. Therefore, early in the course of either infection, an individual may not have immunologic evidence of infection, and tests done during this time may yield false-negative results.

Moreover, false-negative results may occur late in either HIV infection or tuberculosis, when the infection is severe and the immune system is overwhelmed and unable to react sufficiently to produce a positive result in the test. This stage is called **anergy** (from Greek, meaning "not working"). Anergy is frequently seen in HIV-positive individuals, particularly those with symptoms and signs of acquired immunodeficiency syndrome (AIDS). The situation is especially serious in this group, because HIV-related damage to the cell-mediated immune system may cause anergy relatively early in infection, and false-negative results in the tuberculin skin test are frequent in HIV-positive individuals.

The **spectrum of disease** in the study population is important in evaluating a test's potential usefulness in the real world. Both false-negative and false-positive results can be more of a problem than anticipated. In the case of the tuberculin skin test, for example, false-positive results used to be found in persons from the southeastern USA. Exposure to atypical mycobacteria in the soil is common in this region, and because there is some cross-reactivity between the atypical bacteria and the bacteria tested in the tuberculin skin test, equivocal and even false-positive test results were fairly common among this population until the standards were tightened. To accomplish this, the use of an antigen called old tuberculin (OT) was replaced by the use of a purified protein derivative (PPD) of mycobacteria at a standardized strength of 5 tuberculin units (5 TU). Moreover, the diameter of skin induration needed for a positive test result was increased from 5 mm to 10 mm. These tightened criteria worked satisfactorily for decades, until the appearance of AIDS. Now, because of the possibility of anergy in HIV-infected persons, it has been recommended that an induration of 5 mm once again be considered a positive result in the tuberculin test. This reopens the possibility of increased false-positive reactions in people previously exposed to atypical mycobacteria.

False-positive and false-negative results are not limited to tests of infectious diseases, as is illustrated in the following discussion concerning the use of serum calcium values to rule out parathyroid disease, particularly hyperparathyroidism, in new patients seen at an endocrinology clinic. Hyperparathyroidism is a disease of calcium metabolism. In an affected patient, the serum level of calcium is often elevated but will vary from time to time. When the level of calcium is not elevated in a patient who has hyperparathyroidism, the result would be considered falsely negative. Conversely, when the level of calcium is elevated in a patient who does not have hyperparathyroidism (but instead has cancer, sarcoidosis, multiple myeloma, milk-alkali syndrome, or another condition that can also cause a rise in the

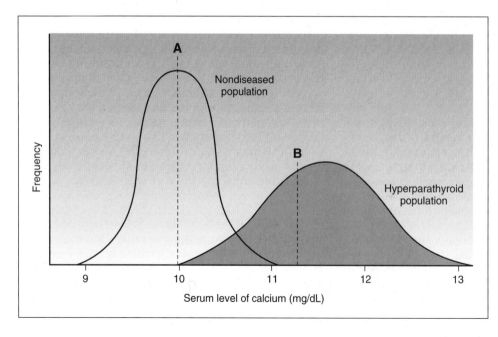

FIGURE 7–3. Overlap in values of randomly taken tests in a population where most of the people are healthy (curve on the left) but some of the people are diseased (curve on the right). A person with a level of calcium below point A would be unlikely to have hyperparathyroidism. A person with a level of calcium above point B would be likely to have an abnormality of calcium metabolism, possibly hyperparathyroidism. A person with a level of calcium between point A and point B may or may not have an abnormality of calcium metabolism. (Note: The normal range of calcium depends on the method used in a specific laboratory. In some laboratories, the range is from 8.5 to 10.5 mg/dL. In others, as in this illustration, it is from 9 to 11 mg/dL.)

calcium level), the result would be considered falsely positive for hyperparathyroidism.

Fig. 7–3 shows two anticipated frequency distributions of serum calcium values, one in a population of healthy people without parathyroid disease and the other in a population of patients with hyperparathyroidism. If the level of calcium were sufficiently low (say, below point A in Fig. 7–3), the patient would be unlikely to have hyperparathyroidism. If the level of calcium were sufficiently high (say, above point B in Fig. 7–3), the patient would be likely to have an abnormality of calcium metabolism, possibly hyperparathyroidism. However, if the level of calcium were in the intermediate range (between point A and point B) in a single calcium test, although the patient probably would not have a disease of calcium metabolism, this possibility could not be ruled out, and if such disease were suspected, serial calcium values should be obtained.

Laboratories usually provide a range of "normal" values for substances that they measure, such as calcium. A value above the "normal" range will require further diagnostic tests for hyperparathyroidism. For many laboratories, the upper limit of normal for serum calcium is stated to be 11 mg/dL. If the **cutoff point** for the upper limit of normal is set too low, considerable time and money would be wasted following up on false-positive results; but if it is set too high, many persons with the disease might be missed. As discussed below, determining the sensitivity, specificity, and predictive values of a test at different cutoff points will help investigators choose the best cutoff point for that test. It would be nice if there were no overlaps between the test results in diseased and nondiseased persons; if this were true, the only errors would be in the performance of the tests. Unfortunately, the distribution of values in nondiseased persons often overlaps with the distribution of values in diseased persons, so the techniques discussed here are necessary.

It is easier to visualize the idea of a false-positive error where there is a clear distinction between diseased and nondiseased states, as in the evaluation of a spot on a mammogram. The area in question either does or does not represent cancer. Even here, however, the situation is not always simple. There may be an abnormality (e.g., fibrocystic disease) without cancer being present. In this case, a radiologist's diagnosis of cancer would be a false-positive for cancer (the big concern), but it would be correct about an abnormality being present. In contrast, a radiologist's diagnosis of normal breast tissue would be a true-negative for cancer but would not have indicated the existence of the abnormality. Radiologists frequently indicate uncertainty by reporting the results as "abnormality present—probably not cancer" and recommending that the mammogram be repeated after a defined number of months. Such readings really are analogous to laboratory values in the indeterminate range, and they are even more difficult to study than results from laboratory analysis (Elmore et al. 1994).

TABLE 7–1. Standard 2 × 2 Table Comparing the Test Results and the True Disease Status of the Subjects Tested

		TRUE DISEASE STATUS		
		Diseased	Nondiseased	Total
TEST RESULT	Positive	a	b	$a+b$
	Negative	c	d	$c+d$
	Total	$a+c$	$b+d$	$a+b+c+d$

Interpretation of the cells is as follows:

a = subjects with a true-positive test result
b = subjects with a false-positive test result
c = subjects with a false-negative test result
d = subjects with a true-negative test result

$a + b$ = all subjects with a positive test result
$c + d$ = all subjects with a negative test result
$a + c$ = all subjects with the disease
$b + d$ = all subjects without the disease

$a + b + c + d$ = all study subjects

Formulas are as follows:

$a/(a + c)$ = sensitivity

$d/(b + d)$ = specificity

$b/(b + d)$ = false-positive error rate (alpha error rate, type I rate)

$c/(a + c)$ = false-negative error rate (beta error rate, type II rate)

$a/(a + b)$ = positive predictive value

$d/(c + d)$ = negative predictive value

$[a/(a + c)]/[b/(b + d)] = (a/b)/[(a + c)/(b + d)]$ = likelihood ratio positive (LR+)

$[c/(a + c)]/[d/(b + d)] = (c/d)/[(a + c)/(b + d)]$ = likelihood ratio negative (LR−)

$(a + c)/(a + b + c + d)$ = prevalence

Sensitivity and Specificity

Sensitivity and specificity are two important measures of test function. To calculate these measures, the data concerning the subjects studied and the test results can be put in a 2×2 table of the type shown in Table 7–1. Note that the cells in this table are labeled *a, b, c,* and *d,* as in Table 6–1, but the measures to be calculated are different.

The first column in Table 7–1 represents all of the diseased subjects, consisting of those with **true-positive results** *(a)* and those with **false-negative results** *(c)*. The second column represents all of the nondiseased subjects, consisting of those with **false-positive results** *(b)* and those with **true-negative results** *(d)*. When the total in the first column is divided by the total of all of the subjects studied, the result represents the **prevalence** of the disease in the study population.

Sensitivity, which refers to the ability of a test to detect a disease when it is present, is calculated as

$a/(a + c)$. If a test is *not* sensitive, it will fail to detect disease in some of the diseased subjects, and these subjects will appear in cell c. The rate at which this occurs is called the **false-negative error rate** and is calculated as $c/(a + c)$. The correct denominator for the false-negative error rate is all of those who are diseased, because only those who are diseased can *falsely* be called nondiseased. The sensitivity and the false-negative error rate add up to 1.0 (100%).

Specificity, which refers to the ability of a test to indicate nondisease when no disease is present, is calculated as $d/(b + d)$. If a test is *not* specific, it will falsely indicate the presence of disease in nondiseased subjects, and these subjects will appear in cell b. The rate at which this occurs is called the **false-positive error rate.** Since only nondiseased subjects are at risk for *falsely* being called diseased, this rate is calculated as $b/(b + d)$. The specificity and the false-positive error rate add up to 1.0 (100%).

First, suppose that 80 consecutive persons entering an endocrine clinic have their serum level of calcium checked and also have a hyperparathyroidism workup to determine whether they have the disease or not. Second, assume the upper cutoff point for "normal" serum calcium is 11 mg/dL, so that levels above 11 mg/dL are presumptively "test positive" and levels of 11 mg/dL or less are "test negative." Third, assume that the results are as shown in Table 7–2. The following observations could be made. Of the 80 persons tested, 20 were ultimately shown to have hyperparathyroidism. Of these 20 persons, 12 had an elevated level of calcium in initial calcium testing. Thus, the sensitivity of the initial test

TABLE 7–2. The Serum Level of Calcium and the True Disease Status of 80 Subjects Tested (Fictitious Data)

		TRUE DISEASE STATUS		
		Diseased	Nondiseased	Total
SERUM LEVEL OF CALCIUM	High	12	3	15
	Normal	8	57	65
	Total	20	60	80

Calculations based on formulas in Table 7–1:

$12/20 = 60\%$ = sensitivity

$57/60 = 95\%$ = specificity

$3/60 = 5\%$ = false-positive error rate (alpha error rate, type I rate)

$8/20 = 40\%$ = false-negative error rate (beta error rate, type II rate)

$12/15 = 80\%$ = positive predictive value

$57/65 = 88\%$ = negative predictive value

$(12/20)/(3/60) = 12.0$ = likelihood ratio positive (LR+)

$(8/20)/(57/60) = 0.42$ = likelihood ratio negative (LR−)

$12.0/0.42 = 28.6$ = ratio of LR+ to LR−

$20/80 = 25\%$ = prevalence

was 60%, and the false-negative error rate was 40% (8/20). This is consistent with the fact that persons with hyperparathyroidism may have serum calcium levels which alternate between the high normal range and definite elevation, so that more than one calcium test is needed to test for the disease. The specificity in Table 7–2 was higher than the sensitivity, with normal levels correctly identified in 57 of 60 nondiseased persons, indicating 95% specificity. The false-positive error rate, therefore, was 5% (3/60).

Predictive Values

Sensitivity and specificity are interesting and are somewhat helpful in themselves, but they do not directly answer two important clinical questions: If a patient's test result is positive, what is the probability that he or she has the disease being tested? If the result is negative, what is the probability that the patient does not have the disease? These questions, which are influenced by both sensitivity and specificity, can be answered by following a different direction of analysis.

In Table 7–1, the formula $a/(a + b)$ is used to calculate the **positive predictive value.** In a study population, this measure indicates what proportion of the subjects who had positive test results had the disease. Likewise, the formula $d/(c + d)$ is used to calculate the **negative predictive value,** which indicates what proportion of the subjects who had negative test results were free of the disease.

In Table 7–2, the positive predictive value is 80% (12/15), and the negative predictive value is 88% (57/65). Based on these numbers, the physician could not be fully confident in either a positive or a negative test result. Why have the predictive values not fulfilled their promise? The predictive values would have been 100% correct if there were no false-positive or false-negative errors. Unfortunately, errors are present in almost any test, and this makes predictive values difficult to interpret, because in the presence of errors the values are influenced profoundly by the prevalence of the condition being sought (Jekel, Greenberg, and Drake 1969).

As shown in Table 7–1, the prevalence is the total number of diseased persons $(a + c)$ divided by the total number of persons studied $(a + b + c + d)$. If, for example, there is a 1% prevalence of the condition (and most conditions are relatively rare), at most there could be an average of 1 true-positive test result out of each 100 persons examined. However, if there is a 5% false-positive rate (not unusual for many tests), 5% of 99 nondiseased persons would have false-positive test results. This would mean 5 false-positive results out of each 100 tests. Therefore, in this example, 5 out of every 6 positive test results could be expected to be falsely positive. It almost seems as though probability is conspiring against the use of screening and diagnostic tests in clinical medicine.

Whenever physicians are testing for *rare* conditions, whether in routine clinical examinations or in large community screening programs, they must be

When a patient presents with complaints of chest pain, the physician begins by obtaining a history, performing a physical examination, and developing a list of diagnoses that might explain the chest pain. The possible diagnoses have the logical status of hypotheses, and the physician must order various tests to screen or "rule out" (discard) the false hypotheses. These tests, which include laboratory analyses and imaging procedures, should be highly sensitive tests. Tests with a high degree of sensitivity have a low false-negative error rate, so they ensure that not many true cases of the disease are missed. Although the physician does not want false-positive results, they are tolerable at this stage, because they can be dealt with by more tests.

After most of the hypothesized diagnoses have been eliminated, the physician begins to consider tests that will "rule in" (confirm) the true diagnosis. These tests should be highly specific. Tests with a high degree of specificity have a small false-positive error rate, so they ensure that not many patients are misdiagnosed as having a particular disease when in fact they have another disease. The physician does not want to treat patients for diseases that they do not have, whether the treatment is surgical or medical.

The principles of testing can therefore be summarized as follows: (1) A **screening test,** which is used to rule out a diagnosis, should have a high degree of **sensitivity.** (2) A **confirmatory test,** which is used to rule in a diagnosis, should have a high degree of **specificity.**

In a similar manner, the **likelihood ratio negative** (LR–) is the ratio of the false-negative error rate divided by the specificity, or $[c/(a+c)]$ divided by $[d/(b+d)]$. In this case, since the LR– is the ratio of something clinicians do *not* want (false-negative error rate) divided by something they *do* want (specificity), the smaller the LR– is—i.e., the closer to 0 the ratio is—the better the test is. In summary, if the LR+ of a test is large and the LR– is small, it is probably a good test.

The LR+ can be calculated from the hypothetical data in Table 7–2. The sensitivity is 12/20, or 60%. The false-positive error rate (1 – specificity) is 3/60, or 5%. The ratio of these is the LR+, which equals 0.60/0.05, or 12.0. Although this looks pretty good, the sensitivity data indicate that, on the average, 40% of the diseased persons would be missed. The LR– here would be 8/20 divided by 57/60, or 0.42, which is much larger than desirable.

Experts in test analysis sometimes calculate the **ratio of LR+ to LR–** to obtain a measure of separation between the positive and the negative test. In this example, LR+/LR– would be 12.0/0.42, which is equal to 28.6, a number not as large as desirable (a desirable number being somewhere around 50 or more). If the data are from a 2×2 table, virtually the same result could have been obtained more simply by calculating the **odds ratio** (ad/bc), which here equals $[(12)(57)]/[(3)(8)]$, or 28.5. For a discussion of the concepts of proportions and odds, see Box 7–2.

prepared for most of the positive test results to be falsely positive. Moreover, they must be prepared to follow up with additional testing in persons who have positive results to determine if the disease is really present. This does not mean that screening tests should be avoided for conditions that have a low prevalence. It still may be worthwhile to do a screening program, because the persons in whom follow-up diagnostic tests are needed will represent a small percentage of the total population. A crucial point to remember is that one test does not make a diagnosis, unless it is a **pathognomonic test**—that is, a test that elicits a reaction that is synonymous with having the disease. Box 7–1 summarizes principles concerning **screening tests** and **confirmatory tests.**

Likelihood Ratios, Odds Ratios, and Cutoff Points

Unlike predictive values, likelihood ratios are not influenced by the prevalence of the disease.

The **likelihood ratio positive** (LR+) is the ratio of the sensitivity of a test to the false-positive error rate of the test. As shown in Table 7–1, the equation is as follows: $[a/(a+c)]$ divided by $[b/(b+d)]$. Since the LR+ is the ratio of something that clinicians *do* want in a test (sensitivity) divided by something they do *not* want (false-positive error rate), the higher the ratio is, the better the test is. For a test to be a good one, the ratio should be much larger than 1. Note that both the sensitivity and the false-positive error rate are independent of the prevalence of the disease. Therefore, the ratio is also independent of the prevalence.

Most people are familiar with proportions (percentages), which take the form $a/(a+b)$. Those who have never gambled are probably less familiar with the idea of an odds, which is simply a/b. In a mathematical sense, a proportion is less pure, because the term a is in both the numerator and the denominator of a proportion, and that is not true of an odds. The odds is the probability that something will occur divided by the probability that it will not occur (or the number of times it occurs divided by the number of times it does not occur). Odds can only describe a variable that is dichotomous (i.e., has only two possible outcomes, such as success and failure).

The odds of a particular outcome (outcome X) can be converted to the probability of that outcome and vice versa, using the following formula:

$$\text{Probability of outcome } X = \frac{\text{Odds of outcome } X}{1 + \text{Odds of outcome } X}$$

Suppose, for example, that the proportion of successful at-bats of a baseball player on a certain night equals 1/3 (a batting average of 0.333). That means there was one success (X) and two failures (Y). The odds of success (number of successes to number of failures) is therefore 1:2, or 0.5. To convert back to a proportion from the odds, put the odds of 0.5 into the equation above, giving 0.5/(1 + 0.5) = 0.5/1.5 = 0.333.

If the player goes 1 for 4 another night, the proportion of success is 1/4 (a batting average of 0.250), and the odds of success is 1:3, or 0.333. The formula above converts the odds (0.333) back into a proportion: 0.333/(1 + 0.333) = 0.333/1.333 = 0.250.

TABLE 7–3.   Calculation of Likelihood Ratios in Analyzing the Performance of a Serum Test
with Multiple Cutoff Points (Multiple Ranges of Results)

| Serum Creatine Kinase Value* | Diagnosis of Myocardial Infarction (MI) | | Likelihood Ratio |
	MI Present	MI Absent	
≥280 IU/L	97	1	(97/1)/(230/130) = 54.8
80–279 IU/L	118	15	(118/15)/(230/130) = 4.45
40–79 IU/L	13	26	(13/26)/(230/130) = 0.28
0–39 IU/L	2	88	(2/88)/(230/130) = 0.013
	230	130	

Source of data: Smith, A. F. Diagnostic value of serum creatine kinase in a coronary care unit. Lancet 2:178, 1967.
*The methods of determining creatine kinase values have changed since the time of this report, so these values cannot be directly applied to patient care today.

The LR+ will look better if a high (more stringent) **cutoff point** is used (e.g., a serum calcium level ≥ 13 mg/dL for hyperparathyroidism), even though choosing a high cutoff also lowers the sensitivity. This improvement in the LR+ occurs because as the cutoff point is raised, true-positive results are eliminated at a slower rate than are false-positive results. Moreover, the ratio of LR+ to LR– increases, despite the fact that more of the diseased individuals will be missed. The high LR+ means that when clinicians do happen to find a high level of calcium in an individual they are testing, they can be reasonably certain that hyperparathyroidism or some other disease of calcium metabolism is present. Similarly, if an extremely low cutoff point is used, when clinicians find a low level in an individual, they can be reasonably certain that the disease is absent.

Although these principles can be used to create value ranges that allow clinicians to be pretty certain about the results in the highest and lowest group, the results in the middle group are problematic. This situation is not necessarily bad, because now clinicians need to pursue additional testing only in those whose values fall in the middle.

Three or more ranges can be used to categorize the values of any test whose results occur along a continuum. In Table 7–3, the results of a serum test are divided into four ranges (Smith 1967). Here, 360 patients who had symptoms suggestive of myocardial infarction had an initial blood sample drawn to determine the level of creatine kinase (CK), an enzyme released into the blood of patients with myocardial infarction. After the final diagnoses were made, the initial CK values were compared with these diagnoses. In this case, there are too many levels to measure the sensitivity and specificity in a 2 × 2 table (as was done in Tables 7–1 and 7–2), but the LR+ and LR– can be calculated.

The reason that the LR+ can be applied to multiple levels is that the LR+ is the ratio of two probabilities: the ratio of sensitivity to (1 – specificity). This can also be expressed as $[a/(a+c)]$ divided by $[b/(b+d)]$. When this equation is rearranged algebraically, it can be rewritten as follows:

$$LR+ = (a/b)/[(a+c)/(b+d)]$$

which is the odds of disease among those in whom the test yielded positive results divided by the odds of disease in the entire population. The LR+, therefore, indicates how much the odds of disease was *increased* if the test result was positive.

Similarly, the LR– is the ratio of two probabilities: the ratio of (1 – sensitivity) to specificity. Alternatively, this can be expressed as $[c/(a+c)]$ divided by $[d/(b+d)]$, and the formula can be rearranged algebraically as follows:

$$LR- = (c/d)/[(a+c)/(b+d)]$$

which is the odds of missed disease among those in whom the test yielded negative results divided by the odds of disease in the entire population. The LR–, therefore, shows how much the odds of disease was *decreased* if the test result was negative.

Does this new way of calculating the LR really work? Compare Table 7–2, where the LR+ can be calculated as follows and will yield exactly the same result as obtained before:

$$LR+ = (12/3)/[(12+8)/(3+57)]$$
$$= (12/3)/(20/60)$$
$$= 4/0.333 = 12.0$$

Likewise, the LR– can be calculated as follows and will yield the same result as before:

$$LR- = (8/57)/[(12+8)/(3+57)]$$
$$= (8/57)/(20/60)$$
$$= 0.140/0.333 = 0.42$$

Therefore, the likelihood ratio can be described as the odds of disease given a specified test value divided by the odds of disease in the study population. This general definition of the likelihood ratio can be used for any number of test ranges. In Table 7–3, it is demonstrated for the four ranges of CK results. If the CK value was 280 IU/L or more, the LR was very large (54.8), making it highly probable that the patient had a myocardial infarction. If the CK was 39 IU/L or less, the LR was very small (0.013), meaning that myocardial infarction was likely absent. The LRs for the two middle ranges of CK values, however, do not elicit as much confidence in the test, so additional tests would be needed to make a diagnosis in patients whose CK values were between 40 and 279 IU/L.

Both in Table 7–2 and in Table 7–3, the **posttest odds** of disease (a/b) equals the **pretest odds** multiplied by the LRs. In Table 7–2, for example, the pretest odds of disease was 20/60, or 0.333; that is all that was known about the distribution of disease in the study population before the test was given. The LR+, as calculated above, turned out to be 12.0. When 0.333 is multiplied by 12.0, the result is 4. This is the same as the posttest odds, which were found to be 12/3, or 4.

Receiver Operating Characteristic (ROC) Curves

In clinical tests used to measure a continuous variable, such as serum calcium, blood glucose, or blood pressure, the choice of a good cutoff point is often difficult. As discussed above, there will be few false-positive results and many false-negative results if the cutoff point is very high, and the reverse will occur if the cutoff point is very low. Moreover, since calcium, glucose, blood pressure, and other values can fluctuate in any individual, whether healthy or diseased, there will be some overlap of values in the "normal" population and values in the diseased population, as shown in Fig. 7–3.

In order to decide on a good cutoff point, investigators could construct a receiver operating characteristic (ROC) curve. Beginning with either new or previously published data that showed both

the test results and the true status for every person tested in a study, the investigators could calculate the sensitivity and false-positive error rate for several possible cutoff points and then plot the points on a square graph.

ROC curves are being seen increasingly in the medical literature. Legend has it that the term originated in England during the Battle of Britain, when the performance of radar receiver operators was evaluated on the following basis: a true-positive consisted of a correct early warning of German planes coming over the English Channel; a false-positive occurred when a receiver operator sent out an alarm but no enemy planes appeared; and a false-negative occurred when German planes appeared without previous warning from the radar operators.

An example of an ROC curve for blood pressure screening is shown in Fig. 7–4. The y-axis shows the **sensitivity** of a test, and the x-axis shows the **false-positive error rate** (1 – specificity). Since the LR+ of a test is defined as the sensitivity divided by the false-positive error rate, the ROC curve can be considered a kind of graph of the LR+.

If a group of investigators wanted to determine the best cutoff for a blood pressure screening program, they might begin by taking a single initial blood pressure measurement in a large number of persons and then performing a workup for persistent hypertension; therefore, each person would have a screening blood pressure value and a diagnosis

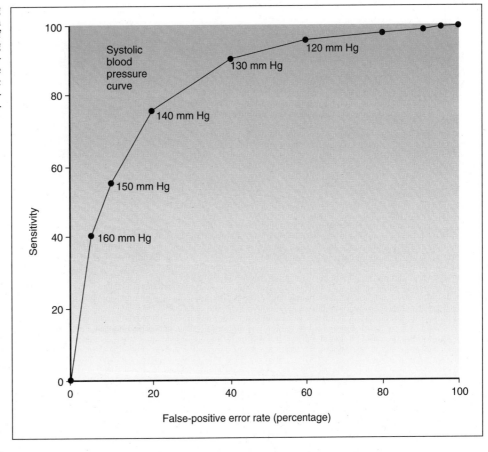

FIGURE 7–4. Receiver operating characteristic (ROC) curve from a study to determine the best cutoff point for a blood pressure screening program (fictitious data). Numbers beside the points on the curve are the cutoffs of systolic blood pressure that gave the corresponding sensitivity and false-positive error rate.

concerning the presence or absence of hypertension. Based on this information, an ROC curve could be constructed. If the cutoff were set at 0 mm Hg (an extreme example used here to help illustrate the procedure), *all* study subjects would be included in the group suspected of having hypertension. This means that all of the persons with hypertension would be detected, and the sensitivity would be 100%. However, all of the normal persons would also screen positive for hypertension, so the false-positive error rate would be 100% and the point would be placed in the upper right (100%–100%) corner of the graph. By similar reasoning, if an extremely high blood pressure, such as 500 mm Hg, were taken as the cutoff, nobody would be detected with hypertension, so sensitivity would be 0%; however, there would be no false-positive results either, so the false-positive error rate would also be 0%. This point would be placed in the lower left (0%–0%) corner of the graph.

Next, the investigators would analyze the data for the lowest reasonable cutoff point—for example, a systolic blood pressure of 120 mm Hg—and plot the corresponding sensitivity and false-positive error rate on the graph. Then they could use 130 mm Hg as the cutoff, determine the new sensitivity and false-positive error rate, and plot the data point on the graph. This would be repeated for 140 mm Hg and for higher values. It is unlikely that the cutoff point for hypertension would be less than 120 mm Hg or higher than 150 mm Hg. When all of the points are in place,

they can be connected to look like Fig. 7–4. Ordinarily, the best cutoff point would be the point closest to the upper left corner (the corner representing a sensitivity of 100% and a false-positive error rate of 0%).

The ideal ROC curve for a test would arise almost vertically from the lower left corner and then move horizontally almost along the upper line, as is shown in the uppermost ROC curve in Fig. 7–5 (the curve labeled "excellent"). If the sensitivity always equaled the false-positive error rate, the result would be a diagonal straight line from the lower left to the upper right corner, as shown in the bottom ROC curve in Fig. 7–5 (the curve labeled "no benefit"). The ROC curve for most clinical tests is somewhere between these two extremes—that is, similar to the curve labeled "good" or "fair" in Fig. 7–5.

The ROC curve in Fig. 7–6 shows the sensitivity and false-positive error rates found by Kinder (1994) in a study of patients with follicular thyroid neoplasms. Kinder sought to use the diameter of the neoplasms to determine the probability of malignancy. Initially, when the ROC curve was plotted using the neoplasm diameters of patients of all ages, the curve was disappointing. But when the patients were divided into two age groups—those under 50 years and those 50 years or older—the diameter of the neoplasms was found to be strongly predictive of cancer in the older group but not in the younger one (Fig. 7–6). It is unusual for the curve to hug the axes as it does for the older group in Fig. 7–6, but that was

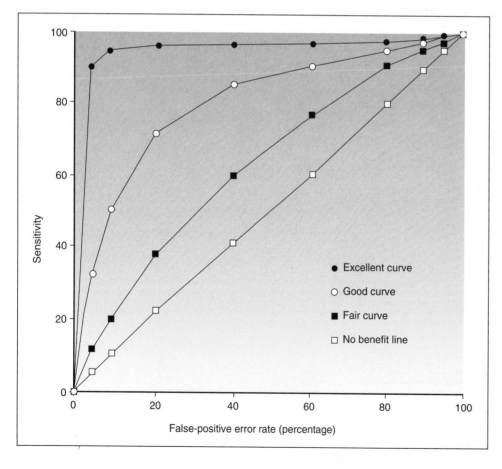

FIGURE 7–5. Examples of receiver operating characteristic (ROC) curves for four tests. The uppermost curve is the best of the four.

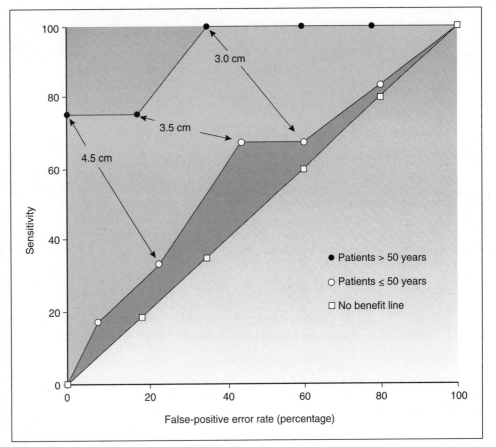

FIGURE 7–6. Receiver operating characteristic (ROC) curves for a test to determine the malignancy status of a follicular thyroid neoplasm on the basis of the diameter of the neoplasm. The upper curve plots the results in patients 50 years or older; the middle curve plots the results in patients under 50 years old; and the bottom curve represents the line of no benefit from the test. Numbers beside the points on the curves are the neoplasm diameters that gave the corresponding sensitivity and false-positive error rate. (Data courtesy of Dr. Barbara Kinder, Department of Surgery, Yale University School of Medicine, New Haven, Conn.)

due to the relatively small number of patients involved (96 patients). In Fig. 7–6, the curve for the older age group can be compared with that for the younger age group. For example, at a false-positive error rate of approximately 20%, the sensitivity is about 30% for the younger group and 75% for the older group. At a sensitivity of 75%, the false-positive error rate is almost 70% for the younger group and is between 0% and 20% for the older group (depending on whether the cutoff point chosen is a diameter of 3.5 cm or above).

Analysis of ROC curves is becoming increasingly more sophisticated and popular in certain fields, such as radiology. One method of comparing different tests is to determine the area under the ROC curve for each test and then to use a statistical test of significance to decide if the area under one curve differs significantly from the area under the other curve.

MEASURING AGREEMENT

An important question both in clinical medicine and in research is the extent to which different observations of the same phenomenon differ. If there is intraobserver agreement or interobserver agreement, as defined at the beginning of this chapter, the data in a study are considered highly reliable and will elicit more confidence. However, reliability is not proof of validity; two observers can report the same readings (i.e., show reliability) but be wrong.

It is not unusual to find imperfect agreement between observers, nor is it unusual to find that the same individual looking at the same data (e.g., an x-ray or a pathology slide) often disagrees with his or her own reading done on a previous occasion. For example, in a study involving the interpretation of a series of chest x-ray films to diagnose the progression of tuberculosis, Yerushalmy et al. (1950) found that two different readers disagreed frequently and that the same person in two independent readings of the same x-ray disagreed with his or her own previous reading almost as frequently.

Overall Percent Agreement

If a test uses a dichotomous variable (i.e., two categories of results, such as positive and negative), the results can be placed in a standard 2 × 2 table, as shown in Table 7–4, so that observer agreement can be calculated. Cells *a* and *d* represent agreement, whereas cells *b* and *c* represent disagreement.

A common way to measure agreement is to calculate the overall percent agreement. Thus, if 90% of the observations are in cells *a* and *d*, the overall percent agreement would be 90%. Nevertheless, merely reporting the overall percent agreement is considered inadequate for a number of reasons. First, the overall percent agreement does not tell the prevalence of the finding in the subjects studied. Second, it does not tell how the disagreements

TABLE 7–4. Standard 2 × 2 Table Comparing the Test Results Reported by Two Observers

		OBSERVER No. 1		
		Positive	Negative	Total
OBSERVER No. 2	Positive	a	b	a + b
	Negative	c	d	c + d
	Total	a + c	b + d	a + b + c + d

Interpretation of the cells is as follows:

    a = positive/positive observer agreement
    b = negative/positive observer disagreement
    c = positive/negative observer disagreement
    d = negative/negative observer agreement

Formulas are as follows:

    $a + d$ = observed agreement (A_o)

    $a + b + c + d$ = maximum possible agreement (N)

    $(a + d)/(a + b + c + d)$ = overall percent agreement

    $[(a + b)(a + c)]/(a + b + c + d)$ = cell a agreement expected by chance

    $[(c + d)(b + d)]/(a + b + c + d)$ = cell d agreement expected by chance

    cell a agreement expected by chance + cell d agreement expected by
        chance = total agreement expected by chance (A_c)

    $(A_o - A_c)/(N - A_c)$ = kappa

occurred: were the positive and negative results evenly distributed between the two observers, or did one observer consistently find more positive results than the other? Third, considerable agreement would be expected by chance alone, and the overall percent agreement does not tell the extent to which the agreement improves on chance.

Kappa Test Ratio

Suppose two physicians examined the same 100 patients during the same hour and recorded the presence or absence of a heart murmur in each patient. Next, suppose that for 7 patients, the first physician reported the absence and the second physician reported the presence of a murmur; for 3 patients, the second physician reported the absence and first physician reported the presence of a murmur; for 30 patients, the physicians agreed that a murmur was present; and for 60 patients, the physicians agreed that a murmur was absent. These results could be arranged in a 2 × 2 table as shown in Table 7–5. Then in addition to calculating the overall percent agreement, the kappa test could be performed to determine the extent to which the agreement between the two physicians improves on chance agreement alone.

As shown in Tables 7–4 and 7–5, the **observed agreement** (A_o) is the sum of the actual number of observations in cells a and d. The **maximum possible agreement** is the total number of observations (N).

The **agreement expected by chance** (A_c) is the sum of the expected number of observations in cells a and d. The method used to calculate the expected agreement for the kappa test is the same method used for the chi-square test (see Chapter 11). For a given cell—for example, cell a—the cell's row total is multiplied by the cell's column total, and the product is then divided by the grand total. Thus, for cell a, the agreement expected by chance is calculated as $[(a + b)(a + c)]$ divided by $(a + b + c + d)$.

Kappa is a ratio: the numerator is the observed improvement over chance agreement (i.e., A_o minus A_c), and the denominator is the maximum possible improvement over chance agreement (i.e., N minus A_c). Thus, the kappa ratio is a proportion that can go from –1 (indicating perfect disagreement) through 0 (representing the agreement expected by chance) to +1 (indicating perfect agreement). Frequently, the results of the kappa test are expressed as a percentage. The following arbitrary divisions for interpreting the results are usually used: under 20% is negligible; from 20% to 40% is minimal; from 40% to 60% is fair; from 60% to 80% is good; and over 80% is excellent. In the example of cardiac murmurs, the kappa test yielded a result of 0.78, or 78%, indicating that the physician ratings were a "good" improvement on the chance expectation.

Although the kappa test described here provides valuable data on observer agreement, two important points should be noted. First, while many studies of

TABLE 7–5. Clinical Agreement between Two Physicians Regarding the Presence or Absence of Cardiac Murmur on Physical Examination of 100 Patients (Fictitious Data)

		PHYSICIAN No. 1		
		Murmur Present	Murmur Absent	Total
PHYSICIAN No. 2	Murmur Present	30	7	37
	Murmur Absent	3	60	63
	Total	33	67	100

Calculations based on formulas in Table 7–4:

    $30 + 60 = 90$ = observed agreement (A_o)

    $30 + 7 + 3 + 60 = 100$ = maximum possible agreement (N)

    $(30 + 60)/(30 + 7 + 3 + 60) = 90/100 = 90\%$ = overall percent agreement

    $[(30 + 7)(30 + 3)]/100 = [(37)(33)]/100 = 12.2$ = cell a agreement expected by chance

    $[(3 + 60)(7 + 60)]/100 = [(63)(67)]/100 = 42.2$ = cell d agreement expected by chance

    $12.2 + 42.2 = 54.4$ = total agreement expected by chance (A_c)

    $(90 - 54.4)/(100 - 54.4) = 35.6/45.6 = 0.78 = 78\%$ = kappa

observer variability involve **dichotomous data** (in which there are two categories of results, such as positive and negative), some studies involve **ordinal data** (in which there are three or more categories of results, such as negative, suspicious, and probable). If the data are ordinal, a **weighted kappa test** must be used. The weighted test is similar in principle to the unweighted test described here but is somewhat more complex (see Cicchetti, Sharma, and Cotlier 1982). Second, in evaluating the accuracy and usefulness of a laboratory assay, imaging procedure, or any other clinical test, comparing the findings of one observer with those of another observer is not as useful as comparing the findings of an observer with the true status of disease in the patients being tested. The true disease status, which is used to determine the sensitivity and specificity of tests, is considered to be the "gold standard," and its use is preferable whenever data concerning the true status are available. Unfortunately, "gold standards" seldom exist in clinical medicine, and even a small error in the "gold standard" can create the incorrect appearance of considerable error in a test (Greenberg and Jekel 1969). Not only are careful studies of the errors of new diagnostic tests urgently needed, but additional studies of many of the older tests that have not been adequately analyzed are also needed in the field of clinical medicine.

SUMMARY

Three important goals of data collection and analysis are the promotion of accuracy and precision (see Figs. 7–1 and 7–2); the reduction of differential and nondifferential errors (that is, nonrandom and random errors); and the reduction in interobserver and intraobserver variability (that is, variability between the findings of two observers or between the findings of one observer on two different occasions).

Various statistical methods are available to study the accuracy and usefulness of screening tests and diagnostic (confirmatory) tests in clinical medicine. In general, tests with a high degree of sensitivity and a corresponding low false-negative error rate are helpful for screening patients, while tests with a high degree of specificity and a corresponding low false-positive error rate are useful for confirming the diagnosis in patients suspected of having a particular disease. Tables 7–1, 7–2, and 7–3 provide definitions of and formulas for calculating sensitivity, specificity, and error rates, as well as predictive values and likelihood ratios. Similarly, Tables 7–4 and 7–5 define measures concerning interobserver agreement and provide formulas for calculating the overall percent agreement and the kappa test ratio.

References Cited

Cicchetti, D. V., Y. Sharma, and E. Cotlier. Assessment of observer variability in the classification of human cataracts. Yale Journal of Biology and Medicine 55:81–88, 1982.

Dosemeci, M., S. Wacholder, and J. H. Lubin. Does nondifferential misclassification of exposure always bias a true effect toward the null value? American Journal of Epidemiology 132:746–748, 1990.

Elmore, J. G., et al. Variability in radiologists' interpretations of mammograms. New England Journal of Medicine 331:1493–1499, 1994.

Greenberg, R. A., and J. F. Jekel. Some problems in the determination of the false positive and false negative rates of tuberculin tests. American Review of Respiratory Disease 100:645–650, 1969.

Jekel, J. F., R. A. Greenberg, and B. M. Drake. Influence of the prevalence of infection on tuberculin skin testing programs. Public Health Reports 84:883–886, 1969.

Kinder, B. [Professor of Surgery, Yale University School of Medicine, New Haven, Conn.] Personal communication, 1994.

Ransohoff, D. F., and A. R. Feinstein. Problems of spectrum and bias in evaluating the efficacy of diagnostic tests. New England Journal of Medicine 299:926–930, 1978.

Smith, A. F. Diagnostic value of serum creatine kinase in a coronary care unit. Lancet 2:178, 1967.

Yerushalmy, J., et al. The role of dual reading in mass radiography. American Review of Respiratory Disease 61:443–464, 1950.

Selected Readings

Ransohoff, D. F., and A. R. Feinstein. Problems of spectrum and bias in evaluating the efficacy of diagnostic tests. New England Journal of Medicine 299:926–930, 1978. [The use of diagnostic tests to rule in and rule out a disease.]

Sackett, D. L., R. B. Haynes, and P. Tugwell. Clinical Epidemiology: A Basic Science for Clinical Medicine, 2nd ed. Boston, Little, Brown, and Company, 1991. [Likelihood ratios, pretest odds, and posttest odds.]

CHAPTER EIGHT

IMPROVING DECISIONS IN

CLINICAL MEDICINE

There are a variety of quantitative tools for understanding the errors in clinical data and for improving the accuracy and precision of clinical tests and measurements. The tools discussed in Chapter 7 are in common use, and there is relatively little debate about the value of using sensitivity, specificity, and predictive values or even of making use of likelihood ratios and kappa tests. The quantitative tools discussed here in Chapter 8 involve the analysis of clinical decisions, and their use is the subject of much debate.

There is no controversy about the need to improve clinical decision making; everyone agrees that this should be done. There is, however, a difference of opinion regarding the extent to which the tools discussed in this chapter are likely to help in actual clinical decision making. Some individuals and medical centers already use these tools to guide the care of individual patients. Others acknowledge that the tools can help to guide in policy formulation, and although they appreciate their use in analyzing the cost-effectiveness of medical interventions such as immunizations (see, for example, Koplan et al. 1979; Bloom et al. 1993), they do not use them for making decisions about individual patients. Regardless of one's philosophic approach to using these tools, they can help physicians and other health care workers understand the quantitative basis for making clinical decisions in the increasingly complex field of medicine.

BAYES' THEOREM

It is useful to know the sensitivity and specificity of a test, but as noted in Chapter 7, once a physician decides to use a certain test, two important clinical questions require answers: If the test results are positive, what is the probability that the patient has the disease? If the test results are negative, what is the probability that the patient does not have the disease? Bayes' theorem provides a way to answer these questions.

Bayes' theorem, which was first described centuries ago by the English clergyman after whom it is named, is one of the most imposing statistical formulas in medicine. Put in symbols more meaningful for physicians, the formula is as follows:

$$p(D+|T+) = \frac{p(T+|D+)p(D+)}{[p(T+|D+)p(D+)] + [p(T+|D-)p(D-)]}$$

where p denotes probability; D+ means that the patient has the disease in question; D− means that the patient does not have the disease; T+ means that a certain diagnostic test for the disease is positive; T− means that the test is negative; and the vertical line (|) means "conditional upon" what immediately follows.

Most clinicians, even those who can deal with sensitivity, specificity, and predictive values, throw in the towel when it comes to Bayes' theorem. This is odd, because a close look at the above equation reveals that Bayes' theorem is merely the formula for

the **positive predictive value,** a value discussed in Chapter 7 and illustrated there in a standard 2×2 table (Table 7–1).

The **numerator of Bayes' theorem** merely describes **cell *a*** (the true-positive results) in Table 7–1. The probability of being in cell *a* is equal to the prevalence times the sensitivity, where $p(D+)$ is the prevalence (the probability of being in the diseased column) and where $p(T+|D+)$ is the sensitivity (the probability of being in the top row, *given the fact of being in the diseased column*). The **denominator of Bayes' theorem** consists of two terms, the first of which once again describes **cell *a*** (the true-positive results) and the second of which describes **cell *b*** (the false-positive results) in Table 7–1. In this second term of the denominator, the probability of the false-positive error rate, or $p(T+|D-)$, is multiplied by the prevalence of nondiseased persons, or $p(D-)$. As outlined in Chapter 7, the true-positive results (a) divided by the true-positive plus false-positive results $(a + b)$ gives $a/(a + b)$, which is the positive predictive value.

In genetics, an even simpler-appearing formula for Bayes' theorem is sometimes used. The numerator is the same, but the denominator is merely $p(T+)$. This makes sense because the denominator in $a/(a + b)$ is equal to all of those who have positive test results, whether they are true-positive or false-positive results.

Now that Bayes' theorem has been demystified, its uses in community screening and in individual patient care can be discussed.

Bayes' Theorem and Community Screening Programs

In a population with a low prevalence of a particular disease, most of the positive results in a screening program for that disease would be falsely positive (see Chapter 7). Although this does not automatically invalidate a screening program, it raises some concerns about cost-effectiveness, and these can be explored using Bayes' theorem.

A program employing the tuberculin tine test to screen children for tuberculosis will be discussed as an example. This test uses small amounts of tuberculin antigen on the tips of tiny prongs called tines. The tines pierce the skin on the forearm and leave some antigen behind. The skin is examined 48 hours later, and the presence of an inflammatory reaction in the area where the tines entered is considered a positive result. If the sensitivity and specificity of the test and the prevalence of tuberculosis in the community are known, Bayes' theorem can be used to predict what proportion of the children with positive test results will have true-positive results (actually be infected with mycobacteria).

Box 8–1 shows how the calculations are made. If the test has a sensitivity of 96% and a specificity of 94% and if the prevalence of tuberculosis in the community is 1%, only 13.9% of those with a positive test result are predicted actually to be infected (Jekel,

---

BOX 8–1.   Use of Bayes' Theorem or a 2 × 2 Table to Determine the Positive Predictive Value of a Hypothetical Tuberculin Screening Program

Part 1. Beginning data:

Sensitivity of tuberculin tine test	$= 96\% = 0.96$
False-negative error rate of the test	$= 4\% = 0.04$
Specificity of the test	$= 94\% = 0.94$
False-positive error rate of the test	$= 6\% = 0.06$
Prevalence of tuberculosis in the community	$= 1\% = 0.01$

Part 2. Use of Bayes' theorem:

$$p(D+\mid T+) = \frac{p(T+\mid D+)p(D+)}{[p(T+\mid D+)p(D+)] + [p(T+\mid D-)p(D-)]}$$

$$= \frac{(\text{Sensitivity})(\text{Prevalence})}{[(\text{Sensitivity})(\text{Prevalence})] + [(\text{False-positive error rate})(1 - \text{Prevalence})]}$$

$$= \frac{(0.96)(0.01)}{[(0.96)(0.01)] + [(0.06)(0.99)]} = \frac{0.0096}{0.0096 + 0.0594} = \frac{0.0096}{0.0690} = 0.139 = \textbf{13.9\%}$$

Part 3. Use of a 2 × 2 table, with numbers based on the assumption that 10,000 persons are in the study:

		TRUE DISEASE STATUS					
		Diseased		**Nondiseased**		**Total**	
		Number	(Percentage)	Number	(Percentage)	Number	(Percentage)
TEST RESULT	Positive	96	(96)	594	(6)	690	(7)
	Negative	4	(4)	9,306	(94)	9,310	(93)
	Total	100	(100)	9,900	(100)	10,000	(100)

Positive predictive value $= 96/690 = 0.139 = \textbf{13.9\%}$

Source of data: Jekel, J.F., R.A Greenberg, and B.M. Drake. Influence of prevalence of infection on tuberculin skin testing programs. Public Health Reports 84:883–886, 1969.

Greenberg, and Drake 1969). Physicians and others involved in community health programs can quickly develop a table that lists different levels of test sensitivity, test specificity, and disease prevalence and shows how these levels affect the proportion of positive results that are likely to be true-positive results. Although this calculation is fairly straightforward and is extremely useful, it has seldom been used in the early stages of planning for screening programs.

Another important point to keep in mind when planning community screening programs is that the first time a previously unscreened population is screened, a considerable number of cases of disease may be found, but repeating the screening program soon afterward may result in finding relatively few cases of new disease. This is because the first screening will detect cases that had their onset during a period of many years (prevalent cases), while the second screening will primarily detect cases that had their onset during the interval since the last screening (incident cases).

Bayes' Theorem and Individual Patient Care

Suppose a clinician is uncertain about a patient's diagnosis and obtains a positive test result for a certain disease. Even if the clinician knows the sensitivity and specificity of the test, that does not solve the problem, because to calculate the positive predictive value, whether using Bayes' theorem or a table like Table 7–1, it is necessary to know the prevalence of the particular disease that the test is designed to detect. In a clinical setting, the prevalence is thought of as the expected prevalence in the population from which the patient comes. The actual prevalence is usually not known, but often a reasonable estimate can be made.

Say, for example, a physician in a general medical clinic sees a male patient who complains of easy fatigability and has a history of kidney stones but has no other symptoms or signs of parathyroid disease on physical examination. The physician considers the probability of hyperparathyroidism and decides that it is low, perhaps 2% (reflecting that in 100 similar patients, probably only 2 of them would have the disease). This probability is called the **prior probability,** reflecting the fact that it is estimated prior to the performance of laboratory tests and is based on the estimated prevalence of a particular disease among patients with similar signs and symptoms. Although the physician believes that the probability of hyperparathyroidism is low, she orders a serum calcium test to "rule out" the diagnosis. Somewhat to her surprise, the results of the test come back positive, with an elevated level of 12.2 mg/dL. She could order more tests for parathyroid disease, but even here, some test results might come back positive and some negative.

Under the circumstances, Bayes' theorem could be used to make a second estimate of probability, which is called the **posterior probability,** reflecting the fact that it is made after the test results are known. Calculation of the posterior probability is based on the sensitivity and specificity of the test that was performed, which in this case was the serum calcium test, and on the prior probability, which in this case was 2%. If the serum calcium test had a 90% sensitivity and a 95% specificity, that means it had a false-positive error rate of 5% (specificity plus the false-positive error rate equals 100%). When this information is used in the Bayes' equation, as shown in Box 8–2, the result is a posterior probability of 27%. This means that the patient is now in a group of patients with a significant possibility of parathyroid disease. In Box 8–2, note that the result is the same (i.e., 27%) when a 2×2 table is used. This is true because, as discussed above, the probability based on the Bayes' theorem is identical to the positive predictive value.

In light of the 27% posterior probability, the physician decides to order a parathyroid hormone radioimmunoassay with simultaneous measurement of serum calcium, even though this test is expensive. If the radioimmunoassay had a sensitivity of 95% and a specificity of 98% and the results turned out to be positive, the Bayes' theorem could again be used to calculate the probability of parathyroid disease. This time, however, the posterior probability for the first test (27%) would be used as the prior probability for

---

BOX 8–2.   Use of Bayes' Theorem or a 2 × 2 Table to Determine the Posterior Probability and the Positive Predictive Value in a Clinical Setting

Part 1. Beginning data:

Sensitivity of the first test $= 90\% = 0.90$
Specificity of the first test $= 95\% = 0.95$
Prior probability of disease $= 2\% = 0.02$

Part 2. Use of Bayes' theorem:

$$p(D+\mid T+) = \frac{p(T+\mid D+)p(D+)}{[p(T+\mid D+)p(D+)] + [p(T+\mid D-)p(D-)]}$$

$$= \frac{(0.90)(0.02)}{[(0.90)(0.02)] + [(0.05)(0.98)]}$$

$$= \frac{0.018}{0.018 + 0.049} = \frac{0.018}{0.067} = 0.269 = \mathbf{27\%}$$

Part 3. Use of a 2 × 2 table:

		TRUE DISEASE STATUS					
		Diseased		Nondiseased		Total	
		Number	(Percentage)	Number	(Percentage)	Number	(Percentage)
TEST RESULT	Positive	18	(90)	49	(5)	67	(6.7)
	Negative	2	(10)	931	(95)	933	(93.3)
	Total	20	(100)	980	(100)	1000	(100.0)

Positive predictive value $= 18/67 = 0.269 = \mathbf{27\%}$

BOX 8–3. Use of Bayes' Theorem or a 2 × 2 Table to Determine the Second Posterior Probability and the Second Positive Predictive Value in a Clinical Setting

---

Part 1. Beginning data:

Sensitivity of the second test	= 95% = 0.95
Specificity of the second test	= 98% = 0.98
Prior probability of disease (see Box 8–2)	= 27% = 0.27

Part 2. Use of Bayes' theorem:

$$p(D+\mid T+) = \frac{p(T+\mid D+)p(D+)}{[p(T+\mid D+)p(D+)] + [p(T+\mid D-)p(D-)]}$$

$$= \frac{(0.95)(0.27)}{[(0.95)(0.27)] + [(0.02)(0.73)]}$$

$$= \frac{0.257}{0.257 + 0.0146} = \frac{0.257}{0.272} = 0.9449^* = \mathbf{94\%}$$

Part 3. Use of a 2 × 2 table:

		TRUE DISEASE STATUS					
		Diseased		Nondiseased		Total	
		Number	(Percentage)	Number	(Percentage)	Number	(Percentage)
TEST RESULT	Positive	256	(95)	15	(2)	271	(27.1)
	Negative	13	(5)	716	(98)	729	(72.9)
	Total	269	(100)	731	(100)	1000	(100.0)

Positive predictive value = 256/271 = 0.9446* = **94%**

---

*The slight difference in the results for the two approaches is due to rounding errors. It is not important clinically.

---

the second test. The result of the calculation, as shown in Box 8–3, is a new probability of 94%. Thus, the patient in all probability does have hyperparathyroidism.

Why did the posterior probability increase so much the second time? One reason was that the prior probability was considerably higher in the second calculation than in the first (27% versus 2%), based on the fact that the first test yielded positive results. Another reason was that the specificity of the second test was quite high (98%), which markedly reduced the false-positive error rate and therefore increased the positive predictive value.

DECISION ANALYSIS

A decision-making tool that recently came into the medical literature from management science is called decision analysis. Its purpose is to improve decision making under conditions of uncertainty. In clinical medicine, decision analysis can be used for an individual patient or for a general class of patients. As a technique, decision analysis is somewhat more popular clinically than Bayes' theorem, and it is being used with increasing frequency in the literature, particularly to make judgments about a class of patients or clinical problems.

The benefit of decision analysis is to help health care workers understand (1) the kinds of data that must go into a clinical decision, (2) the sequence in which decisions have to be made, and (3) the personal values (particularly those of the patients) that must be considered before major decisions are made. As a general rule, decision analysis is more important as a tool to help health care workers take a disciplined approach to decision making than as a tool for making the actual clinical decisions. Nevertheless, as computer programs for using decision analysis become more available, some clinicians are using decision analysis regularly in their clinical work.

Steps in Creating a Decision Tree

There are four logical steps to be taken when setting up a decision tree (see Weinstein and Fineberg

1980): (1) identify and set limits to the problem, (2) diagram the options, (3) obtain information concerning each option, and (4) compare the utility values and perform sensitivity analysis.

Identify the Problem

In identifying the problem, the clinician must determine the possible alternative clinical decisions, the sequence in which the decisions must be made, and the possible patient outcomes of each decision.

Diagram the Options

Fig. 8–1 provides an example of how to diagram the options. The beginning point of a decision tree is the patient's current clinical status. **Decision nodes,** defined as points where clinicians have to make decisions, are represented by squares. **Chance nodes,** defined as points where clinicians have to wait to see the outcomes, are represented by circles. Time goes from left to right, so the first decision is at the left and subsequent decisions are progressively to the right. In Fig. 8–1, the beginning point is the presence of asymptomatic gallstones, and the primary decision at the decision node is whether to operate immediately or to wait (Rose and Wiesel 1983).

Obtain Information Concerning Each Option

First, the **probability of each possible outcome** must either be obtained from studies or estimated. For example, in Fig. 8–1, if the physician waits rather than operating, the probability is 81.5% (0.815) that

the patient will remain asymptomatic, 15% that the patient will have occasional biliary pain, 3% that the patient will develop complications such as acute cholecystitis or common duct obstruction from gallstones, and 0.5% that the patient eventually will develop cancer of the gallbladder. Note that the probabilities of the possible outcomes for a chance node must add up to 100%, as they do in this case.

Second, the **utility of each final outcome** must be obtained. In decision analysis, the term "utility" is used to mean the value or benefit of a chosen course of action. Utility may be expressed in many ways, including in terms of death or illness rates (in which case smaller rates have greater utility), years of disability-free life, or dollars saved. In Fig. 8–1, each final outcome is expressed in terms of a negative utility (i.e., probability of death). If surgery is performed now, the probability of death is 0.4% (0.004). If the surgeon waits and the patient remains asymptomatic, however, the probability of a gallbladder-related death is 0%. Utility values for biliary pain, complications, and cancer are 0.4%, 10%, and 100%, respectively. For many patients, however, other considerations—such as the timing of death and the quality of life in the interim—are of equal or greater importance than the quantity of life. For example, a person who wanted to finish writing a book while he or she was still in relatively good health might prefer a nonaggressive approach to disease treatment. Someone else who was willing to risk everything for the sake of a cure might express a preference for the most aggressive treatment possible. These considerations must always be taken into account.

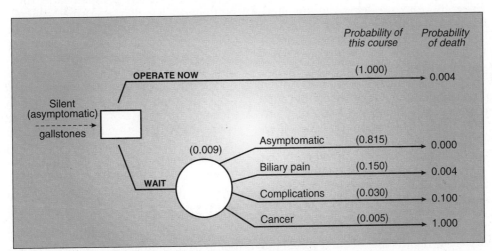

FIGURE 8–1. A decision tree concerning treatment for silent (asymptomatic) gallstones. The decision node, defined as a point where the clinician has to make a decision, is represented by a square. The chance node, defined as a point where the clinician must wait to see the outcome, is represented by a circle. If the clinician decides to operate now, the probability of surgery is 100% (1.000), and the probability of death (the negative utility value) from complications of surgery is 0.04% (0.004, or 1 out of every 250 patients undergoing surgery). If, instead, the clinician decides to wait, there are four possible outcomes, each with a different probability and negative utility value: (1) There is an 81.5% (0.815) probability of remaining asymptomatic, in which case the probability of dying from gallstones would be 0% (0.000). (2) There is a 15% (0.150) probability of developing biliary pain, which would lead to surgery and a 0.4% (0.004) risk of death. (3) There is a 3% (0.030) probability of biliary complications (such as acute cholecystitis or common duct obstruction), with a 10% (0.100) risk of death. (4) There is a 0.5% (0.005) probability of gallbladder cancer, with a 100% (1.000) risk of death. The probabilities of the possible outcomes at the chance node add up to 1 (here, 0.815 + 0.150 + 0.030 + 0.005 = 1.000). (Adapted from Rose, D. N., and J. Wiesel. Letter to the editor. New England Journal of Medicine 308:221–222, 1983. Copyright 1983. Massachusetts Medical Society. All rights reserved.)

Compare the Utility Values and Perform a Sensitivity Analysis

The decision tree can show how a given set of probabilities and utilities will turn out. If the decision tree shows that one or another choice is clearly preferable to any other, that would be strong evidence in favor of that choice. Often, however, the decision analysis will give two or more outcomes with similar utilities, which means either that better data are needed or that there really are options at that decision node. In addition to comparing the utility values, it is sometimes helpful to perform a sensitivity analysis, which consists of varying the probabilities of occurrence of a particular outcome at various points in the decision tree (one at a time) to see how the overall outcomes and clinical decisions would be affected by these changes. This helps both clinician and patient to see which probabilities and utilities have the largest impact on the outcomes through a reasonable range of values. Fig. 8–1 can be used to demonstrate how to compare utility values and to discuss the rationale for performing a sensitivity analysis.

On the decision tree shown in Fig. 8–1, there are two branches from the decision node, one labeled "operate now" and the other labeled "wait." As discussed earlier, the probability of death from operating immediately is 0.004, whereas there are four different probabilities of death from waiting, depending on what happens during the waiting period (patient remains asymptomatic or patient develops pain, complications, or cancer). Before the utility of operating now versus waiting can be compared, it is necessary to "average out" the data associated with waiting. First, the probability of each outcome of waiting is multiplied by the probability that death will ensue following that particular outcome. Next, the four products are summed. In Fig. 8–1, the calculation for averaging out is $(0.815 \times 0.000) + (0.150 \times 0.004) + (0.030 \times 0.100) + (0.005 \times 1.000) = 0.0086 = 0.009$, or a little over twice the risk of operating now.

Based on the above calculations, the best option would seem to be to operate now. However, because these two outcome probabilities are fairly close to each other (0.004 versus 0.009 is only a 0.5% difference), even modest errors in the data, if corrected, might lead to a different conclusion. Therefore, in the absence of better data on the risk of clinical states and the probabilities of death, it would be a good idea to perform a sensitivity analysis on these data, to see which estimates are the most crucial for stability of the decision tree.

The majority of the deaths that occur if surgery is not performed immediately are deaths due to cancer of the gallbladder. It is not fair to make a direct comparison of deaths due to surgery and deaths due to gallbladder cancer, however, because surgical deaths would occur immediately, whereas most of the cancer deaths would occur many years hence. Given the option, many people would choose to avoid immediate surgery (because they are feeling well, have family responsibilities, and so forth), preferring simply to deal with complications if and when they arise.

Although this was a simple example, other decision trees have multiple decision nodes that involve complicated issues and factors such as the passage of time and reevaluation. In these more complex decision analyses, the objective is to find decisions that are clearly less satisfactory than others and to cut off or "prune" the corresponding branches, because they are not rational alternatives. The process of choosing the best branch at each decision node, working back from the right to the left, is called "folding back."

Applications of Decision Trees

Decision trees can be used in the clinical setting, as discussed above in the case of patients with asymptomatic gallstones, but they are also increasingly being applied to public health problems.

Despite the availability of a safe and effective hepatitis B vaccine since 1981, the incidence of hepatitis B in the USA has increased by 37% (Schaffner, Gardner, and Gross 1993). In considering what strategy would be most cost-effective in reversing this trend, Bloom et al. (1993) turned to the use of a decision tree and analyzed data concerning several possible options: no routine hepatitis B vaccination; a screening program followed by hepatitis B vaccination for persons meeting certain criteria; and hepatitis B vaccination for specific populations (newborns, 10-year-olds, high-risk adults, or the general adult population in the USA). Included in the decision tree were the effects of compliance with recommendations.

Bloom et al. (1993) presented a full page of probabilities for various outcomes, combined with the costs of each program and the costs of each outcome. They also performed a sensitivity analysis. They concluded that vaccination of high-risk adults who have not already been vaccinated or do not already have evidence of previous hepatitis B infection would result in a net savings. They recommended that all pregnant women be screened at or near the time of delivery and that the vaccine be given to the infants of those women who are found to have active infection (i.e., those who are HBsAg-positive). In addition, they recommended that all 10-year-olds be routinely vaccinated and that booster doses be given 10 years and 20 years later.

META-ANALYSIS

Meta-analysis (meaning "analysis among") is being used increasingly in medicine to try to obtain a qualitative or quantitative synthesis of the research literature on a particular issue. The technique is usually (but not always) applied to the synthesis of several randomized clinical trials.

Selection of the Studies to Be Analyzed

The issue of study selection is perhaps the most troublesome issue for those doing meta-analysis. Several questions need to be addressed.

(1) Should studies be limited to those which are published? It is well known that negative studies (studies that report little or no benefit from following a particular course of action) are less likely to be published than are positive studies. Therefore, the published literature may be biased toward studies with positive results, and a synthesis of these studies would give a biased estimate of the impact of pursuing some courses of action. Unpublished studies, however, often are of lower quality than are published studies, and poor research methods often produce an underestimate of impact. Moreover, the unpublished studies are often difficult to discover.

(2) Should studies be limited to those which appear in peer-reviewed publications? Peer review is considered the primary method for quality control in medical publishing. Some investigators recommend that only those studies which are published in peer-reviewed publications be considered in meta-analysis. Although this may seem an attractive option, it might produce an even more highly biased selection of studies.

(3) Should studies be limited to those which meet additional quality-control criteria? If investigators impose an additional set of criteria before including a study in meta-analysis, this may further improve the average quality of the studies used, but it introduces still greater concerns about selection bias. Moreover, different investigators might use different criteria for a "good" study and therefore select a different group of studies for meta-analysis.

(4) Should studies be limited to randomized controlled trials? This is a variant of the above question concerning quality control. At one time, rigid quality standards were more likely to be met by randomized controlled trials than by case-control studies. Increasingly, however, case-control methods have been used to evaluate certain kinds of interventions, particularly those for rare diseases. For example, case-control methods have been used to evaluate vaccines for uncommon diseases, because these methods are less costly and provide results more quickly (Shapiro et al. 1991).

(5) Should studies be limited to those using identical methods? For practical purposes, this would mean using only separately published studies from multicenter trials, for which the methods were the same for all and the similarity of methods was monitored. This criterion is very difficult to achieve.

Types of Meta-analysis
Pooled (Quantitative) Analysis

Usually, the main purpose of meta-analysis is quantitative. The goal is to develop better overall estimates of the amount of benefit achieved by particular medical interventions, based on the combining (pooling) of estimates found in the existing studies of the interventions. This type of meta-analysis is sometimes called a pooled analysis (Gerbarg and Horwitz 1988) because the analysts pool the observations of many studies and then calculate parameters such as risk ratios or odds ratios from the pooled data.

Because of the many decisions regarding inclusion or exclusion of studies, different meta-analyses might reach very different conclusions on the same topic. Even after the studies are chosen, there are many other methodologic issues in choosing how to combine means and variances (e.g., what weighting methods should be used). Pooled analyses should report both relative risks and risk reductions as well as absolute risks and risk reductions (Sinclair and Bracken 1994).

Methodologic (Qualitative) Analysis

Sometimes the question to be answered is not how much benefit is derived from the use of a particular intervention but whether there is any benefit at all. In this case, a qualitative meta-analysis may be done, in which the quality of the research concerning the intervention is scored according to a list of objective criteria. The meta-analyst then examines the methodologically superior studies to determine whether or not the question of benefits is answered consistently by them. This qualitative approach has been called methodologic analysis (Gerbarg and Horwitz 1988) or quality scores analysis (Greenland 1994).

In some cases, the methodologically strongest studies agree with one another and disagree with the weaker studies, which may or may not be consistent with one another. An example was provided by a meta-analysis that showed that of the eight major controlled trials of the bacillus Calmette-Guérin (BCG) vaccine against tuberculosis, only three trials met all or almost all of the methodologic criteria and had precise statistical estimates (Clemens, Chuong, and Feinstein 1983). These three trials agreed that BCG vaccine afforded a high level of protection against tuberculosis. The remaining five studies were methodologically weaker and had large confidence intervals (see Chapter 10). Their conclusions varied from showing a weak protective efficacy to actual harm from the vaccine. It should be noted that not everyone believes that this type of methodologic analysis is generally useful (Greenland 1994).

SUMMARY

Although there is general agreement about the need to improve clinical decision making, there is controversy about the methods to be used to achieve this goal. Among the tools available for decision analysis are Bayes' theorem and decision trees. These tools can be applied to individual patient care as well as to community health programs. Bayes' theorem can be used to calculate positive predictive values and posterior probabilities (see Boxes 8–1, 8–2, and 8–3). Decision trees can help health care workers pursue a logical, step-by-step approach to exploring the possible alternative clinical decisions, the sequence in which these decisions must be made, and the probabilities and utilities of each possible outcome (see Fig. 8–1).

Another tool used increasingly in medicine is meta-analysis, a technique to obtain either a quantitative or a qualitative synthesis of the research literature on a specific topic or question. In exploring the question of benefits derived from a particular treatment or vaccine, for example, either pooled analysis or methodologic analysis might be performed. Pooled analysis would focus on providing a quantitative estimate of benefits, based on data derived from many studies. In contrast, methodologic analysis would pursue the issue of whether methodologically superior studies found that the treatment or vaccine provided any benefit at all.

References Cited

Bloom, B. S., et al. A reappraisal of hepatitis B virus vaccination strategies using cost-effectiveness analysis. Annals of Internal Medicine 118:298–306, 1993.

Clemens, J. D., J. J. Chuong, and A. R. Feinstein. The BCG controversy: a methodological and statistical reappraisal. Journal of the American Medical Association 249:2362–2369, 1983.

Gerbarg, Z. B., and R. I. Horwitz. Resolving conflicting clinical trials: guidelines for meta-analysis. Journal of Clinical Epidemiology 41:503–509, 1988.

Greenland, S. Invited commentary: a critical look at some popular meta-analytic methods. American Journal of Epidemiology 140:290–296, 1994.

Jekel, J. F., R. A. Greenberg, and B. M. Drake. Influence of prevalence of infection on tuberculin skin testing programs. Public Health Reports 84:883–886, 1969.

Koplan, J. P., et al. Pertussis vaccine: an analysis of benefits, risks, and costs. New England Journal of Medicine 301:906–911, 1979.

Rose, D. N., and J. Wiesel. Letter to the editor. New England Journal of Medicine 308:221–222, 1983.

Schaffner, W., P. Gardner, and P. A. Gross. Hepatitis B immunization strategies: expanding the target. Annals of Internal Medicine 118:308–309, 1993.

Shapiro, E. D., et al. The protective efficacy of polyvalent pneumococcal polysaccharide vaccine. New England Journal of Medicine 325:1453–1460, 1991.

Sinclair, J. C., and M. B. Bracken. Clinically useful measures of effect in binary analyses of randomized trials. Journal of Clinical Epidemiology 47:881–889, 1994.

Weinstein, M. C., and H. V. Fineberg. Clinical Decision Analysis. Philadelphia, W. B. Saunders Company, 1980.

Selected Reading

Weinstein, M. C., and H. V. Fineberg. Clinical Decision Analysis. Philadelphia, W. B. Saunders Company, 1980.

CHAPTER NINE

DESCRIBING VARIATION

IN DATA

Variation is evident in almost every characteristic of patients, including their physiologic measurements, diseases, diets, environments, and life-styles. A measure of a single characteristic is called a variable. Statistics enables investigators to (1) describe the patterns of variation in single variables, as discussed in this chapter; (2) determine when observed differences are likely to be real differences, as discussed in Chapters 10 and 11; and (3) determine the patterns and strength of association between variables, as discussed in Chapters 11 and 13.

SOURCES OF VARIATION IN MEDICINE

While variation in clinical medicine may be due to biologic differences or the presence or absence of disease, it may also be due to differences in measurement techniques and conditions, errors in measurement, and random variation.

Biologic differences include factors such as differences in genes, nutrition, and environmental exposures. Height provides a good example. Tall parents usually have tall children. Extremely short people may have specific genetic conditions (such as achondroplasia) or a deficiency of growth hormone. While poor nutrition will slow growth and starvation may stop growth altogether, good nutrition allows the full genetic growth potential to be achieved. A polluted environment may cause many infections in children, and this in turn can retard growth.

Variation is seen not only in the **presence or absence of disease** but also in the **stages and manifestations of disease.** For example, cancer of the cervix may be in situ, localized, invasive, or metastatic. In some cases, multiple diseases may be present. Insulin-dependent diabetes mellitus, for instance, may be accompanied by coronary artery disease or renal disease.

Different conditions of measurement often account for the variations observed in medical data and include factors such as time of day, ambient temperature or noise, and the presence of fatigue or anxiety in the patient. Differences in measurement caused by different environments and conditions are not errors of measurement, but standardizing the conditions under which the data are obtained is important to ensure that observed variation is due to factors of interest.

Different methods of measurement can produce different results. For example, the blood pressure measurement derived from the use of an intra-arterial catheter may differ from that derived from the use of an arm cuff. This does not necessarily mean that the measurements are in error. An intra-arterial catheter has a more central location (i.e., is nearer the heart), while a blood pressure cuff on the arm or leg is more distal and thus may yield a lower measurement. Both measurements could be correct but may differ because they are measuring pressure at different points in the arterial tree.

Variations in some cases are due to **measurement error.** Blood pressure cuffs of different sizes may give different readings of the same blood pressure; different blood pressure cuffs of the same size may give different measurements, owing to errors in some cuffs; different laboratory instruments or methods may produce different readings from the same sample; and different x-ray machines may produce films of different quality. Similarly, different observers may report different results. One radiologist may read a mammogram as abnormal and recommend further tests such as a biopsy, while another may read the same mammogram as normal and not recommend any further workup (Elmore et al. 1994). One physician may detect a problem such as a retinal hemorrhage or a heart murmur, and another physician may fail to detect it. Two physicians may both detect a heart murmur in the same patient but disagree on its characteristics. And if two physicians are asked to characterize a dark skin lesion, one may call it a mole, while the other diagnoses it as a malignant melanoma.

Determinists would probably say that if clinicians and investigators only knew enough and measured accurately enough, **random variation** would disappear. Perhaps, but unexplained variation seems to be a ubiquitous phenomenon in clinical medicine and research. Statistics helps investigators to interpret data despite random variation, but statistics cannot correct for errors in the observation or recording of data.

STATISTICS AND VARIABLES

Statistical methods help clinicians and investigators understand and explain the variation in medical data. The first step in understanding variation is to describe the variation. Therefore, this chapter focuses on how to describe variations in medical observations. Statistics can be thought of as a set of tools for working with data, just as brushes are tools used by an artist for painting. One reason for the choice of a specific tool over another is the kind of material on which the tool will be used. One kind of brush is needed for oil paints, another kind for tempera paints, and another kind for water colors. The artist must know the materials to be used in order to choose the correct tools. Similarly, a person who works with data must understand the different types of variables that exist in medicine.

Quantitative and Qualitative Data

The first question to answer before analyzing data is whether the data describe a quantitative or a qualitative characteristic. A **quantitative characteristic,** such as a systolic blood pressure or serum sodium level, can be characterized using a rigid, dimensional measurement scale. A **qualitative characteristic,** such as coloration of the skin, must be described in detail. For example, normal skin can vary in color from pinkish-white through tan to dark brown or black. Medical problems can be evident in changes in skin color, with white denoting pallor, as in anemia; red suggesting rash or a sunburn; blue denoting cyanosis, as in cardiac or lung failure; bluish-purple occurring when blood has been released subcutaneously, as in a bruise; yellow suggesting the presence of jaundice, as in common bile duct obstruction or liver disease; and brown or black characterizing a nevus or mole.

Examples of disease manifestations that have both quantitative and qualitative characteristics are heart murmurs and bowel sounds. Not only does the loudness of a heart murmur vary from patient to patient, but the sound may vary from blowing to harsh or rasping in quality; a bruit may be continuous or intermittent. Bowel sounds may vary from normal gurgling in the absence of disease to an intense cascade of sounds in the presence of intestinal infection or obstruction.

Any kind of information that can vary is called a variable. Thus, the qualitative information on colors just described could form a variable called skin coloration. The quantitative information on blood pressure could be contained in variables called systolic pressure and diastolic pressure.

Types of Variables

Variables can be classified as nominal variables, dichotomous (binary) variables, ordinal (ranked) variables, continuous (dimensional) variables, ratio variables, and risks and proportions.

Nominal Variables

Nominal variables are "naming" or categorical variables that have no measurement scales. Examples are blood groups (O, A, B, and AB), occupations, food groups, and skin coloration. If skin coloration is the variable being examined, a different number is assigned to each color (for example, 1 is bluish-purple, 2 is black, 3 is white, 4 is blue, 5 is tan, and so forth) before the information is entered into a computer data system. Any number could be assigned to any color, and that would make no difference to the statistical analysis. This is because the number is merely a numerical name for a color, and the number given to a particular color has nothing to do with the quality, value, or rank of the color.

Dichotomous Variables (Binary Variables)

If all possible skin colors were included in one nominal variable (as was done just above), there is a problem: this variable does not distinguish between normal and abnormal skin color, which is usually the most important aspect of skin color for both clinical and research purposes. As discussed above, abnormal skin coloration (pallor, jaundice, cyanosis, etc.) may be a sign of any number of health problems (anemia, liver disease, cardiac failure, etc.). Therefore, researchers might choose to create a variable with only two levels: normal skin color (coded as a 1) and abnormal skin color (coded as a 2), for example.

This variable, which has only two levels, is said to be dichotomous (from the Greek language, meaning "cut into two").

Some dichotomous variables—such as well/sick, living/dead, and normal/abnormal—have an implied qualitative direction, with the first option in the pair clearly preferred. Skin color as a dichotomous variable has a directional value, since having normal coloration is preferable to having abnormal coloration. Other dichotomous variables—such as female/male and treatment/placebo—have no a priori qualitative direction. Usually, it makes no difference to the statistical analysis whether or not the dichotomous variable has an implied direction, but the direction may be important for the conclusions drawn from the data.

Dichotomous variables, although common and important, often are not adequate by themselves. For example, in analyzing cancer therapy, it is not only important to know whether the patient survives or dies (a dichotomous variable) but is also crucial to know how long the patient survives (a continuous variable). A survival analysis or life table analysis, as described in Chapter 11, may therefore be done. Similarly, for a study of heart murmurs, various types of data may be needed, such as dichotomous data concerning a murmur's timing (systolic or diastolic); nominal data concerning its location (e.g., aortic valve area) and character (e.g., rough); and ordinal data concerning its loudness (e.g., grade III).

Discrete Variables

Dichotomous variables and nominal variables are sometimes called discrete variables because the different categories are completely separate from each other.

Ordinal Variables (Ranked Variables)

Many types of medical data can be characterized in terms of more than two values and have a clearly implied direction from better to worse, but the data are not measured on a continuous measurement scale. These data form ordinal (ranked) variables.

There are many clinical examples of ordinal variables. The amount of extracellular fluid in a patient's legs is estimated by the physician and is usually reported as "none" or 1+, 2+, 3+, or 4+ pitting edema (puffiness). A patient may have a systolic murmur ranging from 1+ to 6+. Respiratory distress is reported as being absent, mild, moderate, or severe. Although pain also may be reported as being absent, mild, moderate, or severe, in some cases patients are asked to describe their pain on a scale from 0 to 10, with 0 being no pain and 10 being the worst imaginable pain.

None of these variables is measured on an exact measurement scale, but more information is contained in these variables than in nominal variables. This is so because it is possible to see the relationship between ordinal categories and know whether one is more desirable, equally desirable, or less desirable than another. Because ordinal variables contain more information than nominal variables, the ordinal variables enable more robust (certain) conclusions to be drawn. As described in Chapter 11, ordinal variables often require special techniques of analysis.

Continuous Variables (Dimensional Variables)

Many types of medically important data are measured on continuous (dimensional) measurement scales. Patients' heights, weights, systolic and diastolic blood pressures, and serum glucose levels are all examples of data measured on continuous scales. Even more information is contained in continuous data than in ordinal data, because continuous data not only show the position of the different observations relative to each other but also show the extent to which one observation differs from another. Continuous data usually enable investigators to make more detailed inferences than do ordinal or nominal data.

Perhaps surprisingly, relationships between continuous variables are not always linear (in a straight line). For example, there is not a linear relationship between birth weight and survival of newborns (Buehler et al. 1987). As shown in Fig. 9–1, infants weighing under 3000 g and infants weighing over 4500 g are both at greater risk for neonatal death than

are infants weighing between 3000 and 4500 g (between about 6.6 and 9.9 pounds).

Ratio Variables

If a continuous scale has a true 0 point, the variables derived from it can be called ratio variables. The kelvin temperature scale is a ratio scale, because 0 degrees on this scale is absolute 0. The centigrade temperature scale is a continuous scale but not a ratio scale, because 0 degrees on this scale does not mean the absence of heat. For most statistical purposes, however, this distinction is of no importance.

Risks and Proportions as Variables

As discussed in Chapter 6, a risk is the conditional probability of an event (e.g., death or disease) in a defined population. Risks and proportions, which are two important types of variables in medicine, share some characteristics of a discrete variable and some characteristics of a continuous variable. Just as it makes no sense to say that a fraction of a death occurred, it makes no sense to say that a fraction of a person suffered an event. However, it does make sense to say that a discrete event (e.g., death) or a discrete characteristic (e.g., presence of a murmur) occurred in a fraction of a population. Risks and proportions are variables created by the ratio of discrete counts in the numerator to counts in the

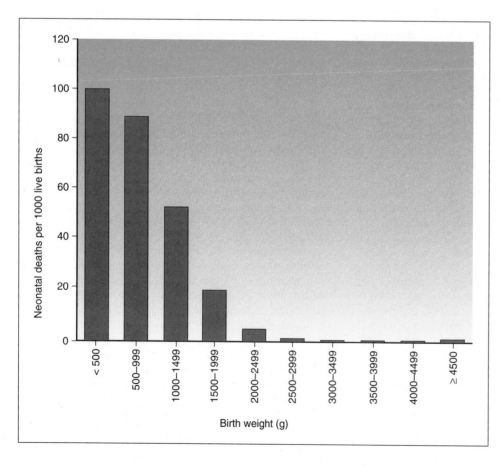

FIGURE 9–1. Histogram showing the neonatal mortality rate by birth weight group, all races, USA, 1980. (Source of data: Buehler, J. W., et al. Birth weight–specific infant mortality, United States, 1960 and 1980. Public Health Reports 102: 151–161, 1987.)

TABLE 9–1. Standard 2 × 2 Table Showing the Gender of 71 Subjects and Whether the Serum Level of Total Cholesterol Was Checked

		CHOLESTEROL LEVEL					
		Checked		Not Checked		Total	
		Number	(Percentage)	Number	(Percentage)	Number	(Percentage)
GENDER	Female	17	(63)	10	(37)	27	(100)
	Male	25	(57)	19	(43)	44	(100)
	Total	42	(59)	29	(41)	71	(100)

Source of data: Unpublished findings in a sample of 71 professional persons in Connecticut.

denominator. Depending on the circumstances, they may be analyzed as discrete variables or as continuous variables.

Counts and Units of Observation

The unit of observation is the source of data. Common examples of units of observation in medical studies are persons, animals, and organisms. The same statistical principles apply in clinical research as in laboratory research. Units of observation may be arranged in a **frequency table,** with one characteristic on the x-axis, some other characteristic on the y-axis, and the appropriate counts in the cells of the table. Table 9–1, which provides an example of this type of 2 × 2 table, shows that among 71 young professional persons studied, 63% of females and 57% of males had previously had their cholesterol level checked. Using these data and a test that will be described in Chapter 11, analysts can determine whether the difference between the percentage of women and the percentage of men with cholesterol checks was likely to have been due to chance variation.

Combining Data

A continuous variable may be converted to an ordinal variable by grouping units with similar values together. For example, the individual birth weights of infants (a continuous variable) can be converted to ranges of birth weights (an ordinal variable), as shown in Fig. 9–1. When the data are presented as categories or ranges (less than 500 g, 500–999 g, 1000–1499 g, and so forth), information is lost, because the individual weights of infants are no longer apparent. However, the advantage is that now percentages can be created, and the relationship of birth weight to mortality is easier to show.

Three or more groups must be formed to convert a continuous variable to an ordinal variable. In the example of birth weight, the result of forming several groups is that it creates a ranked order that goes progressively from lightest to heaviest. By dividing the data into only two groups, it is possible to convert a continuous variable into a dichotomous variable. For example, dividing infants into two groups creates a dichotomous variable of those weighing less than 2500 g (low birth weight) and those weighing 2500 g or more (normal birth weight). However, more information is lost by forming only two groups than by forming more than two.

FREQUENCY DISTRIBUTIONS
Frequency Distributions of Continuous Variables

Observations on one variable may be shown visually by putting the value on one axis and the frequency with which that value appears on the other axis. This is known as a frequency distribution. For example, Table 9–2 and Fig. 9–2 both show the distribution of the levels of total cholesterol among 71 professional persons; the distribution is easier to see in the figure.

Distribution and Range of a Variable

A frequency distribution can be described, albeit imperfectly, using only the lowest and highest numbers in the data set. For example, the cholesterol levels in Table 9–2 vary from a low value of 124 mg/dL to a high value of 264 mg/dL. The distance between the lowest and highest observations is called the range of the variable. Thus, the range of the total cholesterol values in Table 9–2 is the difference between 124 mg/dL and 264 mg/dL, or 140 mg/dL.

Real and Theoretical Frequency Distributions

Real frequency distributions are those obtained from actual data, and theoretical frequency distributions are calculated using certain assumptions. When theoretical distributions are used, they are assumed to describe the underlying populations from which data are obtained. The majority of measurements of continuous data in medicine and biology tend to approximate the theoretical distribution that is known as the **normal distribution** and is also called the **gaussian distribution** (named after Johann Karl Gauss, the person who best described it).

The normal (gaussian) distribution looks something like a bell seen from the side, as shown in Fig. 9–3. In statistical texts, smooth, bell-shaped curves are drawn to describe normal distributions. Real distributions, found by gathering real data, however, are seldom if ever perfectly smooth and bell-shaped.

TABLE 9–2. Serum Levels of Total Cholesterol Reported in 71 Subjects*

Cholesterol Value (mg/dL)	Number of Observations	Cholesterol Value (mg/dL)	Number of Observations	Cholesterol Value (mg/dL)	Number of Observations
124	1	169	1	217	1
128	1	171	4	220	1
132	1	175	1	221	1
133	1	177	2	222	1
136	1	178	2	226	1
138	1	179	1	227	1
139	1	180	4	228	1
146	1	181	1	241	1
147	1	184	2	264	1
149	1	186	1		
151	1	188	2		
153	2	191	3		
158	3	192	2		
160	1	194	2		
161	1	196	2		
162	1	197	2		
163	2	206	1		
164	3	208	1		
165	1	209	1		
166	1	213	1		

*In this data set, the mean is 179.1 mg/dL, and the standard deviation is 28.2 mg/dL.
Source of data: Unpublished findings in a sample of 71 professional persons in Connecticut.

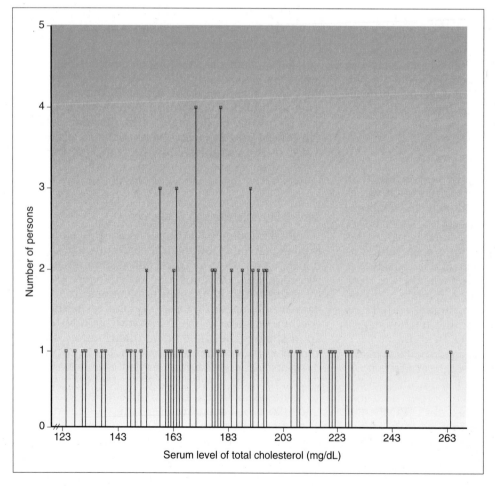

FIGURE 9–2. Histogram showing the frequency distribution of the serum levels of total cholesterol reported in a sample of 71 subjects. The data shown here are the same data listed in Table 9–2. (Source of data: Unpublished findings in a sample of 71 professional persons in Connecticut.)

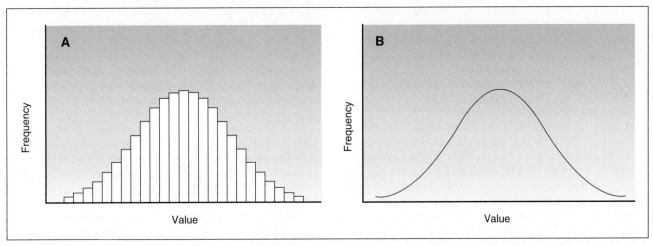

FIGURE 9–3. Illustration of the normal (gaussian) distribution. Diagram A shows a probability distribution of actual data, plotted as a histogram with very narrow ranges, and diagram B shows the way this idea is represented, for simplicity, in textbooks, articles, and tests.

For example, the frequency distribution of total cholesterol values among the 71 young professionals shows peaks and valleys when the data are presented in the manner shown in Fig. 9–2. This should not cause concern, however, if partitioning the same data into reasonably narrow ranges results in a bell-shaped frequency distribution. For example, when the cholesterol levels from Table 9–2 and Fig. 9–2 are partitioned into seven groups with narrow ranges (ranges of 20 mg/dL width), the resulting frequency distribution appears almost perfectly nor-

mal (gaussian), as shown in Fig. 9–4. If the sample size had been much larger than 71, the distribution of raw data (Fig. 9–2) would probably have looked much smoother.

In textbooks, the smooth, bell-shaped curves are often used to represent the **expected frequency of observations** (on the y-axis) according to their observed value on a measurement scale (on the x-axis) (Fig. 9–3). When readers see a perfectly smooth, bell-shaped gaussian distribution, they should remember that the y-axis is really describing the

FIGURE 9–4. Histogram showing the frequency distribution of the serum levels of total cholesterol reported in a sample of 71 subjects, grouped in ranges of 20 mg/dL. Individual values for the 71 subjects are reported in Table 9–2 and Fig. 9–2. The mean is 179.1 mg/dL, and the median is 178 mg/dL.

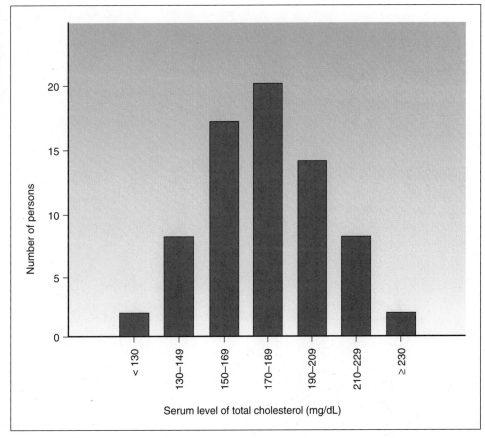

frequency with which the corresponding values in the x-axis are expected to be found. With an intuitive feeling for the meaning of Fig. 9–3, it will be easier to understand advanced statistical textbooks and problems presented on examinations.

Although the term "normal" distribution is used in this book and is used frequently elsewhere in the literature, there is no implication that data which do not strictly follow this distribution are somehow abnormal. Even when data do not form perfectly normal distributions, it is possible to draw powerful inferences (tentative conclusions) about the data by using certain statistical tests that assume the observed data came from a normal (gaussian) distribution. If the sample size is sufficiently large, this assumption usually works well (see the discussion of the central limit theorem and tests of statistical significance in Chapter 10).

Histograms, Frequency Polygons, and Line Graphs

There are several ways to illustrate the characteristics of the frequency distribution of a set of data. Usually, the best way is to create a **histogram,** which is a bar graph in which the number of units of observation (e.g., persons) is shown on the y-axis, the measurement values (e.g., cholesterol levels) are shown on the x-axis, and the frequency distribution is illustrated by a series of bars. In a histogram, the area of each bar represents the relative proportion of all observations that fall in the range represented by that bar. Fig. 9–2 is a histogram in which each bar represents a single number value for the cholesterol level. An extremely large number of observations would be needed to get a smooth curve for single values such as these. The underlying distribution of the data is somewhat clearer when the data are grouped into ranges of cholesterol levels, such as is shown in the histogram in Fig. 9–4.

A shorthand way of presenting a histogram is first to put a dot at the center of the top of each bar and then to connect these dots with a line. In this way, a graph called a **frequency polygon** is created. Fig. 9–5 shows a frequency polygon that was constructed from the histogram shown in Fig. 9–4. Although histograms generally are recommended for presenting frequency distributions, frequency polygons have two advantages. First, the shape of the distribution is more easily seen in a frequency polygram than in a histogram. Second, a linear dose-response relationship (discussed in Chapter 4 and illustrated in Fig. 4–1) is suggested more clearly by a frequency polygon than by a histogram.

Chapter 3 provides numerous examples of graphs depicting relationships between time and incident cases or between time and incidence rates. The **epidemic time curve** (illustrated in Figs. 3–11, 3–12, 3–13, 3–14, and 3–19) is a kind of histogram in which the x-axis is time and the y-axis is the *number of incident cases* in each time interval. When the x-axis represents time and the y-axis presents *rates*, a **line graph** is recommended.

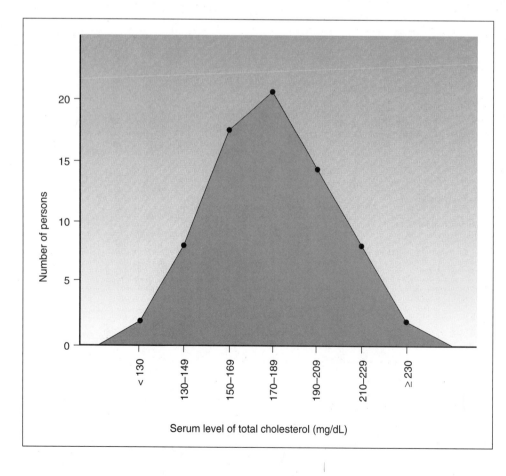

FIGURE 9–5. Frequency polygon showing the frequency distribution of the serum levels of total cholesterol reported in a sample of 71 subjects, grouped in ranges of 20 mg/dL. The data in this polygon are the same as the data in the histogram shown in Fig. 9–4. Individual values for the 71 subjects are reported in Table 9–2 and Fig. 9–2.

Number of persons

Serum level of total cholesterol (mg/dL)

Fig. 3–1, which shows the incidence rates of salmonellosis during several decades, is an example of an **arithmetic line graph,** meaning that both the x-axis and the y-axis use an arithmetic scale. Fig. 3–2, which illustrates the impact that diphtheria vaccine had on the incidence rates of disease and death during several decades, is an example of a **semilogarithmic line graph** in which the x-axis uses an arithmetic scale but the y-axis uses a logarithmic scale in order to amplify the lower end of the scale. Although semilogarithmic line graphs have the disadvantage of making the absolute magnitude of the changes that occurred look less dramatic, they have two advantages. First, they enable the detail of changes in very low rates of disease to be seen, which would be difficult on an arithmetic graph comparing current rates with those decades ago. Second, as shown in Fig. 3–2, they depict proportionately similar changes as parallel lines. The decline in diphtheria deaths was proportionately similar to the decline in reported cases of disease, so that the case fatality ratio remained fairly constant.

Parameters of a Frequency Distribution

Frequency distributions from continuous data are defined by two types of measures, or parameters: measures of central tendency and measures of dispersion. The **measures of central tendency** locate a scale of observations in space and are something like a street address for the variable. The **measures of dispersion** suggest how widely the observations are spread out and can be thought of as indicating the property lines for the variable. In the case of a perfectly normal (gaussian) distribution, the bell-shaped curve can be fully described using only the mean (a measure of central tendency) and the standard deviation (a measure of dispersion).

Measures of Central Tendency. The first step in examining a distribution is to look for the central tendency of the observations. Most types of medical data tend to clump in such a way that the density of observed values is greatest near the center of the distribution. In the case of the observed cholesterol values listed in Table 9–2 and depicted graphically in Fig. 9–2, there appears to be some tendency for the values to cluster near the center of the distribution, but this tendency is much clearer visually when the values from Table 9–2 and Fig. 9–2 are grouped in ranges of 20 mg/dL, as shown in Fig. 9–4.

The next step is to examine the distribution in greater detail and look for the mode, the median, and the mean, which are the three measures of central tendency.

(1) Mode. The most commonly observed value (that is, the value with the highest number of observations) in a data set is called the mode. The mode is of some interest but seldom is of statistical value. It is not uncommon for a distribution to have a mode at more than one value. For example, in Fig. 9–2, the most commonly observed cholesterol values (each with 4 observations) are 171 mg/dL and

180 mg/dL. In this case, although technically the figure shows a **bimodal distribution,** the two modes are close enough together to be considered part of the same central cluster. In other cases, distributions may be truly bimodal, usually because the population contains two subgroups, each of which has a different distribution that peaks at a different point. More than one mode can also be produced artificially by what is known as **digit preference,** when observers tend to favor certain numbers over others. For example, persons who measure blood pressure values tend to favor even numbers, particularly those ending in 0.

(2) Median. The median is the middle observation when data have been arranged in order from the lowest to the highest value. The median value in Table 9–2 is 178 mg/dL. When there is an even number of observations, the median is considered to lie halfway between the two middle observations. For example, in Table 9–3, which shows the high-density lipoprotein (HDL) cholesterol values for 26 persons, the two middle observations are the 13th and 14th observations. The corresponding values for these are 57 and 58 mg/dL, so the median is 57.5 mg/dL.

TABLE 9–3.   Raw Data and Results of Calculations in a Study Concerning Serum Levels of High-Density Lipoprotein (HDL) Cholesterol in 26 Subjects

Parameter	Raw Data or Results of Calculation
Number of observations, or N	26
Initial HDL cholesterol values of the subjects	31, 41, 44, 46, 47, 47, 48, 48, 49, 52, 53, 54, 57, 58, 58, 60, 60, 62, 63, 64, 67, 69, 70, 77, 81, and 90 mg/dL
Highest value	90 mg/dL
Lowest value	31 mg/dL
Mode	47, 48, 58, and 60 mg/dL
Median	$(57 + 58)/2 = 57.5$ mg/dL
Sum of the values, or sum of x_i	1,496 mg/dL
Mean, or $\bar{x}$	$1,496/26 = 57.5$ mg/dL
Range	$90 - 31 = 59$ mg/dL
Interquartile range	$64 - 48 = 16$ mg/dL
Sum of $(x_i - \bar{x})^2$, or TSS	4,298.46 mg/dL squared*
Variance, or s^2	171.94 mg/dL†
Standard deviation, or s	$\sqrt{171.94} = 13.1$ mg/dL

*For a discussion and example of how statisticians measure the total sum of the squares (TSS), see Box 9–3.

†Here, the following formula is used:

$$\text{Variance} = s^2 = \frac{\sum(x_i^2) - \left[\frac{(\sum x_i)^2}{N}\right]}{N-1} = \frac{90,376 - \frac{2,238,016}{26}}{26 - 1}$$

$$= \frac{90,376 - 86,077.54}{25} = \frac{4,298.46}{25} = 171.94$$

BOX 9-1. Properties of the Mean

(1) The mean of a sample is an *unbiased estimator* of the mean of the population from which it came.
(2) The mean is the *mathematical expectation.* As such, it is different from the mode, which is the value observed most often.
(3) The sum of the squared deviations of the observations from the mean is *smaller* than the sum of the squared deviations from any other number.
(4) The sum of the squared deviations from the mean is *fixed* for a given set of observations. This property is not unique to the mean, but it is a necessary property of any good measure of central tendency.

The median HDL value is also called the 50th percentile observation, because 50% of the observations lie below it. Percentiles are frequently used in medicine to describe normal growth standards for children. They are also used to describe the LD_{50} for experimental animals, defined as the dose of an agent, such as a drug, which is lethal for 50% of the animals that are exposed to it. The median length of survival is more useful than the mean (average) length of survival, because it is not strongly influenced by a small number of study subjects with unusually short or unusually long survival periods. Therefore, the median gives a better sense of the survival of most study subjects. The median is seldom used to make complicated inferences from medical data, however, because it does not lend itself to the development of advanced statistics.

(3) Mean. The mean is the average value, or the sum (Σ) of all of the observed values (x_i) divided by the total number of observations (N_i):

$$\text{Mean} = \overline{x} = \frac{\Sigma(x_i)}{N_i}$$

The mean ($\overline{x}$) has both practical and theoretical advantages as a measure of central tendency. It is simple to calculate, and the sum of the deviations of observations from the mean (expressed in terms of negative and positive numbers) should equal 0, which provides a simple check of the calculations. As listed in Box 9–1, the mean also has mathematical properties that enable the development of advanced statistics. Most descriptive analyses of continuous variables and even advanced statistical analyses use the mean as the measure of central tendency. Table 9–3 gives an example of the calculation of the mean.

Measures of Dispersion. After the central tendency of a frequency distribution is determined, the next step is to determine how spread out (dispersed) the numbers are. This can be done by calculating measures based on percentiles or measures based on the mean.

(1) Measures of Dispersion Based on Percentiles. Percentiles, which are sometimes called **quantiles,** are the percentage of observations below the point

indicated when all of the observations are ranked in descending order. The median, discussed above, is the 50th percentile. The 75th percentile is the point below which 75% of the observations lie, while the 25th percentile is the point below which 25% of the observations lie.

In Table 9–3, the **overall range** of HDL cholesterol values is 59 mg/dL, reflecting the distance between the highest value (90 mg/dL) and the lowest value (31 mg/dL) in the data set. In the same table, the 75th and 25th percentiles are 64 mg/dL and 48 mg/dL, respectively, and the distance between them is 16 mg/dL. This distance is called the **interquartile range** (sometimes abbreviated Q3 – Q1). The interquartile range is usually considerably smaller than half the size of the overall range of values.

The advantage of using percentiles is that they can be applied to any set of continuous data, even if the data do not form any known distribution. Percentiles are often used to describe the results of educational testing and to set ranges for growth standards for infants and children. Because few statistical tests of inference have been developed for use with medians and other percentiles, their use in medicine is mostly limited to description, but in this role, percentiles are often useful clinically.

(2) Measures of Dispersion Based on the Mean. Mean deviation, variance, and standard deviation are three measures of dispersion based on the mean. Although mean deviation is seldom used, a discussion of it will provide a better understanding of the concept of dispersion.

(a) Mean Deviation. Because the mean has many advantages, it might seem logical to measure dispersion by taking the "average deviation" from the mean. That proves to be useless, because the sum of the deviations from the mean is 0. However, this inconvenience can easily be solved by computing the mean deviation, which is the average of the absolute value of the deviations from the mean, as shown in the following formula:

$$\text{Mean deviation} = \frac{\Sigma(|x_i - \overline{x}|)}{N}$$

Because the mean deviation does not have mathematical properties that enable many statistical tests to be based on it, the formula has not come into

---

BOX 9-2. Properties of the Variance

(1) When the denominator of the equation for variance is expressed as the number of observations minus 1 ($N - 1$), the variance of a random sample is an *unbiased estimator* of the variance of the population from which it was taken.
(2) The variance of the sum of two independent variables is equal to the *sum* of the variances.
(3) The variance of the difference between two variables is equal to the *sum* of the variances as well. (The importance of this will become clear when the *t*-test is considered in Chapter 10.)

BOX 9–3.   How Do Statisticians Measure Variation?

In statistics, variation is measured as the sum of the squared deviations of the individual observations from an expected value, such as the mean. The mean is the mathematical expectation or expected value of a continuous frequency distribution. The quantity of variation in a given set of observations, therefore, is simply the numerator of the variance, which is the sum of the squares. The sum of the squares (SS) is sometimes called the total sum of the squares (TSS).

For purposes of illustration, assume that the data set consists of the following six numbers: 1, 2, 4, 7, 10, and 12. Assume that x_i denotes the individual observations, $\bar{x}$ is the mean, N is the number of observations, s^2 is the variance, and s is the standard deviation.

Part 1. Tabular representation of the data:

	x_i	$(x_i - \bar{x})$	$(x_i - \bar{x})^2$
	1	−5	25
	2	−4	16
	4	−2	4
	7	+1	1
	10	+4	16
	12	+6	36
Sum, or Σ	36	0	98

Part 2. Graphic representation of the data shown in the third column of the above table—that is, $(x_i - \bar{x})^2$ for each of the six observations:

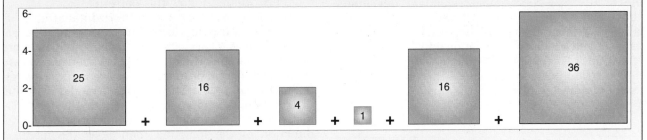

Part 3. Calculation of moments:

$\Sigma(x_i) = 36$ $\Sigma(x_i - \bar{x})^2 = \text{TSS} = 98$

$N = 6$ $s^2 = \text{TSS}/(N - 1) = 98/5 = 19.6$

$\bar{x} = 6$ $s = \sqrt{19.6} = 4.43$

---

popular use. Instead, the variance has become the fundamental measure of dispersion in statistics that are based on the normal distribution.

(b) Variance. The variance for a set of observed data is the sum of the squared deviations from the mean, divided by the number of observations minus 1:

$$\text{Variance} = s^2 = \frac{\Sigma(x_i - \bar{x})^2}{N - 1}$$

The symbol for a variance calculated from observed data, or a sample variance, is s^2. In the above formula, the squaring solves the problem that the deviations from the mean add up to 0. Dividing by $N - 1$ (called the **degrees of freedom**) instead of by N is necessary for the sample variance to be an unbiased estimator of the population variance.

The numerator of the variance (i.e., the sum of the squared deviations of the observations from the mean) is an extremely important entity in statistics. It is usually called either the **sum of squares** (abbreviated SS) or the **total sum of squares** (TSS). The TSS measures the total amount of variation in a set of observations. Box 9–2 lists the mathematical properties of variance that permit the development of statistical tests, and Box 9–3 explains how statisticians measure variation. Understanding what the concept of variation means in statistics will make much of the following discussion easier to grasp. Therefore, readers may wish to refer to these boxes now.

For simplicity of calculation on a pocket calculator, there is another (but algebraically equivalent) formula used to calculate the variance. It is the sum of the squared value of each observation, minus a correction factor (to correct for the fact that it is the absolute values, rather than the deviation from the mean, which are being squared), all divided by $N - 1$:

$$\text{Variance} = s^2 = \frac{\sum(x_i^2) - \left[\frac{(\sum x_i)^2}{N}\right]}{N - 1}$$

Table 9–3 illustrates the calculation of a variance using this second formula.

(c) Standard Deviation. The variance tends to be a large and unwieldy number, and its value falls outside the range of observed values in a data set. Therefore, the standard deviation, which is the square root of the variance, can be used to describe the amount of spread in the frequency distribution. The symbol for the standard deviation of an observed data set is *s*, and the formula is as follows:

$$\text{Standard deviation} = s = \sqrt{\frac{\sum(x_i - \bar{x})^2}{N - 1}}$$

In an observed data set, the term $\bar{x} \pm s$ represents 1 standard deviation above and below the mean, and the term $\bar{x} \pm 2s$ represents 2 standard deviations above and below the mean. One standard deviation falls well within the range of observed numbers in the data set and has a known relationship to the normal (gaussian) distribution, which is given in a table of the *z* distribution (see Appendix). This relationship is useful in drawing inferences in statistics.

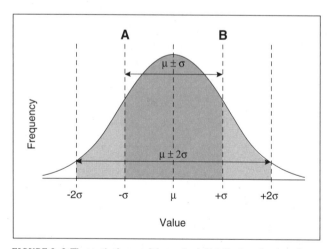

FIGURE 9–6. Theoretical normal (gaussian) distribution showing where 1 and 2 standard deviations above and below the mean would fall. The Greek letter mu (μ) stands for the mean in the theoretical distribution, and the Greek letter sigma (σ) stands for the standard deviation in the theoretical population. (The italic Roman letters $\bar{x}$ and *s* apply to an observed [sample] population.) In this figure, the area under the curve represents all of the observations in the distribution. One standard deviation above and below the mean, shown in dark orange and represented by the distance from point A to point B, is equivalent to 68% of the area under the curve, and therefore 68% of the observations in a normal distribution fall within this range. Two standard deviations above and below the mean, represented by the areas shown in dark and light orange, are equivalent to 95.4% of the area of the curve or 95.4% of the observations in a normal distribution.

In a theoretical normal (gaussian) distribution, as shown in Fig. 9–6, the area under the curve represents all of the observations in the distribution. One standard deviation above and below the mean, represented in Fig. 9–6 by the distance from point A to point B, is equivalent to 68% of the area under the curve, and therefore 68% of the observations in a normal distribution fall within this range. Two standard deviations above and below the mean are equivalent to 95.4% of the area (i.e., 95.4% of the observations) in a normal distribution. Exactly 95% of the observations from a normal frequency distribution lie between 1.96 standard deviations below the mean and 1.96 standard deviations above the mean. The formula $\bar{x} \pm 1.96$ standard deviations is often used in medicine to show the extent of variation in data obtained by research.

Problems in Analyzing a Frequency Distribution

In a normal (gaussian) distribution, the following holds true: mean = median = mode. In an observed data set, there may be skewness, kurtosis, and extreme values, in which case the measures of central tendency will not follow this pattern.

Skewness and Kurtosis. A horizontal stretching of a frequency distribution to one side or the other, so that one tail of observations is longer and has more observations than the other tail, is called **skewness.** When a histogram or frequency polygon has a longer tail on the left side of the diagram, as in Fig. 9–7, the distribution is said to be skewed to the left. If a distribution is skewed, the mean moves farther in the direction of the long tail than does the median, because the mean is more heavily influenced by extreme values. A quick way to get an approximate idea of whether or not a frequency distribution is skewed is to compare the mean and the median. If these two measures are close to each other, the distribution is probably not skewed. For example, in the data from Table 9–2, the mean equals 179.1 mg/dL and the median equals 178 mg/dL. These two values are very close, and as can be seen from Fig. 9–4, the distribution is not skewed very much either.

Kurtosis is characterized by a vertical stretching of the frequency distribution. As shown in Fig. 9–8, a kurtotic distribution could look more peaked or could look more flattened than the bell-shaped normal distribution.

Significant skewness or kurtosis can be detected by statistical tests which reveal that the observed data do not form a normal distribution. Many statistical tests require that the data they analyze be normally distributed, and the tests may not be valid if they are used to compare very abnormal distributions. On the other hand, the statistical tests discussed in this book are relatively robust, meaning that as long as the data are not too badly skewed or kurtotic, the results can be considered valid. Kurtosis is seldom discussed as a problem in the medical literature, although skewness is frequently observed and is treated as a problem.

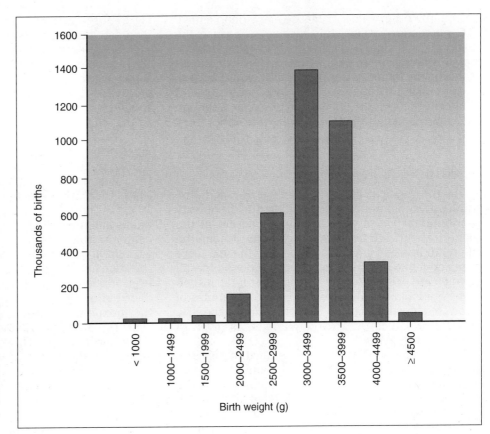

FIGURE 9–7. Histogram showing a skewed frequency distribution. Values are for thousands of births by birth weight group, USA, 1987. Note the long tail on the left. (Source of data: National Center for Health Statistics. Trends in Low Birth Weight: United States, 1975–85. Series 21, No. 48. Washington, D.C., Government Printing Office, 1989.)

Extreme Values (Outliers).   One of the most serious problems for the analysis of data is how to treat a value that is abnormally far above or below the mean. This problem is suggested in the data set of cholesterol values shown in Table 9–2 and Fig. 9–2. The standard deviation of the distribution in the data set is 28.2 mg/dL, so that if the distribution were normal, 95% of the cholesterol values would be expected to be between 123.8 mg/dL and 234.4 mg/dL.

Moreover, 99% of the values would be expected to be found within the range of the mean plus or minus 2.58 standard deviations, which in this case would be between 106.3 mg/dL and 251.9 mg/dL.

When the data are observed visually in Fig. 9–2, everything looks normal below the mean; the lowest value is 124 mg/dL, which is within the 95% limits. The upper value, however, is 264 mg/dL, which is beyond the 99% limits of expectation and looks suspiciously

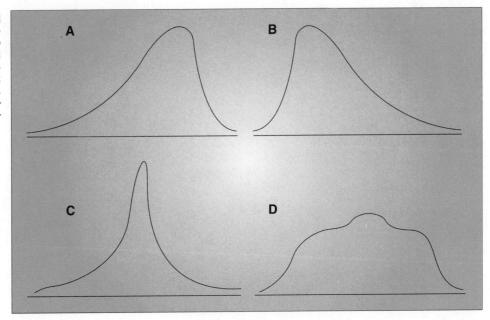

FIGURE 9–8. Examples of skewed and kurtotic frequency distributions. Distribution A is skewed to the left; distribution B is skewed to the right; distribution C is kurtotic, with abnormal peaking; and distribution D is kurtotic, with abnormal flattening in comparison to the normal distribution.

far from the other values. Because many people have total cholesterol values this high and because the observation is almost within the 99% limits, there is probably no reason to be concerned. However, before analyzing the data set, the investigator would want to be sure that this item of data was legitimate and would check the source of data. In this case, although the value is an outlier, it is what the laboratory reported.

Methods of Depicting a Frequency Distribution

In the medical literature, **histograms** and **line graphs** are commonly used to illustrate frequency distributions. These were introduced earlier in the chapter, along with **frequency polygons**. Among the other methods of visually displaying the data are stem and leaf diagrams, quantiles, and boxplots—all of which are printed out by computer programs such as the Statistical Analysis System (SAS). Examples of these are shown in Fig. 9–9. In each example, the HDL cholesterol values for 26 young adults, as given in Table 9–3, are plotted.

Stem and Leaf Diagrams. As shown in Fig. 9–9, the stem and leaf diagram has three components. The **stem**, which is the vertical column of numbers on the left, represents the value of the left-hand digit (in this case, the 10s digit). The **leaf** is the set of numbers immediately to the right of the stem and is sometimes separated from the stem by a vertical line. Each of the numbers in the leaf represents the next digit in one of the 26 observations in the data set of HDL cholesterol values. Thus, the stem and leaf value shown on the first line of the diagram represents 90 mg/dL. The **# symbol** to the right of the leaf tells how many observations were seen in the range indicated (in this case, 1 observation of 90 mg/dL or greater).

Among the observations that can quickly be made from viewing the stem and leaf diagram in

Fig. 9–9 are the following: (1) The highest value in the data set was 90 mg/dL. (2) The lowest value was 31 mg/dL. (3) There were 8 observations in the range of the 40s, consisting of 41, 44, 46, 47, 47, 48, 48, 49. (4) When the diagram is rotated 90 degrees counterclockwise, the distribution looks fairly normal, although it has a long tail to the left (that is, it is skewed to the left).

Quantiles. Below the stem and leaf diagram in Fig. 9–9 is a display of the quantiles (percentiles). Among the data included are the maximum (100% of the values were at this level or below) and minimum (0% of the values were below this); the 99%, 95%, 90%, 10%, 5%, and 1% percentile values; the range; the mode; and the interquartile range (from the 25th percentile to the 75th percentile, abbreviated Q3 – Q1).

Boxplots. The boxplot is shown to the right of the stem and leaf diagram in Fig. 9–9 and provides an even briefer way of summarizing the data in a distribution than the stem and leaf diagram does. In the boxplot, the rectangle formed by four plus signs (+) and the horizontal dashes (----) depicts the interquartile range. The two asterisks (*) connected by dashes depict the median. The mean, shown by the smaller plus sign (+), is very close to the median. Outside of the rectangle, there are two vertical lines, called the "whiskers" of the boxplot. The whiskers show the range where other values might be expected, given the median and interquartile range of the distribution. All of the values except the value of 90 mg/dL might reasonably have been expected; this value, however, is considered an outlier observation, which status is indicated by the 0 near the top, just above the top of the upper whisker. Thus, it takes only a quick look at the boxplot to see how wide the distribution is, whether or not it is skewed, where the interquartile range falls, how close the median is to the mean, and how many (if any) observations might reasonably be considered outliers.

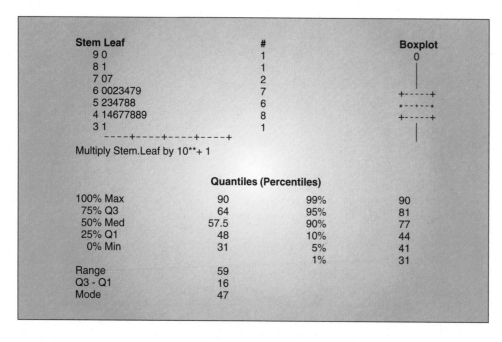

FIGURE 9–9. Stem and leaf diagram, boxplot, and quantiles (percentiles) for the data shown in Table 9–3, as printed out by the Statistical Analysis System (SAS). See the text for a detailed description of how to interpret the data shown here.

Stem	Leaf	#	Boxplot
9	0	1	0
8	1	1	
7	07	2	
6	0023479	7	+-----+
5	234788	6	*--+--*
4	14677889	8	+-----+
3	1	1	

```
----+----+----+----+
```

Multiply Stem.Leaf by 10**+ 1

Quantiles (Percentiles)

100% Max	90	99%	90
75% Q3	64	95%	81
50% Med	57.5	90%	77
25% Q1	48	10%	44
0% Min	31	5%	41
		1%	31
Range	59		
Q3 - Q1	16		
Mode	47		

Use of Unit-Free (Normalized) Data

Data from a normal (gaussian) frequency distribution can be described completely by the **mean** and the **standard deviation.** However, even the same set of data will provide a different value for the mean and standard deviation depending on the choice of **units of measurement.** For example, the same person's height may be expressed as 66 inches or 167.6 cm, and an infant's birth weight may be recorded as 2500 g or 5.5 pounds. Here, the units of measurement differ, even though the true height and weight are the same. To eliminate the distorting effect produced by the choice of units, the data can be put into a unit-free form (normalized).

The first step in normalizing data is to set the mean equal to 0 by subtracting the mean from each observation in whatever units have been used. The next step is to measure each observation in terms of the number of standard deviations it is above or below the mean. As long as the same units are used to calculate the mean and the standard deviation, the same value (in terms of standard deviations) will be obtained for each observation, regardless of which unit of measurement was initially used. The normalized values obtained by this process are called **z values,** and the formula for creating individual z values (z_i) is as follows:

$$z_i = \frac{x_i - \bar{x}}{s}$$

where x_i represents individual observations, $\bar{x}$ represents the mean of the observations, and s is the standard deviation.

Suppose, for example, that the goal is to standardize blood pressure values for a group of patients whose systolic blood pressures were observed to have a mean of 120 mm Hg and a standard deviation of 10 mm Hg. If two of the values to be standardized were 140 mm Hg and 115 mm Hg, the calculations would be as follows:

$$\frac{140 - 120}{10} = +2.0 \qquad \frac{115 - 120}{10} = -0.5$$

A distribution of z values always has a mean of 0 standard deviations and always has a standard deviation of 1 standard deviation. The z values here are called by various names, often **standard normal deviates.**

Clinically, z values are useful for determining how extreme an observed test result is. For example, in Table 9–2, the highest total cholesterol value observed among 71 persons was 264 mg/dL, 23 points higher than the next highest value. Is this cholesterol value suspect? Its z value is $(264 - 179.1)/28.2 = +3.0$. This means that it is 3 standard deviations above the mean. Usually, about 1% of observed values are 2.58 standard deviations away from the mean, and this is the only one of the 71 observed values this far away; therefore, there is no strong reason to suppose it is an error.

Frequency Distributions of Dichotomous Data and Proportions

Dichotomous data can be thought of in terms of flipping a coin. If the coin is flipped in an unbiased manner, on the average it would be expected to land with the heads side up in half of the flips and with the tails side up in half of the flips, so the probability of heads would equal 0.5 and the probability of tails would equal 0.5. The sum of all of the probabilities for all of the possible outcomes must equal 1.0. If a coin if flipped 10 times, the result would very rarely be 10 heads or 10 tails, would somewhat less rarely be a combination of 9 heads plus 1 tail, and would most frequently be a combination of 5 heads and 5 tails.

The probabilities of getting various combinations of heads and tails from flipping a coin can be calculated by expanding the following expression: $(a + b)^n$. In this expression, a is the probability of heads, b is the probability of tails, and n is the number of coin tosses in a trial. The process of calculating the probabilities is called **expanding the binomial,** and the distribution of probabilities for each combination gives the **binomial distribution.**

If n is large (say, hundreds of tosses of the coin) and if the coin is thrown in an unbiased manner, the distribution of the binomial toss would look much like a normal (gaussian) distribution. In fact, if n were infinite, a were 0.5, and b were 0.5, then the binomial distribution would be *identical* to the normal distribution. Therefore, a mean and standard deviation can be calculated for the binomial distribution.

If the probability of heads does not equal 0.5, the binomial distribution would look like a skewed distribution, and the previously mentioned cautions concerning statistical analysis would apply (see Problems in Analyzing a Frequency Distribution, above).

Because of the close relationship between the binomial and the normal distributions, binary data expressed as **proportions** can be analyzed using theory based on the normal distribution.

Frequency Distributions of Other Types of Data

Data from nominal (categorical) and ordinal (ranked) variables are not properly analyzed using theory and tests based on the normal (gaussian) distribution. These data should be analyzed using statistical methods that do not make any assumptions about an underlying frequency distribution. Because they are not based on either the normal or binomial distribution (for which parameters such as means and standard deviations can be calculated), statistical tests for nominal and ordinal variables are called **nonparametric tests.**

Of particular importance, the analysis of the counts in frequency tables (such as Table 9–1) depends on a different distribution, which is known as the chi-square distribution and is discussed in Chapter 11. The chi-square analysis, however, does not require that the data themselves follow any particular distribution, so it is a nonparametric test.

Ordinal data are sometimes analyzed in the medical literature as though they were continuous data, and means and standard deviations are reported. This is usually satisfactory for describing ordinal data, but it is generally not appropriate for testing probabilities. As discussed in Chapter 11, the Wilcoxon test, the Mann-Whitney U test, and other tests for ordinal data have been developed and do not require that the data follow any particular distribution; they require only that the data be ordinal.

SUMMARY

While variation in clinical medicine may be due to biologic differences or the presence or absence of disease, it may also be due to differences in measurement techniques and conditions, errors in measurement, and random variation. Statistics is an aid to describing and understanding the variation and minimizing errors.

Statistical analysis cannot correct for bias (see Chapter 4), and the analysis can only "adjust" for random error in the sense that it can estimate how much of the total variation is due to random error and how much is due to a particular factor being investigated. In this regard, an illustration that students often find useful comes from the concepts of signal and noise in radio broadcast engineering. Listeners who are searching for a particular station on their radio dial will find background noise on every radio frequency. When they reach the station they want to hear, in addition to hearing background noise, they will hear the station's signal. The critical factor is the ratio of signal to noise. The task of the radio is to amplify the signal enough so that the listeners can hear the music clearly without being so annoyed by the background noise that they switch to another channel. In medical studies, the particular factor that is being investigated can be thought of as the signal, and random variation can be thought of as the background noise. Statistical analysis helps to sort out the two by comparing their impact. If the variation due to the particular factor is considerably larger than the variation due to random factors (approximately 1.96 times as large), the difference in impact becomes statistically "detectable" and can be considered real. This is similar to saying that if the strength of the signal is about twice the strength of the noise, the signal can be understood.

Fundamental to any analysis of data is understanding the types of variables or data, including nominal, dichotomous, ordinal, continuous, and ratio data, as well as risks and proportions. Data may be combined into ranges for simplifying analyses, but once this is done, some information is lost.

Continuous (measurement) data have a frequency distribution that can be described in terms of two types of parameters: the measures of central tendency (of which median and mean are the most important) and the measures of dispersion based on the mean (of which variance and standard deviation are the most important). The most common distribution is called the normal (gaussian) distribution and has the shape of a bell when viewed from the side.

In a normal distribution, the mean and the median coincide, and 95% of the observations are within 1.96 standard deviations above and below the mean. Frequently, the normal distribution appears pulled to one side or the other (appears to have a long tail), in which case it is called a skewed distribution. In a skewed distribution, the mean is farther in the direction of the long tail than is the median.

Data may be made unit-free by creating z values, in which the mean is subtracted from each value and the result is divided by the standard deviation. This expresses the value of each observation as the number of standard deviations it is above or below the mean.

The probability distribution for dichotomous data may be described by the binomial distribution. If the probability of success and failure are the same (i.e., 0.5 each) and if the number of trials is very large, the binomial distribution is identical to the normal distribution.

References Cited

Buehler, J. W., et al. Birth weight–specific infant mortality, United States, 1960 and 1980. Public Health Reports 102:151–161, 1987.

Elmore, J. G., et al. Variability in radiologists' interpretations of mammograms. New England Journal of Medicine 331:1493–1499, 1994.

Selected Reading

Dawson-Saunders, B., and R. G. Trapp. Basic and Clinical Biostatistics, 2nd ed. Norwalk, Conn., Appleton and Lange, 1994.

CHAPTER TEN

STATISTICAL INFERENCE

AND HYPOTHESIS TESTING

THE NATURE AND PURPOSE OF STATISTICAL INFERENCE

Inference means the drawing of conclusions from data. Statistical inference can be defined as the drawing of conclusions from quantitative or qualitative information using the methods of statistics to describe and arrange the data and to test suitable hypotheses.

Differences between Deductive Reasoning and Inductive Reasoning

Because data do not come with their own interpretation, the interpretation must be put into the data by **inductive reasoning** (from Latin, meaning "to lead into"). This approach to reasoning is less familiar to most people than is **deductive reasoning** (from Latin, meaning "to lead out from"), which is learned from mathematics, particularly from geometry.

Deductive reasoning proceeds *from the general* (i.e., from assumptions, from propositions, and from formulas considered true) *to the specific* (i.e., to specific members belonging to the general category). Consider, for example, the following two propositions: (1) All Americans believe in democracy. (2) This person is an American. If both propositions are true, then the following deduction must be true: This person must believe in democracy.

Deductive reasoning is of special use in science once hypotheses are formed. Using deductive reasoning, an investigator says, *If* the following hypothesis is true, *then* the following prediction or predictions also should be true. If a prediction can be tested empirically, the hypothesis may be rejected or not rejected on the basis of the findings.

If the data are inconsistent with the predictions from the hypothesis, they force a rejection or modification of the hypothesis. If the data are consistent with the hypothesis, they cannot prove that the hypothesis is true, although they do lend support to the hypothesis. To reiterate, even if the data are consistent with the hypothesis, they do not prove the hypothesis, as was discussed in Chapter 4 and demonstrated with regard to Fig. 4–3.

Physicians often proceed from formulas accepted as true and from observed data to determine the values that variables must have in a certain clinical situation. For example, if the amount of a medication that can be safely given per kilogram of body weight (a constant) is known, then it is simple to calculate how much of that medication can be given to a patient weighing 50 kg. This is deductive reasoning, because it proceeds from the general (a constant and a formula) to the specific (the patient).

Inductive reasoning, in contrast, seeks to find valid generalizations and general principles from data. Statistics, the quantitative aid to inductive reasoning, proceeds *from the specific* (that is, from data) *to the general* (that is, to formulas or conclusions). For example, by sampling a population and determining both the age and the blood pressure of the persons in the sample (the specific data), an investigator using statistical methods can determine the general relationship between age and blood pressure (e.g., that, on the average, blood pressure increases with age).

Differences between Mathematics and Statistics

The differences between mathematics and statistics can be illustrated by showing that they form the basis for very different approaches to the same basic equation:

$$y = mx + b$$

This equation is the formula for a straight line in analytic geometry. It is also the formula for simple regression analysis in statistics, although the letters used and their order customarily are different.

In the mathematical formula above, the b is a constant, and it stands for the y-intercept (i.e., the value of y when the variable x equals 0). The value m also is a constant, and it stands for the slope (the amount of change in y for a unit increase in the value of x). The important thing to note is that in mathematics, one of the variables (either x or y) is unknown (i.e., to be calculated), while the formula and the constants are known.

In statistics, however, just the reverse is true: the variables, x and y, are known for all observations, and the investigator usually wishes to determine whether or not there is a linear (straight line) relationship between x and y, by estimating the slope and the intercept. This can be done using the form of analysis called linear regression, which is discussed in Chapter 11.

As a general rule, what is known in statistics is unknown in mathematics, and vice versa. In statistics, the investigator starts from specific observations (data) to induce or estimate the general relationships between variables.

THE PROCESS OF TESTING HYPOTHESES

The following discussion introduces the basic concepts underlying the usual tests of statistical significance. These tests determine the probability that a finding (such as a difference between means or proportions) represents a true deviation from what was expected (i.e., from the model, which is often a hypothesis that there will be no difference between the means or proportions). The discussion in this chapter focuses on the justification for and interpretation of the p value, which is designed to minimize false-positive error. False-negative error is discussed more fully in Chapter 12 under sample size.

False-Positive and False-Negative Errors

Science is based on the following set of principles: (1) previous experience serves as the basis for developing hypotheses; (2) hypotheses serve as the basis for developing predictions; (3) and predictions must be subjected to experimental or observational testing. In deciding whether data are consistent or inconsistent with the hypotheses, investigators are subject to two types of error. They could assert that the data support the hypotheses when in fact the hypotheses are false; this would be a **false-positive error,** which is also called an **alpha error** or a **type I error.** Conversely, they could assert that the data do not support the hypotheses when in fact the hypotheses are true; this would be a **false-negative error,** which is also called a **beta error** or a **type II error.**

Based on the knowledge that scientists become attached to their own hypotheses and based on the conviction that the proof in science, as in the courts, must be "beyond reasonable doubt," investigators have historically been particularly cautious in avoiding the false-positive error. Probably this is best for theoretical science. In medicine, however, where a false-negative error in a diagnostic test may mean missing a disease until it is too late to institute therapy and where a false-negative error in the study of a medical intervention may mean overlooking an effective treatment, investigators cannot feel comfortable about false-negative errors either.

The Null Hypothesis and the Alternative Hypothesis

The process of significance testing involves three basic steps: (1) asserting the null hypothesis, (2) establishing the alpha level, and (3) accepting the null hypothesis or the alternative hypothesis.

The first step consists of asserting the **null hypothesis,** which is the hypothesis that there is no real (true) difference between means or proportions of the groups being compared or that there is no real association between two continuous variables. For example, the null hypothesis for the data discussed in Chapter 9 and presented in Table 9–1 is that there is no real difference between the percentage of men and the percentage of women who had previously had their serum cholesterol levels checked. It may seem strange to begin the process by asserting that something is not true, but it is far easier to reject an assertion than to prove that something is true. (If the data are not consistent with a hypothesis, the hypothesis can be rejected. If the data are consistent with a hypothesis, this still does not prove the hypothesis, because other hypotheses may fit the data equally well.)

The second step is to determine the probability of being in error if the null hypothesis is rejected. This step requires that an alpha level be established, as described below.

If the null hypothesis is unlikely, the third step is to accept the **alternative hypothesis,** which is the hypothesis that there is in fact a real difference or association. Although it may seem awkward, this process is now standard in medical science and has yielded considerable scientific benefits.

As an example, consider a hypothetical clinical trial of a drug designed to lower high blood pressure among patients with essential hypertension (hypertension occurring without a discoverable organic cause). One group of patients would receive the ex-

perimental drug, and the other group (the control group) would receive a placebo. The null hypothesis might be that following the intervention, the average change in blood pressure in the treatment group will not differ from the average change in blood pressure in the control group. If a test of significance (such as a *t*-test on the average change in systolic blood pressure) forces rejection of the null hypothesis, then the alternative hypothesis—namely, the hypothesis that there was a true difference in the average change in blood pressure in the two groups—will be accepted.

The Alpha Level and *p* Value

Before doing any calculations to test the null hypothesis, the investigator must establish a criterion called the **alpha level,** which is the maximum probability of making a false-positive error that the investigator is willing to accept. By custom, the level of alpha is usually set at $p = 0.05$. This says that the investigator is willing to run a 5% risk (but no more) of being in error when asserting that the treatment and control groups truly differ. In choosing an alpha level, value judgment is inserted into the process. However, when that is done before the data are collected, at least the post hoc bias of being tempted to adjust the alpha level to make the data show statistical significance is avoided.

The **p value** obtained by a statistical test (such as the *t*-test described later in this chapter) gives the probability that the observed difference could have been obtained by chance alone, given random variation and a single test of the null hypothesis. Usually, if the observed *p* value is ≤ 0.05, members of the scientific community who read about an investigation will accept the difference as being a real difference. Although setting alpha at ≤ 0.05 is somewhat arbitrary, that level has become so customary that it is wise to provide explanations for choosing another alpha level or for choosing not to perform tests of significance at all, which may be the best approach in some descriptive studies.

Once the alpha level is established, the *p* value for the data can be obtained. In this process, the first step is to calculate a critical ratio (such as the *t, z, F,* or chi-square value) from the data. The second step is to consult a standard table of the possible values of *p* (see the Appendix). If the *p* value determined from the table is less than or equal to the preselected alpha level (in this example, $p \leq 0.05$), the null hypothesis is rejected and the alternative hypothesis is accepted. If the *p* value is greater than the alpha level (in this example, $p > 0.05$), the investigator fails to reject the null hypothesis. Note that failing to reject the null hypothesis is *not* the same as accepting the null hypothesis. Rather, it is similar to a jury's finding that the evidence did not prove the guilt (or in the example here, did not prove the difference) beyond a reasonable doubt. A court trial is not designed to prove innocence. The defendant's innocence is assumed and must be disproved beyond a reasonable doubt.

An everyday analogy may help to simplify the logic of the level of alpha and the process of significance testing. Suppose that a young couple was given instructions to buy a silver bracelet for a friend during a trip if one could be bought for $50 or less. If a suitable bracelet is found, it would be bought only if it could be obtained for $50 or less. Any more would be too high a price to pay. Alpha is like the price limit in the analogy. Once it has been set (say, at 0.05), an investigator would "buy" the alternative hypothesis of a true difference or association if the cost (in the probability of being wrong) were no greater than 1 in 20 (0.05). The alpha, therefore, is the price that an investigator is willing to pay in the probability of being wrong if he or she rejects the null hypothesis.

Variation in Individual Observations and in Multiple Samples

Most tests of significance relate to a difference between means or proportions. They help investigators decide whether an observed difference is real, which in statistical terms is defined as whether the difference is greater than would be expected by chance alone. In the example of the experimental drug to lower blood pressure in hypertensive patients, the experimenters would measure the mean blood pressures of the study subjects under experimental conditions both before and after the new drug or placebo is given. They would determine the average change seen in the treatment group and the average change seen in the control group and then pursue tests to determine whether the difference was large enough to be unlikely to have occurred by chance alone. Therefore, the fundamental process in this test of significance would be to see if the mean blood pressure changes in the two study groups were different.

Why not just inspect the means to see if they were different? This is not adequate, because it is not known whether the observed findings were unusual or whether they would probably have been found repeatedly if the experiment were repeated. Although the investigators examine the findings in particular patients, their real interest is determining whether the findings of the study could be generalized to other, similar hypertensive patients. To generalize beyond the particular subjects in the single study, the investigators must know the extent to which the differences discovered in the study are reliable. The estimate of reliability is given by the standard error, which is not the same as the standard deviation discussed in Chapter 9 and below.

Standard Deviation and Standard Error

Chapter 9 focused on individual observations and the extent to which they varied from the mean. One of the assertions discussed in the chapter was that a normal (gaussian) distribution could be completely described by its mean and **standard deviation.** Fig. 9–6 demonstrated that 68% of observations

fall within the range described as the mean plus or minus 1 standard deviation, 95.4% fall within the range of the mean plus or minus 2 standard deviations, and 95% fall within the range of the mean plus or minus 1.96 standard deviations. This information is useful in describing individual observations (raw data), but it is not useful in determining how close a sample mean is to the mean for the underlying population (which is also called the true mean or the population mean). This determination must be made on the basis of the standard error.

The **standard error** is related to the standard deviation, but it differs from it in important ways. Basically, the standard error is the standard deviation of a population of sample means, rather than of individual observations. Therefore, the standard error refers to the variability of means, rather than the variability of individual observations, so that it provides an idea of how variable a single estimate of the mean is likely to be.

The data shown in Table 10–1 can be used to explore the concept of standard error. The table lists the systolic and diastolic blood pressures of 26 young, healthy, adult subjects. To determine the probable error of the estimate of the mean blood pressure obtained from the 26 subjects, an unbiased estimate is needed of the variation in the underlying population. How can this be done with only one rather small sample? The solution requires a bit of

TABLE 10–1.   **Systolic and Diastolic Blood Pressure Values of 26 Young, Healthy, Adult Subjects**

Subject	Blood Pressure		Sex
	Systolic (mm Hg)	Diastolic (mm Hg)	
1	108	62	Female
2	134	74	Male
3	100	64	Female
4	108	68	Female
5	112	72	Male
6	112	64	Female
7	112	68	Female
8	122	70	Male
9	116	70	Male
10	116	70	Male
11	120	72	Male
12	108	70	Female
13	108	70	Female
14	96	64	Female
15	114	74	Male
16	108	68	Male
17	128	86	Male
18	114	68	Male
19	112	64	Male
20	124	70	Female
21	90	60	Female
22	102	64	Female
23	106	70	Male
24	124	74	Male
25	130	72	Male
26	116	70	Female

Source of data: Unpublished findings in a sample of 26 professional persons in Connecticut.

statistical theory. Suppose instead of the single sample, there were 100 different samples, each consisting of 26 individuals, from the same underlying population. (This supposition is not as farfetched as it might seem; the same research is often funded in many different medical centers, using strictly comparable criteria.) Then 100 mean blood pressure values could be determined from the 100 different samples.

The frequency distribution of the 100 different means could be plotted, treating each mean as a single observation. These sample means will form a truly normal (gaussian) frequency distribution, the mean of which would be very close to the true mean for the underlying population. More important for this discussion, the standard deviation of this distribution of sample means is an unbiased estimate of the standard deviation of the underlying population and is called the standard error of the distribution. (Technically, the variance is an unbiased estimator of the population variance, and the standard deviation, although not quite unbiased, is close enough to being unbiased that it works well.)

The standard error is a parameter that enables the investigator to do two things that are central to the function of statistics. One is estimating the probable amount of error around the quantitative assertions. The other is performing tests of statistical significance. If only the standard deviation and sample size are known, however, they can be converted to a standard error so that these functions can be pursued.

Although the proof will not be shown here, an unbiased estimate of the standard error can be obtained from the standard deviation of a single sample if the standard deviation was originally calculated using the degrees of freedom ($N - 1$) in the denominator (see Chapter 9). The formula for converting a standard deviation (SD) to a standard error (SE) is as follows:

$$\text{Standard error} = \text{SE} = \frac{\text{SD}}{\sqrt{N}}$$

The larger the sample size (N), the smaller the standard error will be, and the better the estimate of the population mean will be. At any given point, the height of the bell-shaped curve of the sample means represents the relative probability that a single sample mean would fall at that point. Most of the time, the sample mean would be near the true mean. Less often, it would be farther away.

In the medical literature, means or proportions are often reported either as the mean plus or minus 1 SD or as the mean plus or minus 1 SE. Reported data must be examined carefully to determine whether the SD or the SE is shown. Either is acceptable in theory, because an SD can be converted to an SE and vice versa if the sample size is known. However, many journals have a policy stating whether the SD or SE must be reported. The sample size should also be shown.

BOX 10–1.   Calculation of the Standard Error and the 95% Confidence Interval for Systolic Blood Pressure Values of 26 Subjects

Part 1. Beginning data (see Table 10–1):

Number of observations, or $N = 26$
Mean, or $\bar{x}$ $\quad\quad\quad = 113.1$ mm Hg
Standard deviation, or SD $\quad = 10.3$ mm Hg

Part 2. Calculation of the standard error, or SE:

$$\text{SE} = \frac{\text{SD}}{\sqrt{N}} = \frac{10.3}{\sqrt{26}} = \frac{10.3}{5.1} = 2.02 \text{ mm Hg}$$

Part 3. Calculation of the 95% confidence interval, or 95% CI:

$$95\% \text{ CI} = \text{mean} \pm 1.96 \text{ SE}$$
$$= 113.1 \pm (1.96)(2.02)$$
$$= 113.1 \pm 3.96$$
$$= \text{between } 113.1 - 3.96 \text{ and } 113.1 + 3.96$$
$$= 109.1, 117.1 \text{ mm Hg}$$

Confidence Intervals

Whereas the SD shows the variability of individual observations, the SE shows the variability of means. Whereas the mean plus or minus 1.96 SD estimates the range in which 95% of individual observations would be expected to fall, the mean plus or minus 1.96 SE estimates the range in which 95% of the means of repeated samples would be expected to fall. Moreover, if the value for the mean plus or minus 1.96 SE is known, it can be used to calculate the 95% confidence interval, which is the range of values in which the investigator can be 95% confident that the true mean of the underlying population falls. Other confidence intervals, such as the 99% confidence interval, can easily be determined as well.

Box 10–1 shows the calculation of the SE and the 95% confidence interval for the systolic blood pressure data in Table 10–1.

Confidence intervals alone can be used as a test to see whether a mean or proportion differs significantly from a **fixed value.** The most common situation for this is testing to see whether a risk ratio or an odds ratio differs significantly from the ratio of 1.0 (which means no difference). Thus, if a risk ratio of 1.7 had a 95% confidence interval between 0.92 and 2.70, it would not be significantly different from 1.0 if the alpha was chosen to be 0.05. However, if the same risk ratio had a 95% confidence interval between 1.02 and 2.60, it would be significantly different from a risk ratio of 1.0, because 1.0 does not fall within the confidence interval shown.

TESTS OF STATISTICAL SIGNIFICANCE

The tests described below allow investigators to compare two parameters, such as means or proportions, and to determine whether the difference between them is statistically significant. The various **t-tests** (the one-tailed Student's t-test, the two-tailed Student's t-test, and the paired t-test) compare differences between **means,** while **z-tests** compare differences between **proportions.** All of these tests make comparisons possible by calculating the appropriate form of a ratio, called a **critical ratio** because it permits the investigator to make a decision. This is done by comparing the ratio obtained from whatever test is performed (e.g., a t-test) with the values in the appropriate statistical table (e.g., a table of t values) for different degrees of freedom. Before individual tests are discussed in detail, the concepts of critical ratios and degrees of freedom are defined. The statistical tables of t values and z values are included at the end of the book (see the Appendix).

Critical Ratios

Critical ratios are a class of tests of statistical significance that depend on dividing some parameter (such as a difference between means) by the standard error (SE) of that parameter. The general formula for tests of significance is as follows:

$$\text{Critical ratio} = \frac{\text{Parameter}}{\text{SE of that parameter}}$$

When applied to the Student's t-test, the formula becomes:

$$\text{Critical ratio} = t = \frac{\text{Difference between two means}}{\text{SE of the difference between two means}}$$

When applied to a z-test, the formula becomes:

$$\text{Critical ratio} = z = \frac{\text{Difference between two proportions}}{\text{SE of the difference between two proportions}}$$

The value of the critical ratio (e.g., t or z) is then looked up in the appropriate table (of t or z) to determine the corresponding value of p. For any critical ratio, the larger the ratio is, the more likely it is that the difference between means or proportions is due to more than random variation (i.e., the more likely it is that the difference can be considered statistically significant and, hence, real). Unless the total sample size is small (say, under 30), the finding of a critical ratio of greater than about 2 usually indicates that the difference is real and enables the investigator to reject the null hypothesis. The statistical tables adjust the critical ratios for the sample size by means of the degrees of freedom.

The reason that a critical ratio works is somewhat complex and can best be explained through the use of an illustration. Assume that an investigator conducted 1000 different clinical trials of the same *ineffective* antihypertensive drug and that each of the trials had a large sample size. In each trial, assume that the investigator obtained an average value for the change in blood pressure in the experimental group ($\bar{x}_E$) and an average value for the change in blood pressure in the control group ($\bar{x}_C$). Therefore, for each trial, there would be two means, and the difference between the means could be expressed as $\bar{x}_E$ minus $\bar{x}_C$. In this study, the null hypothesis would be that the difference between the means was not a real difference.

If the null hypothesis were true, chance variation would cause $\bar{x}_E$ to be greater than $\bar{x}_C$ about half the time, despite the drug's lack of effect. The reverse would be true, also by chance, about half the time. In a rare trial, $\bar{x}_E$ would exactly equal $\bar{x}_C$. On the average, however, the differences between the two means would be near 0, reflecting the drug's lack of effect.

If the values representing the difference between the two means in each of the 1000 clinical trials were plotted on a graph, the distribution curve would appear normal (i.e., gaussian), with an average difference of 0, as in Fig. 10–1A. Chance variation would cause 95% of the values to fall within the large central zone, which covers the area of 0 ± 1.96 standard errors and is colored light orange in Fig. 10–1A. This is the zone for *failing to reject* the null hypothesis. Outside of this zone is the zone for *rejecting* the null hypothesis, which consists of two areas colored in dark orange in Fig. 10–1A.

Therefore, if only one clinical trial were performed and if the ratio of the difference between the means of the two groups was outside the area of 0 ± 1.96 standard errors of the difference, either the study was a rare (i.e., ≤ 0.05) example of a false-positive difference or there was a true difference between the groups. By setting alpha at 0.05, the investigator is willing to take a 5% risk (i.e., a 1-in-20 risk) of a false-positive assertion but is not willing to take a higher risk. This implies that if alpha is set at 0.05 and if 20 sets of two groups that are *not* truly different are compared, one "statistically significant" difference would be expected by chance alone.

Degrees of Freedom

The term "degrees of freedom" refers to the number of observations that are free to vary. The idea behind this important statistical concept is presented in Box 10–2. For simplicity, the degrees of freedom for any test are considered to be the total sample size minus 1 degree of freedom for each mean that is calculated. In the Student's t-test, 2 degrees of freedom are lost because two means are calculated (one mean for each group whose means are to be compared). The general formula for the degrees of freedom for the Student's t-test is $N_1 + N_2 - 2$, where N_1 is the sample size in the first group and N_2 is the sample size in the second group.

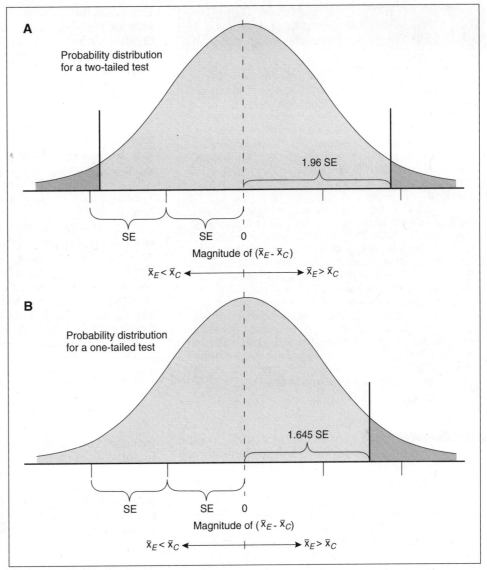

FIGURE 10–1. Probability distribution of the difference between two means when the null hypothesis is actually true (i.e., when there is no real difference between the two means). Dark orange indicates the zone for rejecting the null hypothesis, and light orange indicates the zone for failing to reject the null hypothesis. When a two-tailed test is used, there is a rejection zone on each side of the distribution. When a one-tailed test is used, there is a rejection zone on only one side. SE is the standard error, $\bar{x}_E$ is the mean for the experimental group, and $\bar{x}_C$ is the mean for the control group.

Use of t-Tests

In medical research, t-tests are among the three or four most commonly used statistical tests (Emerson and Colditz 1983). The purpose of a t-test is to compare the means of a continuous variable in two samples in order to determine whether or not the difference between the two observed means exceeds the difference that would be expected by chance.

Sample Populations and Sizes

If the two samples come from two different groups (e.g., a group of men and a group of women), the Student's t-test is used. If the two samples come from the same group (e.g., pretreatment and post-treatment values for the same study subjects), the paired t-test is used.

Both types of t-test depend on certain assumptions, including the assumption that the data in the continuous variable are normally distributed (i.e., have a bell-shaped distribution). Very seldom, how-

ever, will observed data be perfectly normally distributed. Does this invalidate the t-test? Fortunately, it does not. There is a convenient theorem, called the central limit theorem, that rescues the t-test (and much of statistics as well). The **central limit theorem** can be derived theoretically or observed by experimentation. According to the theorem, for reasonably large samples (say, 30 or more), the distribution of the means of many samples is normal (gaussian), even though the data in individual samples may have skewness, kurtosis, or unevenness. Because the critical theoretical requirement for the t-test is that the sample means be normally distributed, a t-test may be computed on almost any set of continuous data, if the observations can be considered a random sample and the sample size is reasonably large.

The t Distribution

The t distribution was described by William Gosset, who used the pseudonym "Student" when he

---

BOX 10–2. The Idea behind the Degrees of Freedom

The term "degrees of freedom" refers to the number of observations *(N)* that are free to vary. A degree of freedom is lost every time a mean is calculated. Why should this be?

Before putting on a pair of gloves, a person has the freedom to decide whether to begin with the left or right glove. However, once the person puts on the first glove, he or she loses the freedom to decide which glove to put on last. If centipedes put on shoes, they would have a choice to make for the first 99 shoes but not for the 100th shoe. Right at the end, the freedom to choose (vary) is restricted.

In statistics, if there are two observed values, only one estimate of the variation between them is possible. Something has to serve as the basis against which other observations are compared. The mean is the most "solid" estimate of the expected value of a variable, so it is assumed to be "fixed." This implies that the numerator of the mean (the sum of individual observations, or the sum of x_i), which is based on N observations, is also fixed. Once $N - 1$ observations (each of which was, presumably, free to vary) have been added up, the last observation is not free to vary, because the total values of the N observations must add up to the sum of x_i. For this reason, 1 degree of freedom is lost each time a mean is calculated. The proper average of a sum of squares when calculated from an observed sample, therefore, is the sum of squares divided by the degrees of freedom $(N - 1)$.

---

wrote the description. (For an explanation of how the *t*-test received its name and for other humorous perspectives on statistics, see Smith 1993.)

The normal distribution is the *z* distribution. The *t* distribution looks similar to it, except that its tails are somewhat wider and its peak is slightly less high, depending on the sample size. The *t* distribution is necessary because when sample sizes are small, the observed estimates of the mean and variance are subject to considerable error. The larger the sample size is, the smaller the errors are, and the more the *t* distribution looks like the normal distribution. In the case of an infinite sample size, the two distributions are identical. For practical purposes, when the combined sample size of the two groups being compared is larger than 120, the difference between the normal distribution and the *t* distribution is negligible.

Student's *t*-Test

There are two types of Student's *t*-test: the one-tailed and the two-tailed type. Their common features will be discussed before their differences are outlined.

Calculation of the Value of *t*. In both types of Student's *t*-test, *t* is calculated by taking the observed difference between the means of the two groups (the numerator) and dividing this difference by the standard error of the difference between the means of the two groups (the denominator). Before *t* can be calculated, then, the **standard error of the difference between the means** (SED) must be determined.

The basic formula for this is the square root of the sum of the respective population variances, each divided by its own sample size.

In theoretical terms, the correct equation for the SED would be as follows:

$$\text{SED of } \mu_E - \mu_C = \sqrt{\frac{\sigma_E^2}{N_E} + \frac{\sigma_C^2}{N_C}}$$

where the Greek symbol μ is the population mean, E is the experimental population, C is the control population, σ^2 is the variance of the population, and N is the number of observations in the population. The rationale behind this formula is discussed in Box 10–3.

The theoretical formula requires that the population variances be known, which usually is not true with experimental data. Nevertheless, if the sample sizes are large enough (e.g., if the total of the two samples is 30 or greater), the above formula can be used with the sample variances substituted for the population variances. In this case, instead of using Greek letters in the formula, the italic Roman symbol $\bar{x}$ is used to indicate the mean of the sample and the italic Roman symbol s^2 is used to indicate the variance:

$$\begin{array}{c}\text{Estimate of the}\\\text{SED of } \bar{x}_E - \bar{x}_C\end{array} = \sqrt{\frac{s_E^2}{N_E} + \frac{s_C^2}{N_C}}$$

Because the *t*-test is usually used to test a null hypothesis of no difference between two means, the assumption is generally made that there is no difference between the variances either, so that a **pooled estimate of the SED** (SED$_p$) is used instead. In this case, if the sample sizes are approximately equal in the two groups and if the combined sample size is

---

BOX 10–3. The Formula for the Standard Error of the Difference between Means

The standard error equals the standard deviation (σ) divided by the square root of the sample size *(N)*. Alternatively, this can be expressed as the square root of the variance (σ^2) divided by *N*:

$$\text{Standard error} = \frac{\sigma}{\sqrt{N}} = \sqrt{\frac{\sigma^2}{N}}$$

As mentioned in Chapter 9, Box 9–3, the variance of a difference is equal to the sum of the individual variances. Therefore, the variance of the difference between the mean of an experimental group (μ_E) and the mean of a control group (μ_C) could be expressed as follows: $\sigma_E^2 + \sigma_C^2$.

As shown above, a standard error can be written as the square root of the variance divided by the sample size, allowing the equation to be expressed as:

$$\text{Standard error of } \mu_E - \mu_C = \sqrt{\frac{\sigma_E^2}{N_E} + \frac{\sigma_C^2}{N_C}}$$

large enough (say, more than 30 in the combined sample), the above formula for the standard error of the difference becomes:

$$\text{SED}_p \text{ of } \overline{x}_E - \overline{x}_C = \sqrt{s_p^2 \left(\frac{1}{N_E} + \frac{1}{N_C}\right)}$$
$$= \sqrt{s_p^2 [(1/N_E) + (1/N_C)]}$$

The s_p^2, which is called the **pooled estimate of the variance,** is a kind of average of s_E^2 and s_C^2. The s_p^2 is calculated as the sum of the two sums of squares, divided by the combined degrees of freedom:

$$s_p^2 = \frac{\sum(x_E - \overline{x}_E)^2 + \sum(x_C - \overline{x}_C)^2}{N_E + N_C - 2}$$

If one sample size is much greater than the other or if the variance of one sample is much greater than the variance of the other, more complex formulas are needed (see Mosteller, Fienberg, and Rourke 1983).

When the Student's t-test is used to test the null hypothesis in research involving an experimental group and a control group, it usually takes the general form of the following equation:

$$t = \frac{\overline{x}_E - \overline{x}_C - 0}{\sqrt{s_p^2 [(1/N_E) + (1/N_C)]}}$$
$$df = N_E + N_C - 2$$

The 0 in the numerator of the equation for t was added for correctness, because the t-test determines if the difference between the means is significantly different from 0. However, because the 0 does not affect the calculations in any way, it is usually omitted from t-test formulas.

The same formula, recast in terms to apply to any two independent samples (e.g., samples of men and women), is as follows:

$$t = \frac{\overline{x}_1 - \overline{x}_2 - 0}{\sqrt{s_p^2 [(1/N_1) + (1/N_2)]}}$$
$$df = N_1 + N_2 - 2$$

in which $\overline{x}_1$ is the mean of the first sample, $\overline{x}_2$ is the mean of the second sample, s_p^2 is the pooled estimate of the variance, N_1 is the size of the first sample, N_2 is the size of the second sample, and df is the degrees of freedom. The 0 in the numerator indicates that the null hypothesis states that the difference between the means will not be significantly different from 0. The df is needed to enable the investigator to refer to the correct line in the table of the values of t and their relationship to p (see the Appendix).

Box 10-4 shows the use of a t-test to compare the mean systolic blood pressures of the 14 men and 12 women whose data were given in Table 10-1. A different and more visual way of understanding the t-test is presented in Box 10-5.

Interpretation of the Results. If the value of t is large, the p value will be small, because it is unlikely that a large t ratio will be obtained by chance alone. If the p value is 0.05 or less, it is customary to assume that there is a real difference. Conceptually, the p value is the probability of being in error if the null hypothesis of no difference between the means is rejected and the alternative hypothesis of a true difference is accepted.

One-Tailed and Two-Tailed t-Tests. The conceptual diagram in Fig. 10-1 shows the theory behind the acceptance and rejection regions for the two different types of Student's t-test. These tests are sometimes called the one-sided test and the two-sided test.

In the two-tailed test, alpha is equally divided at the ends of the two tails of the distribution (Fig. 10-1A). The two-tailed test is generally recommended, because differences in either direction are usually important to document. For example, it is obviously important to know if a new treatment is significantly better than a standard or placebo treatment, but it is also important to know if a new treatment is significantly worse and should therefore be avoided. In this situation, the two-tailed test provides an accepted criterion for when a difference shows the new treatment to be either better or worse.

Sometimes, however, only a one-tailed test is needed. Suppose, for example, that a new therapy is known to cost much more than the currently used therapy. Obviously, it would not be used if it were worse than the current therapy, but it would also not be used if it were merely as good as the current therapy. It would be used only if it were significantly better than the current therapy. Under the circumstances, some investigators consider it acceptable to use a one-tailed test. When this occurs, the 5% rejection region for the null hypothesis is all put on one tail of the distribution (Fig. 10-1B), instead of being evenly divided between the extremes of the two tails.

In the one-tailed test, the null hypothesis nonrejection region extends only to 1.645 standard errors above the "no difference" point. In the two-tailed test, it extends to 1.96 standard errors above and below the "no difference" point. This makes the one-tailed test more robust—that is, more able to detect a significant difference. Many investigators dislike one-tailed tests, because they believe that if an intervention is significantly worse than the standard therapy, that should be documented scientifically. Most reviewers and editors require that the use of a one-tailed significance test be justified.

Paired t-Test

In many medical studies, individuals are followed over time to see if there is a change in the value of some continuous variable. Typically, this occurs in a "before and after" experiment, such as one testing to see if there was a drop in average blood pressure following treatment or to see if there was a drop in weight following the use of a special diet. In this type of comparison, an individual patient serves as his or her own control. The appropriate statistical test for this kind of data is the paired t-test. The paired t-test is more robust than the Student's t-test because it

---

BOX 10–4.   Calculation of the Results of the Student's *t*-Test Comparing the Systolic Blood Pressure Values of 14 Male Subjects with Those of 12 Female Subjects

---

Part 1. Beginning data (see Table 10–1):

Number of observations, or $N = 14$ for males, or M
12 for females, or F

Mean, or $\bar{x} =$ 118.3 mm Hg for males
                           107.0 mm Hg for females

Variance, or $s^2 =$ 70.1 mm Hg for males
                           82.5 mm Hg for females

Sum of $(x_i - \bar{x})^2$, or TSS =   911.3 mm Hg for males
                                       907.5 mm Hg for females

Alpha value for the *t*-test =   0.05

Part 2. Calculation of the *t* value based on the pooled variance ($s_p^{\,2}$) and the pooled standard error of the difference (SED$_p$):

$$s_p^{\,2} = \frac{TSS_M + TSS_F}{N_M + N_F - 2} = \frac{911.3 + 907.5}{14 + 12 - 2} = \frac{1818.8}{24} = 75.78 \text{ mm Hg}$$

$$SED_p = \sqrt{s_p^{\,2}[(1/N_M) + (1/N_F)]}$$

$$= \sqrt{75.78(1/14 + 1/12)}$$

$$= \sqrt{75.78(0.1548)} = \sqrt{11.73} = 3.42 \text{ mm Hg}$$

$$t = \frac{\bar{x}_M - \bar{x}_F - 0}{\sqrt{s_p^{\,2}[(1/N_M) + (1/N_F)]}} = \frac{\bar{x}_M - \bar{x}_F - 0}{SED_p}$$

$$= \frac{118.3 - 107.0 - 0}{3.42} = \frac{11.30}{3.42} = 3.30$$

Part 3. Alternative calculation of the *t* value based on the SED equation using the observed variances for males and females, rather than on the SED$_p$ equation using the pooled variance:

$$SED = \sqrt{\frac{s_M^{\,2}}{N_M} + \frac{s_F^{\,2}}{N_F}} = \sqrt{\frac{70.1}{14} + \frac{82.5}{12}}$$

$$= \sqrt{5.01 + 6.88} = \sqrt{11.89} = 3.45 \text{ mm Hg}$$

$$t = \frac{\bar{x}_M - \bar{x}_F - 0}{SED}$$

$$= \frac{118.3 - 107.0 - 0}{3.45} = \frac{11.30}{3.45} = 3.28$$

Note that the results here ($t = 3.28$) are almost identical to those above ($t = 3.30$), even though the sample size is small.

Part 4. Calculation of the degrees of freedom (*df*) for the *t*-test and interpretation of the *t* value:

$$df = N_M + N_F - 2 = 14 + 12 - 2 = 24$$

For a *t* value of 3.30, with 24 degrees of freedom, p is less than 0.01, as indicated in the table of the values of *t* (see Appendix). This means that the male subjects have a significantly different (higher) systolic blood pressure than do the female subjects in this data set.

BOX 10–5.   Does the Eye Naturally Perform *t*-Tests?

The paired diagrams below show three patterns of overlap between two frequency distributions (e.g., a treatment group and a control group). These distributions can be thought of as the frequency distributions of systolic blood pressure values among hypertensive patients following randomization and treatment either with the experimental drug or with a placebo. The treatment group's distribution is shown in gray, the control group's distribution is shown in orange, and the area of overlap is gray and orange combined. The means are indicated by the vertical dotted lines. The three different pairs show variation in the spread of systolic blood pressure values.

Take a look at the three diagrams. Then try to guess whether each pair was sampled from the *same* universe (i.e., was not significantly different) or was sampled from two *different* universes (i.e., was significantly different).

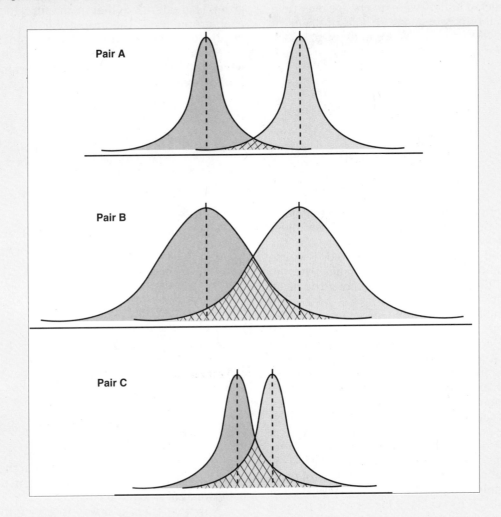

Most observers believe that the distributions in pair A look as though they were sampled from different universes. When asked why they think so, they usually state that there is little overlap between the two frequency distributions. Most observers are not convinced that the distributions in either pair B or pair C were sampled from different universes. They say that there is considerable overlap in each of these pairs, and this makes them doubt that there is a real difference. Their visual impressions are indeed correct.

It is not the absolute distance between the two means which leads most observers to say "different" for pair A and "not different" for pair B, because the distance between the means was drawn to be exactly the same in pairs A and B. Nor is it the absolute amount of dispersion that causes them to say "different" for pair A and "not different" for pair C, because the dispersions were drawn to be exactly the same in pairs A and C. Rather, the essential point, which the eye notices, is the ratio of the distance between the means to the variation around the means. The greater the distance between the means for a given amount of dispersion, the less likely it is that the samples were from the same universe. This ratio is exactly what the *t*-test calculates:

$$t = \frac{\text{Distance between the means}}{\text{Variation around the means}}$$

where the variation around the means is expressed as the standard error of the difference between the means. Therefore, the eye naturally does a *t*-test, although it does not quantify the relationship as precisely as does the *t*-test.

considers the variation from only one group of people, whereas the Student's *t*-test considers variation from two groups. Any variation that is detected in the paired *t*-test is attributable to the intervention or to changes over time in the same person.

Calculation of the Value of *t*. To calculate a paired *t*-test, a new variable is created. This variable, called *d*, is the difference between the values before and after the treatment for each individual studied. The paired *t*-test is a test of the null hypothesis that, on the average, the difference is equal to 0, which is what would be expected if there were no change over time. Using the symbol $\bar{d}$ to indicate the mean observed difference between the before and after values, the formula for the paired *t*-test is as follows:

$$t_{\text{paired}} = t_p = \frac{\bar{d} - 0}{\text{Standard error of } \bar{d}}$$

$$= \frac{\bar{d} - 0}{\sqrt{\frac{s_d^2}{N}}}$$

$$df = N - 1$$

The numerator contains a 0 because the null hypothesis says that the observed difference will not differ from 0; however, the 0 does not enter into the calculation and therefore can be omitted. Because the 0 in the above formula is a constant, it has no variance, and the only error in estimating the mean difference is its own standard error.

The formulas for the Student's *t*-test and the paired *t*-test are similar: the ratio of a difference to the variation around that difference (the standard error). In the Student's *t*-test, each of the two distributions to be compared contributes to the variation of the difference, and the two variances must be added. But in the paired *t*-test, there is only one frequency distribution, that of the before-after difference in each person. In the paired *t*-test, because only one mean is calculated $(\bar{d})$, only 1 degree of freedom is lost; therefore, the formula for the degrees of freedom is $N - 1$.

Interpretation of the Results. The values of *t* and their relationship to *p* are shown in a statistical table in the Appendix. If the value of *t* is large, the *p* value will be small, because it is unlikely that a large *t* ratio will be obtained by chance alone. If the *p* value is 0.05 or less, it is customary to assume that there is a real difference (i.e., that the null hypothesis of no difference can be rejected).

Use of *z*-Tests

In contrast to *t*-tests, which compare differences between means, *z*-tests compare differences between proportions. In medicine, examples of proportions that are frequently studied are sensitivity, specificity, positive predictive value, risks, percentages of people with a given symptom, percentages of people who are ill, and percentages of ill people who survive their illness. Frequently, the goal of research

is to see if the proportion of patients surviving is different in a treated group than in an untreated group.

Calculation of the Value of *z*. As discussed earlier in this chapter (see Critical Ratios), *z* is calculated by taking the observed difference between the two proportions (the numerator) and dividing it by the standard error of the difference between the two proportions (the denominator). For purposes of illustration, assume that research is being conducted to see if the proportion of patients surviving in a treated group is greater than that in an untreated group. For each group, if *p* is the proportion of successes (survivals), then $1 - p$ is the proportion of failures (non-survivals). If *N* represents the size of the group on which the proportion is based, the parameters of the proportion could be calculated as follows:

$$\text{Variance} = \frac{p(1-p)}{N}$$

$$\text{Standard error} = \text{SE} = \sqrt{\frac{p(1-p)}{N}}$$

$$95\% \text{ Confidence interval} = 95\% \text{ CI} = p \pm 1.96 \text{ SE}$$

If there is a 0.60 (60%) survival rate following a given treatment, the calculations of SE and CI, based on a sample of 100 study subjects, would be as follows:

$$\text{SE} = \sqrt{(0.6)(0.4)/100}$$

$$= \sqrt{0.24/100}$$

$$= 0.49/10$$

$$= 0.049$$

$$95\% \text{ CI} = 0.6 \pm (1.96)(0.049)$$

$$= 0.6 \pm 0.096$$

$$= \text{between } 0.6 - 0.096 \text{ and } 0.6 + 0.096$$

$$= 0.504, 0.696$$

The result of the CI calculation means that in 95% of cases, the "true" proportion surviving in the universe is between 50.4% and 69.6%.

Now that there is a way to obtain the standard error of a proportion, the **standard error of the difference between proportions** also can be obtained, and the equation for the *z*-test can be expressed as follows:

$$z = \frac{p_1 - p_2 - 0}{\sqrt{\bar{p}(1-\bar{p})[(1/N_1) + (1/N_2)]}}$$

in which p_1 is the proportion of the first sample, p_2 is the proportion of the second sample, N_1 is the size of the first sample, N_2 is the size of the second sample, and $\bar{p}$ is the mean proportion of successes in all observations combined. The 0 in the numerator indicates that the null hypothesis states that the difference between the proportions will not be significantly different from 0.

Interpretation of the Results. Note that the above formula for z is similar to the formula for t in the Student's t-test, as described earlier. However, because the variance and the standard error of the proportion are based on a theoretical distribution (the binomial approximation to the z distribution), the z distribution is used instead of the t distribution in determining whether the difference is statistically significant. If the z ratio is large, the difference is more likely to be a real difference.

The computations for the z-test appear different from the computations for the chi-square test (see Chapter 11), but when the same data are set up as a 2×2 table, technically the computations for the two tests are identical. Most persons find it easier to do a chi-square test than to do a z-test for proportions.

Use of Other Tests

Chapter 11 discusses other statistical significance tests used in the analysis of two variables (bivariate analysis), and Chapter 13 discusses tests used in the analysis of multiple independent variables (multivariable analysis).

SPECIAL CONSIDERATIONS

Variation between Groups versus Variation Within Groups

If the differences between two groups are found to be statistically significant, it is appropriate to wonder why the groups are different and how much of the total variation is explained by the variable defining the two groups. Here, a straightforward comparison of the heights of men and women can be used to illustrate the considerations involved in answering the following question: Why are men taller than women? While biologists might respond that genetic, hormonal, and perhaps nutritional factors explain the differences in height, a biostatistician would take a different approach. After first pointing out that individual men are not always taller than individual women but the average height of men is greater than that of women, the biostatistician would seek to determine the amount of the total variation in height that is explained by the gender difference and also determine whether or not the difference is more than would be expected by chance.

For purposes of this discussion, suppose that the heights of 200 university students were measured, that 100 of these students were men and 100 were women, and that the unit of measure was centimeters. As discussed in Chapter 9, the **total variation** would be equal to the sum of the squared deviations, which is usually called the **total sum of squares** (TSS) but is sometimes referred to as the **sum of squares** (SS). In the total group of 200 students, suppose that the total SS was found to be 10,000 cm^2. The biostatistician would begin by seeking to determine how much of this variation was actually due to gender and how much was due to other factors.

Fig. 10–2 shows a hypothetical frequency distribution of the heights of a sample of women (black marks) and a sample of men (orange marks), indicating the density of observations at the different heights. An approximate normal curve is drawn over each of the two distributions, and the overall mean (grand mean) is indicated, along with the mean height for women (a gender mean) and the mean height for men (a gender mean).

Although measuring the TSS from the grand mean yielded a result of 10,000 cm^2, measuring the SS from the gender means would yield a much smaller amount—say, about 6,000 cm^2. This leaves 60% of the variation to be explained. The other 40% of the variation is explained by the variable gender. Therefore, from a statistical perspective, explaining variation implies reducing the unexplained SS. If more explanatory variables (such as age, height of father, height of mother, and nutritional status) are analyzed, the unexplained SS can be reduced still further, and even more of the variation can be explained.

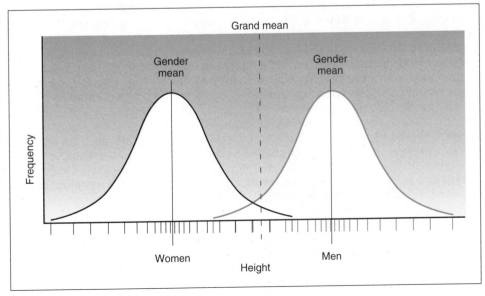

FIGURE 10–2. Hypothetical frequency distribution of the heights of a sample of women (black marks along the x-axis) and a sample of men (orange marks along the x-axis), indicating the density of observations at the different heights. An approximate normal curve is drawn over each of the two distributions, and the overall mean (grand mean) is indicated, along with the mean height for women (a gender mean) and the mean height for men (a gender mean).

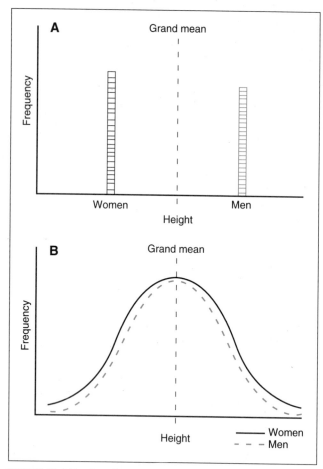

FIGURE 10–3. Two hypothetical frequency distributions of the heights of a sample of women (black lines) and a sample of men (orange lines). Diagram A shows how the distribution would appear if all women were of equal height, all men were of equal height, and men were taller than women. Diagram B shows how the distribution would appear if women varied in height, men varied in height, and the mean heights of the men and women were the same.

The following question is even more specific: Why is the shortest woman shorter than the tallest man? Statistically, there are two parts to the explanation: (1) She is a member of the class (group) of individuals (women) who have a shorter mean height than that of men. (2) She is the shortest of her group of women, and the man selected is the tallest of the group of men, so they are at the opposite extremes of height within their respective groups.

The greater the distance between the means for men and women, the greater is the proportion of the variation that is likely to be explained by **variation between groups.** The larger the standard deviations of heights of women and of men, the greater the proportion of the variation that is likely to be explained by **variation within groups.** The within-groups variation, however, might be reduced still further if other independent variables were added.

Suppose that all women were of equal height, that all men were of equal height, and that men were taller than women (see Fig. 10–3A). Then what percentage of the variation in height would be explained

by gender, and what percentage would be unexplained? The answer is that all of the variation would be due to gender (between-groups variation), and none would be left unexplained.

Suppose that women varied in height, that men varied in height, and that the mean heights of the men and women were the same (see Fig. 10–3B). Now what percentage of the variation in height would be explained by gender, and what percentage would be unexplained? None of the variation would be due to gender, and all of it would be left unexplained.

This simple example demonstrates what statistics ultimately tries to do: divide the total variation into a part that is explained by the independent variables (the model) and a part that is still unexplained. This activity is called **analyzing variation** or analyzing the TSS. A specific method for doing this under certain circumstances and testing hypotheses at the same time is called **analysis of variance,** or **ANOVA** (see Chapter 13).

Clinical Importance and External Validity versus Statistical Significance

A frequent error made by investigators has been to find a statistically significant difference, reject the null hypothesis, and recommend the finding as being useful for determining disease etiology, making a clinical diagnosis, or treating disease, without considering whether the finding is really clinically important and whether it has external validity.

There is no doubt that testing for statistical significance is important, because it helps investigators reject assertions that are not true. But even if a finding is **statistically significant,** it may not be **clinically or scientifically important.** For example, with a very large sample size, it is possible to show that a 2 mm Hg average drop in blood pressure with a certain blood pressure medication is statistically significant, but such a small drop in blood pressure would not be of much clinical use and therefore is not clinically important.

In addition, before the findings of a study can be put to general clinical use, the issue of whether the study has **external validity,** or **generalizability,** must be addressed. For example, in a clinical trial of a new drug, whether the **sample** (the patients in the study) is representative of the **universe** (the patients for whom the new drug might eventually be used) depends on questions concerning the spectrum of disease and the spectrum of individual characteristics in the sample group.

Was the **spectrum of disease** in the sample of patients representative of the spectrum of disease in the universe of patients? Types, stages, and severity of disease can all vary. The spectrum must be clearly defined in terms of the criteria for including or excluding patients, and these criteria must be reported when the findings are reported. For example, if patients with a severe form of the disease were excluded from the study, this **exclusion criterion** must be reported, since the results of the study would not be generalizable to those with severe disease.

Was the **spectrum of individual characteristics** in the sample of patients representative of the spectrum of individual characteristics in the universe of patients? Ages, genders, income levels, ethnic backgrounds, and a whole host of characteristics such as these can vary. An appropriate sampling technique (see Chapter 12) is needed for the selection of the individual study subjects. The sampling method should always be reported along with the findings, because the generalizability of results will depend on both the sampling techniques and the spectrum of characteristics in the sample of patients.

SUMMARY

Statistics is an aid to inductive reasoning, which is the effort to find generalizable relationships and differences in observed data. It is the reverse process from mathematics, which is the attempt to apply known formulas to specific data in order to predict an outcome.

Statistics helps investigators to make reasonable conclusions and estimations from observed data and to provide approximate limits to the probability of being in error in making conclusions and estimations. Significance testing starts with the stating of a null hypothesis, such as the hypothesis that there is no real (true) difference between the mean found in an experimental group and the mean found in the control group. The test of statistical significance (a critical ratio) then provides a p value that gives the probability of being wrong if the null hypothesis is rejected. If the results of the significance test allow the investigator to reject the null hypothesis, then the investigator can accept the alternative hypothesis that a true difference exists.

The Student's t-test enables the investigator to compare the means of a continuous variable from two different groups of study subjects in order to determine whether the difference in means is greater than would be expected by chance alone. The paired t-test enables the investigator to compare the average score on a continuous variable in a group of study subjects before and after some intervention was given. Unlike t-tests, which compare the difference between means, z-tests compare the difference between proportions.

References Cited

Emerson, J. D., and G. A. Colditz. Use of statistical analysis. New England Journal of Medicine 309:709–713, 1983.
Mosteller, F., S. E. Fienberg, and R. E. Rourke. Beginning Statistics with Data Analysis. Reading, Mass., Addison-Wesley Publishing Company, 1983.
Smith, R. P. Statistically speaking. Journal of Clinical Epidemiology 46:1293–1294, 1993.

Selected Readings

Dawson-Saunders, B., and R. G. Trapp. Basic and Clinical Biostatistics, 2nd ed. Norwalk, Conn., Appleton and Lange, 1994.
Inglefinger, J. A., et al. Biostatistics in Clinical Medicine, 2nd ed. New York, Macmillan Publishing Company, 1987.

CHAPTER ELEVEN

BIVARIATE ANALYSIS

A variety of statistical tests can be used to analyze the relationship between two or more variables. This chapter, like the previous chapter, focuses on **bivariate analysis,** which is the analysis of the relationship between one independent variable and one dependent variable. Chapter 13 will focus on **multivariable analysis,** or the analysis of the relationship of more than one independent variable to a single dependent variable. **Multivariate analysis,** a term that is frequently used incorrectly, refers to methods for analyzing more than one dependent variable as well as more than one independent variable.

CHOOSING AN APPROPRIATE STATISTICAL TEST

Among the factors involved in choosing an appropriate statistical test are the goals and research design of the study and the type of data being gathered.

In some studies, the investigators are interested in descriptive information, such as the sensitivity or specificity of a laboratory assay, in which case there may be no reason to perform a test of statistical significance. In other studies, the investigators are interested in determining whether the difference between two means is real, in which case testing for statistical significance is appropriate.

As shown in Table 11–1, numerous tests of statistical significance are available for bivariate analysis. However, the types of variables and the research design set the limits to statistical analysis and determine which test or tests are appropriate. The four **types of variables** shown in the table are continuous data (e.g., levels of glucose in blood samples), ordinal data (e.g., rankings of very satisfied, satisfied, and unsatisfied), dichotomous data (e.g., survival versus death), and nominal data (e.g., ethnic group). An investigator's knowledge of the types of variables and appropriate statistical tests is analogous to a painter's knowledge of the types of media (oils, tempera, water colors, and so forth) and the appropriate brushes and techniques to be used. If the **research design** involves before and after comparisons in the same study subjects or involves comparisons of matched pairs of study subjects, a paired test of statistical significance—such as the paired *t*-test, the Wilcoxon test, or the McNemar chi-square test—would be appropriate. Moreover, if the sampling procedure in a study is not random, statistical tests that assume random sampling, such as most of the parametric tests, may not be valid.

MAKING INFERENCES FROM CONTINUOUS (PARAMETRIC) DATA

Studies often involve one variable that is continuous and another variable that is not. As shown in Table 11–1, a *t*-test is appropriate for analyzing the relationship between one continuous and one dichotomous variable, while a one-way analysis of variance (ANOVA) is appropriate for analyzing the relationship between one continuous and one nomi-

TABLE 11–1. Choice of an Appropriate Statistical Significance Test To Be Used in Bivariate Analysis (Analysis of One Independent Variable and One Dependent Variable)

First Variable	Second Variable	Appropriate Test or Tests of Significance
Continuous	Dichotomous, unpaired	Student's *t*-test
Continuous	Dichotomous, paired	Paired *t*-test
Continuous	Nominal	One-way analysis of variance (ANOVA)
Continuous	Continuous	Pearson correlation coefficient *(r)*; linear regression
Ordinal	Dichotomous, unpaired	Mann-Whitney *U* test; chi-square test for linear trend
Ordinal	Dichotomous, paired	Wilcoxon test
Ordinal	Nominal	Kruskal-Wallis test
Ordinal	Ordinal	Spearman correlation coefficient (rho); Kendall correlation coefficient (tau)
Ordinal	Continuous	Group the continuous variables and calculate Spearman correlation coefficient (rho), Kendall correlation coefficient (tau), or chi-square test
Dichotomous	Dichotomous, unpaired	Chi-square test; Fisher exact probability test
Dichotomous	Dichotomous, paired	McNemar chi-square test
Dichotomous	Nominal	Chi-square test
Nominal	Nominal	Chi-square test

Characterization of Variables To Be Tested*

*For tests other than linear regression analysis, it makes no difference whether the first variable or the second variable is the independent variable.

nal variable. Chapter 10 discusses the Student's and paired *t*-tests in detail (see the section entitled Use of *t*-Tests) and introduces the concept of ANOVA (see the section entitled Variation between Groups versus Variation within Groups).

If a study involves two continuous variables, such as systolic blood pressure and diastolic blood pressure, the following questions may be answered: (1) Is there a real relationship between the variables or not? (2) If there is a real relationship, is it positive or negative linear relationship (a straight line relationship), or is it more complex? (3) If there is a real relationship, how strong is it? (4) How likely is the relationship to be generalizable? The best way to answer these questions is first to plot the continuous data on a joint distribution graph and then to perform correlation analysis and simple linear regression analysis.

The Joint Distribution Graph

The raw data concerning the systolic and diastolic blood pressures of 26 young, healthy, adult subjects were introduced in Chapter 10 and listed in

Table 10–1. These same data can be plotted on a joint distribution graph, as shown in Fig. 11–1. The data do not form a perfectly straight line, but they do appear to lie along a straight line, going from the lower left to the upper right on the graph, and the observations are fairly close to the line.

As indicated in Fig. 11–2, the correlation between two variables, labeled x and y, can range from nonexistent to strong. If the value of y increases as x increases, the correlation is positive; if y decreases as x increases, the correlation is negative. It appears from the graph in Fig. 11–1 that the correlation between diastolic and systolic blood pressure is strong and is positive.

Therefore, based on Fig. 11–1, the answer to the first question above is that there is a real relationship between diastolic and systolic blood pressure. The graph, however, does not reveal the probability that such a relationship could have occurred by chance. The answer to the second question is that the relationship is positive and is linear. The graph does not provide quantitative information about how strong the association is (although it looks strong to the eye), and the graph certainly does not provide any information about the potential generalizability of the relationship. To answer these questions more precisely, it is necessary to use the techniques of correlation and simple linear regression.

The Pearson Correlation Coefficient

Even without plotting the observations for two variables (variable x and variable y) on a graph, the extent of their linear relationship can be determined by calculating the **Pearson product-moment correlation coefficient**, which is given the symbol r and is referred to as the **r value**. This statistic varies from -1 to $+1$, going through 0. A finding of -1 indicates that the two variables have a perfect negative linear relationship; $+1$ indicates that they have a perfect positive linear relationship; and 0 indicates that the two variables are totally independent of each other. The r value is rarely found to be -1 or $+1$. Frequently, there is an imperfect correlation between the two variables, resulting in r values between 0 and 1 or between 0 and -1.

The formula for the correlation coefficient r is shown below. The numerator is the sum of the covariances. The **covariance** is the product of the deviation of an observation from the mean of the x variable multiplied by the same observation's deviation from the mean of the y variable. (When marked on a graph, this usually gives a rectangular area, in contrast to the sum of squares, in which the areas generated are squares of the deviation from the mean.) The denominator is the square root of the sum of the squared deviations from the mean of the x variable multiplied by the sum of the squared deviations from the mean of the y variable:

$$r = \frac{\sum(x_i - \bar{x})(y_i - \bar{y})}{\sqrt{\sum(x_i - \bar{x})^2 \sum(y_i - \bar{y})^2}}$$

Using statistical computer programs, investigators can determine whether the value of r is greater than would be expected by chance alone (i.e., whether the two variables are statistically associated). Most statistical programs provide the p value

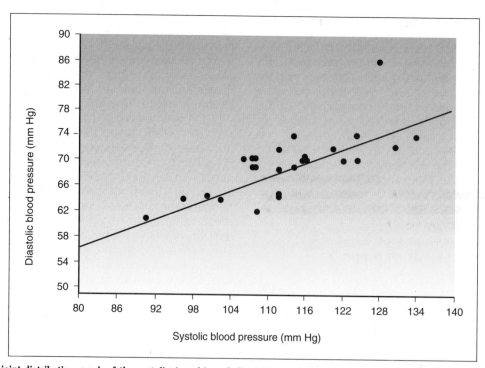

FIGURE 11–1. A joint distribution graph of the systolic (x-axis) and diastolic (y-axis) blood pressure values of 26 young, healthy, adult subjects. The raw data for these subjects are listed in Table 10–1. The correlation between the two variables is strong and is positive.

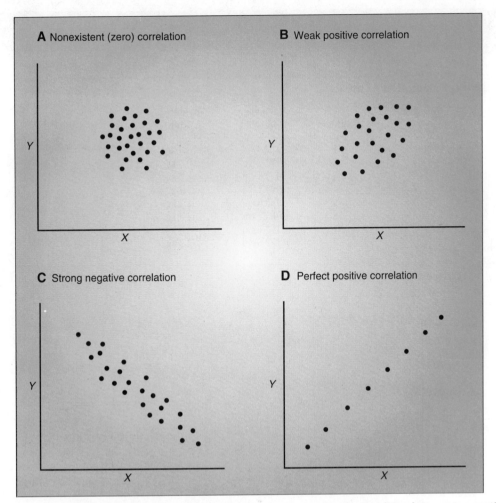

FIGURE 11–2. Four possible patterns in joint distribution graphs. As seen in these examples, the correlation between two continuous variables, labeled *x* and *y,* can range from nonexistent to perfect. If the value of *y* increases as *x* increases, the correlation is positive. If *y* decreases as *x* increases, the correlation is negative.

along with the correlation coefficient, but the *p* value of the correlation coefficient can easily be calculated. Its associated *t* can be calculated from the following formula, and then the *p* value can be determined from a table of *t* (Phillips 1978).

$$t = \frac{r\sqrt{N-2}}{\sqrt{1-r^2}}$$

$$df = N - 2$$

As is the case in every test of significance, for a fixed level of strength of association, the larger the sample size, the more likely it is to be statistically significant. A weak correlation in a large sample might be statistically significant, despite the fact that it was not etiologically or clinically important.

There is no perfect statistical way to estimate clinical importance, but with continuous variables a valuable concept is the **strength of the association,** measured by the square of the correlation coefficient, or r^2. The **r^2 value** is the proportion of variation in *y* explained by *x* (or vice versa). It is an important parameter in advanced statistics. Looking at the strength of association is analogous to looking at the

size and clinical importance of an observed difference, as discussed in Chapter 10.

For purposes of demonstrating the calculation of *r* and r^2, a small set of data is introduced in Box 11–1. The data, consisting of the observed heights (variable *x*) and weights (variable *y*) of 8 subjects, are presented first in tabular form and then in graph form. When *r* is calculated, the result is 0.96 (+0.96), which indicates a strong positive linear relationship and provides quantitative information to confirm what is visually apparent in the graph. Given that *r* is 0.96, then r^2 is $(0.96)^2$, or 0.92. A 0.92 strength of association means that 92% of the variation in weight is "explained" by height. Therefore, the remaining 8% of the variation must be due to factors other than height.

Linear Regression Analysis

Linear regression is related to correlation analysis, but its purposes are more basic. Linear regression seeks to quantify the linear relationship that may exist between an independent variable *x* and a dependent variable *y.*

**BOX 11–1.   Analysis of the Relationship between Height and Weight (Two Continuous Variables)
in a Study of 8 Subjects**

Part 1. Tabular representation of the data:

Subject	Variable x (Height)	Variable y (Weight)
1	182.9 cm	78.5 kg
2	172.7 cm	60.8 kg
3	175.3 cm	68.0 kg
4	172.7 cm	65.8 kg
5	160.0 cm	52.2 kg
6	165.1 cm	54.4 kg
7	172.7 cm	60.3 kg
8	162.6 cm	52.2 kg

Part 2. Graphic representation of the data:

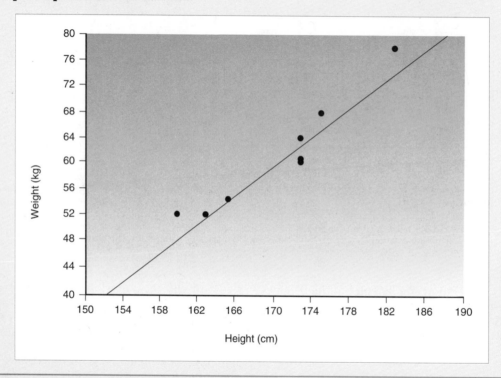

Part 3. Calculation of moments:

$\Sigma(x_i) = 1364.0$ cm

$\Sigma(y_i) = 492.2$ kg

$N = 8$

$\bar{x} = 1364.0/8 = 170.50$ cm

$\bar{y} = 492.2/8 = 61.53$ kg

$\Sigma(x_i - \bar{x})(y_i - \bar{y}) = 456.88$

$\Sigma(x_i - \bar{x})^2 = 393.1$

$\Sigma(y_i - \bar{y})^2 = 575.1$

Continued

**BOX 11–1.   Analysis of the Relationship between Height and Weight (Two Continuous Variables)
in a Study of 8 Subjects** *(Continued)*

**Part 4. Calculation of the Pearson correlation coefficient *(r)* and the strength of
the association of the variables *(r²)*:**

$$r = \frac{\sum(x_i - \bar{x})(y_i - \bar{y})}{\sqrt{\sum(x_i - \bar{x})^2 \sum(y_i - \bar{y})^2}}$$

$$= \frac{456.88}{\sqrt{(393.1)(575.1)}} = \frac{456.88}{\sqrt{226,071.8}} = \frac{456.88}{475.47} = \mathbf{0.96}$$

$$r^2 = (0.96)^2 = \mathbf{0.92} = \mathbf{92\%}$$

Interpretation: The two variables are highly correlated. The association is strong, with 92% of variation in weight *(y)* explained by variation
in height *(x)*.

Part 5. Calculation of the slope *(b)* for a regression of weight *(y)* on height *(x)*:

$$b = \frac{\sum(x_i - \bar{x})(y_i - \bar{y})}{\sum(x_i - \bar{x})^2} = \frac{456.88}{393.1} = \mathbf{1.16}$$

Interpretation: There is a 1.16-kg increase in weight *(y)* for each 1-cm increase in height *(x)*. The *y*-intercept, which indicates the value
of *x* when *y* is 0, is not meaningful in the case of these two variables; therefore, it is not calculated here.

Source of data: Unpublished findings in a sample of 8 professional persons in Connecticut..

Recall that the formula for a straight line is
$y = a + bx$. Linear regression is used to estimate two
parameters: the slope of the line *(b)* and the
y-intercept *(a)*. Most fundamental is the slope, which
determines the strength of the impact of variable *x* on
y. For example, the slope can tell how much weight
will increase, on the average, for each additional
centimeter of height.

When the usual statistical notation is used for a
regression of *y* on *x*, the formulas for the slope *(b)* and
y-intercept *(a)* are as follows:

$$b = \frac{\sum(x_i - \bar{x})(y_i - \bar{y})}{\sum(x_i - \bar{x})^2}$$

$$a = \bar{y} - b\bar{x}$$

Box 11–1 shows the calculation of the slope *(b)*
for the observed heights and weights of 8 subjects.
The graph in Box 11–1 shows the linear relationship
between the height and weight data, with the regression line inserted. In these 8 subjects, the slope was
1.16, meaning that there was an average increase of
1.16 kg of weight for every 1 cm increase in height.
Note that the slope does not appear greater than 45
degrees, as would be expected from a slope of 1.16,
because the scale is compressed more tightly on the
y-axis.

Linear regression analysis enables investigators
to predict the value of *y* from the values that *x* takes.
In other words, the formula for linear regression is a
form of statistical modeling, and the adequacy of the
model is determined by how closely the value of *y* can

be predicted from the other data in the model. Just as
it is possible to set confidence intervals around
parameters such as means and proportions (see
Chapter 10), it is possible to set confidence intervals
around the slope and the intercept, using computations based on linear regression formulas. Most
statistical computer programs perform these computations, and moderately advanced statistics books
provide the formulas (see, for example, Kleinbaum
and Kupper 1978).

Multiple linear regression and other methods
involved in the analysis of more than two variables
are discussed in Chapter 13.

MAKING INFERENCES FROM ORDINAL DATA

Many medical data are ordinal data, which are
ranked from the lowest value to the highest value but
are not measured on an exact scale. In some cases,
investigators will assume that ordinal data meet the
criteria for continuous (measurement) data and will
treat the ordinal data as though they had been
obtained from a measurement scale. For example, if
the patients' satisfaction with the care in a given
hospital were being studied, the investigators might
assume that the conceptual distance between "very
satisfied" (say, coded as a 3) and "fairly satisfied"
(coded as a 2) is equal to the difference between
"fairly satisfied" (coded as a 2) and "unsatisfied"
(coded as a 1). If the investigators are willing to make
these assumptions, the data can be analyzed using
the parametric statistical methods discussed in this

and the previous chapter, such as t-tests, analysis of variance, and analysis of the Pearson correlation coefficient. However, sometimes clinical investigators make this assumption when it is inappropriate, because the statistics are easier to obtain and are more robust.

If the investigator is unwilling to make such assumptions, statistics for discrete (nonparametric) data, such as a chi-square test (see below), can be used. However, analysis using chi-square would require discarding the information about the rank of each observation. Fortunately, there are a number of bivariate statistical tests for ordinal data that can be used. These tests are listed in Table 11–1 and described briefly below. For more details, see Dawson-Saunders and Trapp (1994) or Siegel (1956).

The Mann-Whitney U Test

The test for ordinal data that is similar to the Student's t-test is the Mann-Whitney U test. U, like t, designates a probability distribution. In the Mann-Whitney test, all of the observations in a study of two samples are ranked numerically from the smallest to the largest, without regard to whether the observations came from the first sample (e.g., the control group) or from the second sample (e.g., the experimental group). Next, the observations from the first sample are identified, the ranks in this sample are summed, and the average rank for the first sample is determined. The process is repeated for the observations from the second sample. If the null hypothesis is true (i.e., if there is no real difference between the two samples), the average ranks of the two samples should be similar. If the average rank of one sample is considerably greater or considerably smaller than that of the other sample, the null hypothesis can be rejected. Looking up the value of U in an appropriate table will indicate the p value associated with this test.

The Wilcoxon Test

The rank-order test that is comparable to the paired t-test is the Wilcoxon test, which is also called the **Wilcoxon matched-pairs signed-ranks test.** In this test, all of the observations in a study of two samples are ranked numerically from the largest to the smallest, without regard to whether the observations came from the first sample (e.g., the pretreatment sample) or from the second sample (e.g., the posttreatment sample). After pairs of data are identified (e.g., pretreatment and posttreatment samples are matched), the difference in rank is identified for each pair. If in a given pair the pretreatment observation scored 7 ranks higher than the posttreatment observation, the difference would be noted as −7. If in another pair the pretreatment observation scored 5 ranks lower than the posttreatment observation, the difference would be noted as +5. Each pair would be scored in this way. If the null hypothesis is true (i.e., if there is no real difference between the samples),

the sum of the positive scores and negative scores should be close to 0. If the sum of differences is considerably different from 0, the null hypothesis can be rejected.

The Kruskal-Wallis Test

If the investigators in a study involving continuous data want to compare the means of three or more groups simultaneously, the appropriate test is a one-way analysis of variance (a one-way ANOVA), usually called an F-test. The comparable test for ordinal data is called the Kruskal-Wallis test or the **Kruskal-Wallis one-way ANOVA.** As in the Mann-Whitney U test (see above), in the Kruskal-Wallis test all of the data are ranked numerically, and the rank values are summed in each of the groups to be compared. The Kruskal-Wallis test seeks to determine if the average ranks differ more than would be expected by chance alone.

The Spearman and the Kendall Correlation Coefficients

When relating two continuous variables to each other, investigators can use regression analysis or correlation analysis. For ordinal variables, there is no test comparable to regression, because it is difficult to see how a "slope" could be measured without assuming an underlying measurement scale. However, there are several tests comparable to correlation, the two most common of which are briefly described here. The first is the **Spearman rank correlation coefficient,** which is symbolized by **rho** and is similar to r. The second is the **Kendall rank correlation coefficient,** which is symbolized by **tau.** The tests for rho and tau will usually give similar results, but the tau may be slightly preferable because it works better with small sample sizes.

The Sign Test

Sometimes an experimental intervention produces positive results in many areas, but few if any of the individual outcome variables show a statistically significant improvement. In this case, the sign test can be extremely helpful in comparing the results in the experimental group with those in the control group. If the null hypothesis is true (i.e., there is no real difference between the groups), then, by chance, for half of the outcome variables the experimental group should perform better, and for half of the outcome variables the control group should perform better.

The only data needed for the sign test are the record of whether, on the average, the experimental subjects or the control subjects scored "better" on each outcome variable (by what amount is not important). If the average score in the experimental group is better, the result is recorded as a plus sign (+); if the average score in the control group is better, the result is recorded as a minus sign (−); and if the average score in the two groups is exactly the same, no result is recorded and the variable is omitted from the analysis. For the sign test, "better" can be determined from a continuous variable, an ordinal variable, a dichotomous variable, a clinical score, or a component of a score. Because under the null hypothesis, the expected proportion of plus signs is 0.5 and of minus signs is 0.5, the test compares the observed proportion of successes with the expected value of 0.5.

MAKING INFERENCES FROM DICHOTOMOUS AND NOMINAL (NONPARAMETRIC) DATA

As indicated in Table 11–1, the chi-square test, the Fisher exact probability test, and the McNemar chi-square test can be used in the bivariate analysis of dichotomous nonparametric data. Usually, the data are first arranged in a 2×2 table, and the goal is to test the null hypothesis that the variables are independent.

The 2 × 2 Contingency Table

Data arranged as in Box 11–2 form what is known as a contingency table because it is used to determine whether the distribution of one variable is conditionally dependent (contingent) upon the other variable. More specifically, Box 11–2 provides an example of a 2×2 contingency table, meaning that it has two cells in each direction. In this case, the table shows the data for a study of 91 patients who had a myocardial infarction (Snow 1965). One variable is treatment (propranolol versus a placebo), and the other is outcome (survival for at least 28 days versus death within 28 days).

In a contingency table, a **cell** is a specific location in the matrix created by the two variables whose relationship is being studied. Each cell shows the observed number, the expected number, and the percentage of study subjects in each treatment group who lived or died. For example, in Box 11–2, the top left cell indicates that 38 patients who were treated with propranolol survived the first 28 days of observation, that the 38 patients represented 84% of all patients who were treated with propranolol, and that 33.13 patients treated with propranolol were expected to survive the first 28 days of observation. The methods for calculating the percentages and expected counts are discussed below.

The other three cells indicate the same type of data (observed number, expected number, and percentage) for those who died after propranolol treatment, those who survived after placebo treatment, and those who died after placebo treatment. The bottom row shows the column totals, and the right-hand column shows the row totals.

If there are more than two cells in each direction of a contingency table, the table is called an $R \times C$ table, where R stands for the number of rows and C stands for the number of columns. Although the principles of the chi-square test are valid for $R \times C$ tables, the discussion below focuses on 2×2 tables.

The Chi-Square Test of Independence

After t-tests, the most basic and common form of statistical analysis in the medical literature is the chi-square test of the independence of two variables in a contingency table (Emerson and Colditz 1983). The chi-square test is an example of a common approach to statistical analysis known as **statistical modeling,** which seeks to develop a statistical expression (the model) that predicts the behavior of a dependent variable on the basis of knowledge of one or more independent variables. The process of comparing the **observed counts** with the **expected counts**—that is, of comparing O with E—is called a **goodness-of-fit test,** because the goal is to see how well the observed counts in a contingency table "fit" the counts expected on the basis of the model. Usually, the model in such a table is the null hypothesis that the two variables are independent of each other. If the chi-square value is small, the fit is good. If, however, the chi-square value is large, the data do not fit the hypothesis well.

Box 11–2 will be used here to illustrate the steps and considerations involved both in constructing a 2×2 contingency table and in calculating the chi-square value. For the data presented in Box 11–2, the **null hypothesis** is that the method of treating the myocardial infarction patients did not influence the proportion of patients who survived for at least 28 days. The **alternative hypothesis** is that the outcome (survival or death) depended on the treatment, meaning that the outcome was the **dependent variable** and the treatment was the **independent variable.**

Calculation of Percentages

Each of the four cells of Box 11–2 shows an observed count (or O) and a percentage. The percentage in the first cell of the contingency table was calculated by dividing the number of propranolol-treated patients who survived (38) by the total number of propranolol-treated patients (45), with the result being 84%. Thus, the percentage was calculated as the frequency distribution of the dependent variable, which in this case was survival, reflecting the fact that survival was contingent (dependent) on treatment.

If treatment depended on survival, rather than vice versa, the percentage would be calculated by dividing the number of propranolol-treated patients who survived (38) by the total number of survivors (67). Although the way in which the percentages are calculated does not affect the chi-square test, it does affect the way in which people think about and interpret the data. Therefore, the appropriate way to calculate the percentages in a contingency table is to determine which of the variables is the dependent one and then calculate the frequency distribution of that variable within each level of the independent variable.

BOX 11–2. Chi-Square Analysis of the Relationship between Treatment and Outcome (Two Nonparametric Variables, Unpaired) in a Study of 91 Subjects

---

Part 1. Beginning data, presented in a 2 × 2 contingency table, where O denotes observed counts and E denotes expected counts:

		OUTCOME					
		Survival for at Least 28 Days		Death		Total	
		Number	(Percentage)	Number	(Percentage)	Number	(Percentage)
	Propranolol (O)	38	(84)	7	(16)	45	(100)
	Propranolol (E)	33.13		11.87		45	
TREATMENT	Placebo (O)	29	(63)	17	(37)	46	(100)
	Placebo (E)	33.87		12.13		46	
	Total	67	(74)	24	(26)	91	(100)

Part 2. Calculation of the chi-square (χ^2) value:

$$\chi^2 = \sum \left[\frac{(O-E)^2}{E} \right]$$

$$= \frac{(38-33.13)^2}{33.13} + \frac{(7-11.87)^2}{11.87} + \frac{(29-33.87)^2}{33.87} + \frac{(17-12.13)^2}{12.13}$$

$$= \frac{(4.87)^2}{33.13} + \frac{(-4.87)^2}{11.87} + \frac{(-4.87)^2}{33.87} + \frac{(4.87)^2}{12.13}$$

$$= \frac{23.72}{33.13} + \frac{23.72}{11.87} + \frac{23.72}{33.87} + \frac{23.72}{12.13}$$

$$= 0.72 + 2.00 + 0.70 + 1.96 = \mathbf{5.38}$$

Part 3. Calculation of the degrees of freedom (df) for a contingency table, based on the number of rows (R) and columns (C):

$$df = (R-1)(C-1) = (2-1)(2-1) = 1$$

Part 4. Determination of the p value:

Value from the chi-square table for 5.38 on 1 df: $0.01 < p < 0.025$ (statistically significant)

Exact p from a computer program: 0.0205 (statistically significant)

Interpretation: The statistically significant result indicates that it is highly probable (only 1 chance in about 50 of being wrong) that the investigator can reject the null hypothesis of independence and accept the alternative hypothesis that propranolol does affect the outcome of myocardial infarction in a positive direction.

Source of data: Snow, P. J. Effect of propranolol in myocardial infarction. Lancet 2:551–553, 1965.

Calculation of Expected Counts

In Box 11–2, the propranolol-treated group consists of 45 patients, the placebo-treated group consists of 46 patients, and the total for the study is therefore 91 patients. While the observed counts indicate how many of each group actually survived, the expected counts indicate how many of each group would be expected to survive if the method of treatment made no difference whatsoever (i.e., if survival were independent of treatment).

The general formula for calculating the expected count in the top left cell of a contingency table is as follows:

$$E_{1,1} = \frac{\text{Row}_1 \text{ total}}{\text{Study total}} \times \text{Column}_1 \text{ total}$$

where $E_{1,1}$ is defined as the cell in row$_1$, column$_1$.

In Box 11–2, for example, if survival were independent of the treatment group, 45/91 (or 49.45%) of the observations in each column would be expected to be in the top row, because that is the overall proportion of patients who received propranolol. It follows that 0.4945×67 (or 33.13) observations (the total in column$_1$) would be expected in the top left cell, while 0.4945×24 (or 11.87) observations (the total in column$_2$) would be expected in the top right cell. Note that the expected counts may include fractions and that the sum of the expected counts in a given row will equal the sum of the observed counts in that row $(33.13 + 11.87 = 45)$. By the same logic, 50.55% of observations would be expected to be in the bottom row, with 33.87 in the left bottom cell and 12.13 in the right bottom cell, so that the row total equals the sum of the observed counts $(33.87 + 12.13 = 46)$. Finally, as shown in Box 11–2, the column totals for expected counts should add up to the column totals for observed counts.

The expected counts in each cell of a 2×2 contingency table should equal five or more or the assumptions and approximations inherent in the chi-square test may break down. For a study involving a larger contingency table (an $R \times C$ table), the investigator can usually compromise on this slightly by allowing 20% of the expected counts to be less than five but at the same time making sure that none of the expected counts is less than two. If these conditions are not met and the table is a 2×2 table, the Fisher exact probability test (see below) should be used instead of the chi-square test. If the conditions are not met and the table is larger than a 2×2 table, the best solution is to combine (collapse) categories. For example, if the variable were "ethnic group" and it had seven categories, for many geographic areas of the USA there might be few persons other than African-Americans, Caucasians, or Hispanics. Under the circumstances, the Asians, Native Americans, Pacific Islanders, and members of other ethnic groups might be combined into one category called "other." This might give enough numbers in the revised "other" category that the expected counts would be large enough to use the chi-square test.

Calculation of the Chi-Square Value

Once the observed (O) and expected (E) counts are known, the chi-square (χ^2) value can be calculated. One of two methods can be used, depending on the size of the counts.

Method for Large Numbers. In Box 11–2, the investigators begin by calculating the chi-square value for each cell in the table, using the following formula:

$$\frac{(O-E)^2}{E}$$

Here, the numerator is the square of the deviation of the observed count in a given cell from the count that would be expected in that cell if the null hypothesis were true. This is similar to the numerator of the variance, which is expressed as $(x_i - \overline{x})^2$, where x_i represents the observed value and $\overline{x}$ (the mean) is the expected value (see Chapter 9). However, whereas the denominator for variance is the degrees of

freedom $(N-1)$, the denominator for chi-square is the expected number (E).

To obtain the total chi-square value, the investigators then add up the chi-square values for the four cells:

$$\chi^2 = \sum \left[\frac{(O-E)^2}{E} \right]$$

Thus, the basic statistical method for measuring the total amount of variation in a data set, the total sum of squares (TSS), is rewritten for the chi-square test as the sum of $(O-E)^2$.

Box 11–2 shows how chi-square is calculated for the study of 91 patients with myocardial infarction. Before the result (chi-square value = 5.38) can be interpreted, the degrees of freedom must be determined (see below).

Method for Small Numbers. Because the chi-square test is based on the normal approximation of the binomial distribution (which is discontinuous), many statisticians believe that a correction for continuity is needed in the equation for calculating chi-square, while others believe that this is unnecessary. The correction, originally described by F. Yates and called the **Yates correction for continuity,** makes little difference if the numbers in the table are large, but in tables with small numbers it probably is worth doing. The only change in the chi-square test formula given above is that in the continuity-corrected chi-square test, the number 0.5 is subtracted from the absolute value of the $(O-E)$ in each cell before squaring. The formula is as follows:

$$\text{Yates } \chi^2 = \sum \left[\frac{(|O-E| - 0.5)^2}{E} \right]$$

Clearly, the use of this formula reduces the size of the chi-square value somewhat and reduces the chance of finding a statistically significant difference, so that correction for continuity makes the test more conservative.

Determination of the Degrees of Freedom

As discussed in Chapter 10 and Box 10–2, the term "degrees of freedom" refers to the number of observations that are free to vary. According to the null hypothesis, the best estimate of the expected distribution of counts in the cells of a contingency table is provided by the row and column totals. Therefore, the row and column totals are considered to be "fixed." An observed count can be entered "freely" into one of the cells of a 2×2 table (e.g., the top left cell), but once that count is entered, none of the other three cells are free to vary. This means that a 2×2 table has only 1 degree of freedom.

Another look at Box 11–2 will help explain why there is only 1 degree of freedom in a table with two rows and two columns. If 38 is entered freely in the top left cell, the only possible number that can go in the cell immediately to the right of it is 7, because the two numbers in the top row must equal the fixed row total of 45. Similarly, the only possible number that

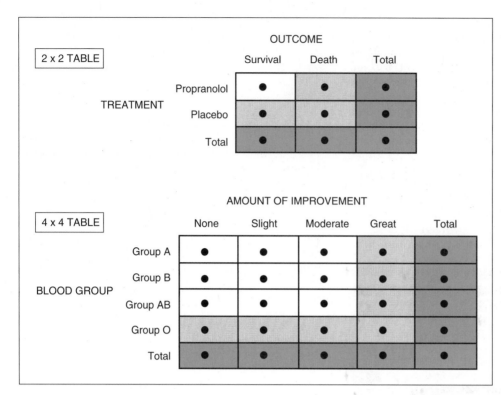

FIGURE 11–3. Conceptualization of the calculation of the degrees of freedom *(df)* in a 2 × 2 contingency table (top) and in a 4 × 4 contingency table (bottom). A white cell is free to vary; a light orange cell is not free to vary; and a dark orange cell is a row or column total. The formula is *df* = (*R* – 1) (*C* – 1), where *R* denotes the number of rows and *C* denotes the number of columns. For the 2 × 2 table, *df* = 1. For the 4 × 4 table, *df* = 9.

can go in the cell below the one containing 38 is the number 29, because the column must add up to 67. Finally, the only possible number that can go in the remaining cell is 17, because the row total must equal 46 and the column total must equal 24.

The same principle applies to tables with more than two rows and columns. In $R \times C$ contingency tables, imagine that the right-hand column and the bottom row are never free to vary, because they must consist of the numbers that make the totals come out right. This is illustrated in Fig. 11–3, where the cells that are free to vary are shown in white, the cells that are not free to vary are shown in light orange, and the fixed row and column totals are shown in dark orange. Therefore, the formula for degrees of freedom in a contingency table of any size is as follows:

$$df = (R - 1)(C - 1)$$

where *df* denotes degrees of freedom, *R* is the number of rows, and *C* is the number of columns.

Interpretation of the Results

After the chi-square value and the degrees of freedom are known, a standard table of chi-square values (see the Appendix) can be consulted to determine the corresponding *p* value. The *p* value indicates the probability that a chi-square value that large would have resulted from chance alone. For data shown in Box 11–2, the chi-square value was 5.38 on 1 degree of freedom, and the *p* value listed in the standard table for a two-tailed test was between 0.01 and 0.025 ($0.01 < p < 0.025$). Most computer programs will provide the exact *p* value when calculating a

chi-square; for the data in Box 11–2, the *p* value was 0.0205. Because the observed *p* was less than alpha (alpha = 0.05), the results were statistically significant.

If the chi-square value for the data in Box 11–2 had been calculated using the Yates correction, the result would have been 4.32, instead of 5.38, and the corresponding *p* value would have been somewhat larger (0.0376). Nevertheless, the results still would be statistically significant at the alpha = 0.05 level.

For the study of 91 patients reported in Box 11–2, the null hypothesis was that the outcome (survival versus death) was not related to the method of treatment (propranolol versus placebo). Because 24 of the 91 patients (26%) died, if the treatment had had no effect, the investigator would expect about 26% of the propranolol-treated patients and 26% of the placebo-treated patients to have died. Because the proportion who survived in each treatment group differed significantly from this expectation, the null hypothesis of independence between the variables can be rejected, and the alternative hypothesis that treatment had an effect on the survival rate can be accepted.

Note that the alternative hypothesis tested does not state whether the effect of the treatment would be to increase or decrease survival. This is because the null hypothesis was only that there would be no difference. In other words, the null hypothesis as stated required a two-tailed test of statistical significance (see Chapter 10). The investigator could have tested the null hypothesis that the propranolol-treated group would show a higher survival rate than the placebo-treated group, but this would have required interpreting the chi-square value as a one-tailed test of statistical significance. The choice of a one-tailed versus a two-tailed test does not affect the performance of a statistical test but does affect how the critical ratio thus obtained is converted to a *p* value in a statistical table. The direction of difference is obvious by inspection.

The Chi-Square Test for Paired Data (McNemar Test)

The chi-square test above was useful for comparing the distribution of a categorical variable in two or more different groups, but a new test is needed to compare before and after findings in the same

individual or to compare findings in a matched analysis. The McNemar chi-square test does this for dichotomous variables.

The McNemar Test of Before and After Comparisons

In the discussion of *t*-tests in Chapter 10, it was noted that a study subject in a before and after study serves as his or her own control. For this reason, it was appropriate to use the paired *t*-test, instead of the Student's *t*-test. In the case of chi-square analysis, it would be appropriate to use the McNemar test, which is a modified chi-square test of data with 1 degree of freedom (Fleiss 1981).

BOX 11–3. McNemar Chi-Square Analysis of the Relationship between Data before and Data after an Event (Two Dichotomous Variables, Paired) in a Study of 200 Subjects (Fictitious Data)

Part 1. Standard 2 × 2 table format on which equations are based:

FINDINGS AFTER EVENT

		Positive	Negative	Total
FINDINGS BEFORE EVENT	Positive	a	b	a + b
	Negative	c	d	c + d
	Total	a + c	b + d	a + b + c + d

Part 2. Data for a study of the opinions of medical school faculty toward second-year medical students before and after seeing a show presented by the students:

POSTSHOW OPINION

		Positive	Negative	Total
PRE-SHOW OPINION	Positive	150	22	172
	Negative	8	20	28
	Total	158	42	200

Part 3. Calculation of the McNemar chi-square (χ^2) value:

$$\text{McNemar } \chi^2 = \frac{(|b-c|-1)^2}{b+c}$$

$$= \frac{(|22-8|-1)^2}{22+8} = \frac{(13)^2}{30} = \frac{169}{30} = 5.63$$

Part 4. Calculation of the degrees of freedom (*df*) for a contingency table, based on the number of rows (*R*) and columns (*C*):

$$df = (R-1)(C-1) = (2-1)(2-1) = 1$$

Part 5. Determination of the *p* value:

Value from the chi-square table for 5.63 on 1 *df*: $p < 0.025$ (statistically significant)
Interpretation: If faculty changed their attitude toward second-year medical students after the show, most of these changes were from a positive attitude to a negative attitude, rather than vice versa.

Suppose, for example, that an investigator wanted to compare the attitudes of the faculty of a certain medical school toward the second-year medical students before and after the "Second-Year Show," an event in which students traditionally perform skits about medical school life, often portraying favorite faculty with gentle humor and less-liked faculty with negative humor. Next, suppose that 200 faculty were asked to fill out questionnaires about their feelings toward the second-year medical students before and after attending the performance and that their responses were recorded as either positive or negative (i.e., dichotomous responses). The data could be set up in a 2×2 table with the preshow opinion on the left axis and the postshow opinion at the top, as shown in Box 11–3, and with each of the four cells representing one of the following four possible combinations: cell a = positive opinion before and after (no change); cell b = change from positive to negative opinion; cell c = change from negative to positive opinion; and cell d = negative opinion before and after (no change).

According to the hypothetical data from 200 faculty who participated in the study, the overall percentage reporting a favorable opinion of second-year students dropped from 86% (172/200) before the show to 79% (158/200) after the show, presumably reflecting a change in those faculty who were not treated kindly in the show. The null hypothesis to be tested is that the show produced no true change in faculty opinion about students, and the following formula would be used:

$$\text{McNemar } \chi^2 = \frac{(|b - c| - 1)^2}{b + c}$$

Note that the formula uses only cells b and c in the 2×2 table. This is because cells a and d do not change and therefore do not contribute to the standard error. Note also that the formula tests data with 1 degree of freedom, using a correction for continuity.

The McNemar chi-square value for the data shown in Box 11–3 is 5.63. This result is statistically significant ($p < 0.025$), so that the null hypothesis is rejected. Care must be taken in interpreting these data, however, because the test of significance only says the following: Among those faculty who *changed* their opinion, significantly more changed from positive to negative than vice versa.

The McNemar Test of Matched Data

In medical research, the McNemar chi-square test is often used in case-control studies, where the cases and controls are matched on the basis of some characteristics such as age, sex, and residence and then are compared for the presence or absence of a specific risk factor. Under these circumstances, the data can be set up in a 2×2 table similar to that shown in the first part of Box 11–4.

For purposes of illustrating the use of the McNemar test in matched data, the observations made by Cohen (1977) in a case-control study are discussed here and reported in the second part of Box 11–4. In this study, the investigator wanted to examine the association between mycosis fungoides (a type of lymphoma that begins in the skin and eventually spreads to internal organs) and a history of employment in an industrial environment with exposure to cutting oils. After matching 54 subjects who had the disease (the cases) with 54 subjects who did not have the disease (the controls), Cohen recorded whether or not the study subjects had a history of this type of industrial employment.

When the McNemar chi-square formula was used to test the null hypothesis that prior occupation was not associated with the development of mycosis fungoides (see Box 11–4), the chi-square value was 5.06. Because the result was statistically significant ($p = 0.021$), the null hypothesis could be rejected, and the alternative hypothesis that industrial exposure was associated with mycosis fungoides could be accepted.

Note that for Cohen's data, a **matched odds ratio** can also be calculated (see Chapter 6). When the data are set up as in Box 11–4, the ratio is calculated as b/c. Here, the ratio is 13/3, or 4.33, indicating that the odds of acquiring mycosis fungoides was over 4 times as great in those with a history of industrial exposure as in those without such a history.

The Fisher Exact Probability Test

When one or more of the expected counts in a 2×2 table is small (i.e., less than two), the chi-square test cannot be used. However, it is possible to calculate the exact probability of finding the observed numbers by using the Fisher exact probability test. The formula is as follows:

$$\text{Fisher } p = \frac{(a+b)!\,(c+d)!\,(a+c)!\,(b+d)!}{N!\,a!\,b!\,c!\,d!}$$

where p is probability; a, b, c, and d denote values in the top left, top right, bottom left, and bottom right cells, respectively, in a 2×2 table; N is the total number of observations; and ! is the symbol for factorial. (The factorial of $4 = 4! = 4 \times 3 \times 2 \times 1$.)

The Fisher exact probability is extremely tedious to calculate unless the investigator has a calculator with a function key that determines factorials. Moreover, unless one of the four cells contains a 0, the sum of more than one calculation is needed. For this reason, it is strongly recommended that the calculation be done using a computer statistical package. Most commercially available statistical packages now calculate the Fisher probability automatically when an appropriate situation arises in a 2×2 table.

Standard Errors for Data in 2×2 Tables

Standard errors for proportions, risk ratios, and odds ratios are sometimes calculated for data in 2×2 tables, although they are not used for data in larger tables.

Standard Error for a Proportion

In a 2×2 table, the proportion of success (defined, for example, as survival) can be determined

BOX 11–4.   McNemar Chi-Square Analysis of the Relationship between Data from Cases and Data from Controls (Two Dichotomous Variables, Paired) in a Case-Control Study of 54 Subjects

Part 1. Standard 2 × 2 table format on which equations are based:

		CONTROLS		
		Risk Factor Present	Risk Factor Absent	Total
CASES	Risk Factor Present	a	b	$a + b$
	Risk Factor Absent	c	d	$c + d$
	Total	$a + c$	$b + d$	$a + b + c + d$

Part 2. Data for a case-control study of the relationship between mycosis fungoides (the disease) and a history of exposure to an industrial environment containing cutting oils (the risk factor):

		CONTROLS		
		History of Industrial Exposure	No History of Industrial Exposure	Total
CASES	History of Industrial Exposure	16	13	29
	No History of Industrial Exposure	3	22	25
	Total	19	35	54

Part 3. Calculation of the McNemar chi-square (χ^2) value:

$$\text{McNemar } \chi^2 = \frac{(\mid b - c \mid - 1)^2}{b + c}$$

$$= \frac{(\mid 13 - 3 \mid - 1)^2}{13 + 3} = \frac{(9)^2}{16} = \frac{81}{16} = \textbf{5.06}$$

Part 4. Calculation of the degrees of freedom (df) for a contingency table, based on the number of rows (R) and columns (C):

$$df = (R - 1)(C - 1) = (2 - 1)(2 - 1) = \textbf{1}$$

Part 5. Determination of the p value:

Value from the chi-square table for 5.06 on 1 df: $p = 0.021$ (statistically significant)

Interpretation: The cases (subjects with mycosis fungoides) were more likely than expected by chance alone to have been exposed to an industrial environment with cutting oils than were the controls (subjects without mycosis fungoides).

Part 6. Calculation of the odds ratio (OR):

$$OR = b/c = 13 \: / \: 3 = \textbf{4.33}$$

Source of data: Cohen, S. R. Mycosis fungoides: clinicopathologic relationships, survival, and therapy in 54 patients, with observation on occupation as a new prognostic factor. Master's thesis, Yale University School of Medicine, New Haven, Conn., 1977.

for each of the two levels (categories) of the independent variable, and the standard error can be calculated for each of these proportions. This is of value when the primary study objective was to estimate the true proportions of success in each of the two groups, rather than to compare the rates of success.

For example, in Box 11–2, the proportion of 28-day survivors in the propranolol-treated group was 0.84 (shown as 84% in the percentage column), and the proportion of 28-day survivors in the placebo-treated group was 0.63. Knowing this information allows the investigator to calculate both the standard error and the 95% confidence interval for each survival percentage by the methods described earlier (see Use of z-Tests, under Tests of Statistical Significance in Chapter 10). When the calculations are performed for the proportions surviving in Box 11–2, the 95% confidence interval for the propranolol-treated group is expressed as (0.73, 0.95), meaning that the true proportion probably is between 0.73 and 0.95, while the confidence interval for the placebo-treated group is expressed as (0.49, 0.77).

Standard Error for a Risk Ratio

If a 2 × 2 table is used to compare the proportion of disease in two different exposure groups or is used to compare the proportion of success in two different treatment groups, the relative risk or relative success can be expressed as a risk ratio. Standard errors can be set around the risk ratio, and if the 95% confidence limits exclude the value of 1.0, there is a statistically significant difference between the risks, at an alpha level of 5%.

For example, in Box 11–2, because the proportion of 28-day survivors in the propranolol-treated group was 0.84 and the proportion of 28-day survivors in the placebo-treated group was 0.63, the risk ratio was 0.84/0.63, or 1.34. This ratio indicates that for the myocardial infarction patients studied, the 28-day survival probability with propranolol was 34% better than that with placebo.

There are several approaches to computing the standard error of a risk ratio. All of the methods are complicated, and they produce somewhat different estimates, so the methods will not be shown here. One or another of these methods is provided in every major statistical computer package. When the risk ratio in Box 11–2 is analyzed by the Taylor series approach used in the EPIINFO 5.01 computer package (Dean et al. 1991), for example, the 95% confidence interval around the risk ratio of 1.34 is reported as (1.04, 1.73). This confirms the chi-square test finding of statistical significance, because the confidence interval does not include a risk ratio of 1.0 (which means no difference between the groups).

Standard Error for an Odds Ratio

If a 2 × 2 table provides data from a case-control study, the odds ratio can be calculated. Even though Box 11–2 is best analyzed by a risk ratio, because the study method is a cohort study (randomized control

trial) rather than a case-control study, the odds ratio can also be examined. Here the odds of surviving in the propranolol-treated group are 38/7, or 5.43, and the odds of surviving in the placebo-treated group are 29/17, or 1.71. The odds ratio is therefore 5.43/1.71, or 3.18, which is much larger than the risk ratio. As was emphasized in Chapter 6, the odds ratio is a good estimate of the risk ratio only if the risk being studied by a case-control study is rare. Since the risk event (mortality) in Box 11–2 is not rare, the odds ratio is not a good estimate of the risk ratio.

Calculating the standard error for an odds ratio is also a complicated process and will not be discussed here. When the odds ratio in Box 11–2 is analyzed by the Cornfield approach used in the EPIINFO 5.01 computer package (Dean et al. 1991), the 95% confidence interval around the odds ratio of 3.18 is reported as (1.06, 9.85). The lower limit estimate of 1.06 with the odds ratio is close to the lower limit estimate of 1.04 with the risk ratio, so this approach also confirms statistical significance. However, the upper limit estimate for the odds ratio is much larger than that for the risk ratio, because the odds ratio itself is much larger than the risk ratio.

Strength of Association of Data in 2 × 2 Tables

Earlier in this chapter, the strength of association between two continuous variables was measured as r^2. For the data shown in 2 × 2 tables, an alternative method is used to estimate the strength of association. A fictitious scenario and set of data will be used here to illustrate how to determine strength of association and why it is important to examine associations for strength as well as statistical significance.

Assume that an eager male student was pursuing a master's degree and based his thesis on a study to determine if there was a true difference between the results of a certain blood test in males and the results in females. After obtaining the data shown in the first part of Box 11–5, he calculated the chi-square value and found that the difference between findings in males and findings in females was not statistically significant ($p = 0.572$). His advisor pointed out that even if the difference had been statistically significant, the data would not have been clinically useful because of the small gender difference in the proportion of subjects with positive findings in the blood test (52% of males versus 48% of females).

This eager student, however, decided to obtain a Ph.D. and to base his dissertation on a continued study of the same topic. Believing that small numbers were the problem with the master's thesis, he decided to obtain blood test findings this time in 20,000 subjects, half from each gender. As shown in the second part of Box 11–5, the difference in proportions was the same as before (52% of males versus 48% of females), so the results were still clinically unimportant (i.e., trivial). However, now the student had obtained (perhaps felt "rewarded" with) a statistical association that was highly significant ($p < 0.0001$).

Findings can have statistical significance and at the same time be of no clinical value, especially if the

BOX 11–5. **Analysis of the Strength of Association (phi) between Blood Test Results and Gender (Two Nonparametric Variables, Unpaired) in an Initial Study of 200 Subjects and a Subsequent Study of 20,000 Subjects (Fictitious Data)**

Part 1. Data and calculation of the phi coefficient for the initial study (the master's thesis):

		GENDER				Total	
		Male		Female			
		Num-ber	(Percent-age)	Num-ber	(Percent-age)	Num-ber	(Percent-age)
BLOOD TEST RESULT	Positive	52	(52)	48	(48)	100	(50)
	Negative	48	(48)	52	(52)	100	(50)
	Total	100	(100)	100	(100)	200	(100)

chi-square (χ^2) value: 0.32
degrees of freedom (df): 1
p value: **0.572** (not statistically significant)

$$\text{phi} = \sqrt{\frac{\chi^2}{N}} = \sqrt{\frac{0.32}{200}} = \sqrt{0.0016} = \mathbf{0.04}$$

Interpretation: The association between gender and the blood test result was neither statistically significant nor clinically important.

Part 2. Data and calculation of the phi coefficient for the subsequent study (the Ph.D. dissertation):

		GENDER				Total	
		Male		Female			
		Num-ber	(Percent-age)	Num-ber	(Percent-age)	Num-ber	(Percent-age)
BLOOD TEST RESULT	Positive	5,200	(52)	4,800	(48)	10,000	(50)
	Negative	4,800	(48)	5,200	(52)	10,000	(50)
	Total	10,000	(100)	10,000	(100)	20,000	(100)

chi-square (χ^2) value: 32.0
degrees of freedom (df): 1
p value: **<0.0001** (highly statistically significant)

$$\text{phi} = \sqrt{\frac{\chi^2}{N}} = \sqrt{\frac{32}{20,000}} = \sqrt{0.0016} = \mathbf{0.04}$$

Interpretation: The association between gender and the blood test result was statistically significant but was clinically unimportant (i.e., it was trivial).

study involves a large number of subjects. This example shows an interesting point: because the sample size in the Ph.D. study was 100 times as large as that in the master's study, the chi-square value for the data in the Ph.D. study was also 100 times as large. It would be helpful to measure the strength of the association in Box 11–5, in order to show that the magnitude of the association was not important, even though it was statistically significant.

In 2 × 2 tables, the strength of association is measured using the **phi coefficient,** which basically adjusts the chi-square value for the sample size and can be considered the correlation coefficient (r) for the data in a 2 × 2 table. The formula is as follows:

$$\text{phi} = \sqrt{\frac{\chi^2}{N}}$$

The phi value in the first part of Box 11–5 is the same as that in the second part (i.e., 0.04) because the strength of the association is the same (i.e., very small). If phi is squared (like r^2), the proportion of variation explained by gender in this example is less than 0.2%, which is extremely small. Note that although phi is not accurate in larger $(R \times C)$ tables, a similar test, called **Cramer's V,** can be used in these tables (see Blalock 1972).

Every association should be examined for strength of association and clinical utility as well as statistical significance. Strength of association can be shown by a risk ratio, a risk difference, an odds ratio, an r^2 value, a phi value, or a Cramer's V value. A **statistically significant association** implies that the association is real (i.e., is not due to chance alone) but not necessarily that it is important. A **strong association** is likely to be important if it is real. Therefore, looking for both statistical significance and strength of association is as important as having both the right and left wings on an airplane.

There is, however, a danger of automatically rejecting as unimportant a statistically significant association that showed only limited strength of association. As discussed in Chapter 6, both the risk ratio (or odds ratio if from a case-control study) and the prevalence of the risk factor determine the population attributable risk. Thus, for a prevalent disease such as myocardial infarction, a common risk factor that showed a risk ratio of only 1.3 could be responsible for a large number of preventable infarctions.

Survival Analysis

In clinical studies of medical or surgical interventions for cancer, for example, success usually is measured in terms of the length of time that some desirable outcome (such as survival or remission of disease) is maintained. An analysis of the time-related patterns of survival commonly involves using life tables and techniques that were first developed in the insurance field, and survival analysis requires that the dependent (outcome) variable be dichotomous (e.g., survival/death, success/failure, or presence/absence of improvement).

The mere reporting of the proportion of patients who are alive at the termination of a study's observation period is obviously inadequate, because it does not account for how long the individual patients were observed, nor does it consider when they died or how many were lost to follow-up. Among the techniques that statisticians use to control for these problems are person-time methods and life table analysis using the actuarial method or the Kaplan-Meier method.

Person-Time Methods

In a survival study, some subjects are lost to follow-up and others die during the observation period. To control for the fact that the length of observation varies from subject to subject, the person-time methods introduced in an earlier discussion of **incidence density** (see Chapter 2) can be used

in calculating risks and rates of death. Briefly, if one person is observed for 3 years and another for 1 year, the **duration of observation** would be equal to 4 **person-years.** Calculations can be made on the basis of years, months, weeks, or any other unit of time. The results can then be reported as the number of events (e.g., deaths or remissions) per person-time of observation.

Person-time methods are useful if the risk of death does not change greatly over the period of follow-up. If the risk of death does depend strongly on the amount of time since baseline (e.g., amount of time since diagnosis of a disease or since entry in a study), as is true with certain cancers that tend to kill quickly if they are going to be fatal, the overall risk using person-time methods will depend on the relative proportion of study subjects in the early versus late follow-up period, and the incidence density will not be useful. As mentioned in Chapter 2, person-time methods are especially useful for studies of phenomena that can occur repeatedly over time, such as otitis media and other acute infections.

Life Table Analysis

In follow-up studies of a single dichotomous outcome such as death, a major problem is that some subjects may be lost to follow-up (unavailable for examination) and some may be censored (when the time of study of a patient is terminated early because the patient entered late and the study is ending). The most popular solution to this problem is to use life table analysis. The two main methods of life table analysis—the actuarial method and the Kaplan-Meier method—handle losses to follow-up and censorship in slightly different ways, but both methods make it possible to base the analysis on the findings in all of the subjects for whom there are data.

Both methods require the following information for each patient: (1) the date of entry in the study; (2) the reason for withdrawal (death, loss to follow-up, or censorship); and (3) the date of withdrawal (date of death for those who died, the last time seen alive for those who were lost to follow-up, and the date withdrawn alive for those who were censored).

The Actuarial Method. The actuarial method, which was developed to calculate risks and premium rates for life insurance companies and retirement plans, was one of the earlier methods used in life table analysis. In medical studies, the actuarial method is used to calculate the survival rates of patients during *fixed* intervals, such as years. First, it determines the number of people surviving to the beginning of each interval. Next, it assumes that those who were censored or lost to follow-up during the interval were observed for only half of that interval. Then the method calculates the mortality rate for that interval (m_x in life tables) by dividing the number of deaths in the interval by the total person-years for all those who began the interval.

The survival rate for an interval (p_x) is 1.0 minus

the mortality rate. The rate of survival of the study group to the end of, say, three of the fixed intervals (P_3) is the product of the survival of each of the three component intervals. Thus, if the intervals were years and if the survival to the end of the first interval (p_1) was 0.75, p_2 was 0.80, and p_3 was 0.85, the numbers would be multiplied to arrive at a 3-year survival rate of 0.51, or 51%.

An example of a study in which this method was used is the Veterans Administration study of the long-term effects of coronary artery bypass grafts (CABG) versus medical treatment of patients with stable angina (see Veterans Administration Coronary Artery Bypass Surgery Cooperative Study Group 1984). Fig. 11–4 shows the 11-year cumulative survival for surgically and medically treated patients who did not have left main coronary artery disease but were nevertheless at high risk according to angiographic analysis in the study.

The actuarial method can also be used in studies of outcomes other than death or survival. Currie, Jekel, and Klerman (1972), for example, used the method in a study of subsequent pregnancies among two groups of teenage mothers. The teenage mothers in one group were enrolled in special programs to help them complete their education and delay subse-

quent pregnancies, while those in the other group had access to the services that are usually available. The actuarial method was used to analyze data concerning the number and timing of subsequent pregnancies in each group, and when tests of significance were performed, the observed differences between the groups were found to be statistically significant.

The actuarial method continues to be used if there are large numbers of study subjects, but another method called the Kaplan-Meier method has many advantages, particularly if the sample size is small.

The Kaplan-Meier Method. The Kaplan-Meier method (Kaplan and Meier 1958) has become the most commonly used approach to survival analysis in medicine. In the medical literature, it is usually referred to as the **Kaplan-Meier life table method.** It is also sometimes referred to as the **product-limit method,** because it takes advantage of the fact that the N year survival rate (P_N) is equal to the product of all of the survival rates of the individual intervals (p_1, p_2, and so forth) leading up to year N.

The Kaplan-Meier method is different from the actuarial method in that it calculates a new line of the life table every time a new death occurs. Because deaths occur unevenly over time, the intervals are *uneven* and there are many of them. For this reason, the graph of a Kaplan-Meier life table analysis often looks like uneven stair steps.

In a Kaplan-Meier analysis, the deaths are not conceived of as occurring during an interval. Rather, they are seen as instantaneously terminating one interval and beginning a new interval at a lower survival rate. The periods of time between when deaths occur are death-free periods, and therefore the proportion surviving between deaths does not change, and the curve of the proportion surviving is flat rather than sloping downward. A death produces an instantaneous drop in the proportion surviving, and then another death-free period begins.

To illustrate the method, the following example was taken from Kaplan and Meier's original (1958) article and is analyzed in Box 11–6. The study began with eight patients, four of whom died and the remaining four of whom were lost to follow-up or censored. The four deaths occurred at 0.8, 3.1, 5.4, and 9.2 months. The four losses occurred at 1.0, 2.7, 7.0, and 12.1 months. Because losses to follow-up and censored patients are removed from the study group after the between-death interval in which they occur, they do not appear in the denominator when the next death occurs.

In Box 11–6, p_x is the proportion surviving interval x (i.e., from the time of the previous death to just before the next death), and P_x is the proportion surviving from the beginning of the study to the end of that interval. (P_x is obtained by multiplying together the p_x values of all of the intervals up to and including the row of interest.) The p_x of the first interval is always 1.0, because the first death ends the first study interval and all of the patients not lost to follow-up survive until the first death.

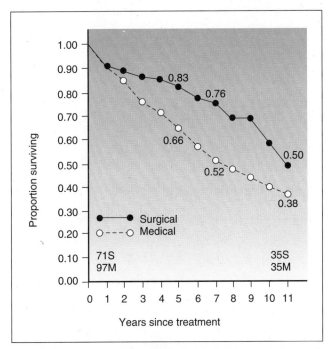

FIGURE 11–4. Graph showing results of survival analysis using the actuarial method in a study of the long-term effects of coronary artery bypass grafts (CABG) versus medical treatment of patients with stable angina. Depicted here is the 11-year cumulative survival for surgically and medically treated patients who did not have left main coronary artery disease but were nevertheless at high risk according to angiographic analysis in the study. Numbers of patients at risk are given at the bottom of the figure, where S denotes surgical and M denotes medical. (Adapted from Veterans Administration Coronary Artery Bypass Surgery Cooperative Study Group. Eleven-year survival in the Veterans Administration randomized trial of coronary bypass surgery for stable angina. New England Journal of Medicine 311:1333–1339, 1984. Copyright 1984. Massachusetts Medical Society. All rights reserved.)

BOX 11–6. Survival Analysis by the Kaplan-Meier Method in a Study of 8 Subjects

Part 1. Beginning data:

Timing of deaths in 4 subjects:
0.8, 3.1, 5.4, and 9.2 months
Timing of loss to follow-up or censorship in 4 subjects:
1.0, 2.7, 7.0, and 12.1 months

Part 2. Tabular representation of the data:

Number of Months at Time of Subject's Death	Number Living Just before Subject's Death	Number Living Just after Subject's Death	Number Lost to Follow-Up between This and Next Subject's Death	p_x	Interval for p_x	P_x to End of Interval
—	—	—	—	1.000	$0 < 0.8$	1.000
0.8	8	7	2	0.875	$0.8 < 3.1$	0.875
3.1	5	4	0	0.800	$3.1 < 5.4$	0.700
5.4	4	3	1	0.750	$5.4 < 9.2$	0.525
9.2	2	1	0	0.500	$9.2 < 12.1$	0.263
No deaths	1	1	1	1.000	> 12.1	0.263

Note: p_x is the proportion surviving interval x (i.e., from the time of the previous death to just before the next death), and P_x is the proportion surviving from the beginning of the study to the end of that interval.

Part 3. Graphic representation of the data:

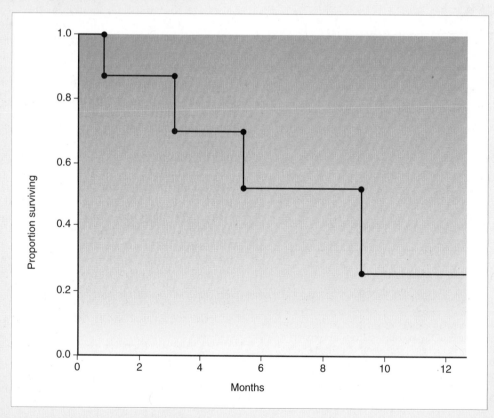

Source of data: Kaplan, E. L., and P. Meier. Nonparametric estimation from incomplete observations. Journal of the American Statistical Association 53:457–481, 1958.

To illustrate the use of Kaplan-Meier analysis in practice, Fig. 11–5 shows a Kaplan-Meier life table of the probability of remaining relapse-free over time for two groups of patients who had cancer of the bladder (Esrig et al. 1994). All of the patients had organ-confined transitional-cell cancer of the bladder with deep invasion into the muscularis propria (i.e., stage 3a disease) but without regional lymph node metastases. One group consisted of 14 patients with negative results in a test for p53 protein in the nuclei of tumor cells, and the other group consisted of 12 patients with positive results in the same test (Esrig et al. 1994). Despite small numbers, the difference in the survival curves for the p53-positive group and the p53-negative group was found to be statistically significant ($p = 0.030$).

Life table methods do not eliminate the bias that occurs if the losses to follow-up happen more frequently in one group than in another, particularly if the characteristics of the patients lost from one group differ greatly from those of the patients lost from the other group. However, the life table method is a powerful tool if the losses are few, if the losses represent a similar percentage of the starting numbers in the groups to be compared, and if the characteristics of those lost to follow-up are similar. The life table method is usually considered the method of choice for describing dichotomous outcomes in longitudinal studies.

In statistics, it is always crucial to look at the raw data, and nowhere is this more important than in survival analysis, where examining the pattern of survival differences may be more important for making a clinical decision than examining whether the difference is statistically significant. For example, a new cancer therapy may result in a greater initial mortality but a higher 5-year survival (i.e., the therapy is a "kill or cure" method), whereas a more traditional therapy results in a lower initial mortality but also a lower 5-year survival. It might be important for patients to know this difference in choosing between these therapies.

Tests of Significance for Differences in Survival

Two or more life table curves can be tested to see if they are significantly different. Statistical computer packages do this using some rather complicated tests, such as the Breslow test and the Cox test. However, reasonably good tests of significance between actuarial curves (such as the z-test for proportions) and between Kaplan-Meier curves (such as the logrank test) can be done by hand.

Significance Tests for Proportions. See Chapter 10 for a discussion of t-tests and z-tests. The t-test for a difference between actuarial method curves depends on the Greenwood formula for the standard error of a proportion. For details, see Cutler and Ederer (1958) or Dawson-Saunders and Trapp (1994).

The Logrank Test. Despite its name, the logrank test does not deal with logarithms or with ranked data. The test is often used to compare data in studies involving treatment and control groups and to test the null hypothesis that each group has the same force of mortality.

In the logrank test, each time a death occurs, the investigator calculates the probability that the observed death would have occurred in the treatment group and the probability that it would have occurred in the control group. These probabilities are proportional to the number of survivors to that point in time in each group. For example, suppose the study started with 100 patients in each group, but at a certain point there were 60 left in the treatment group and 40 in the control group. Under the null hypothesis, the probability that the next death would occur in the treatment group is 0.6, and the probability that the next death would occur in the control group is 0.4.

Within each study group, the expected probabilities for each death are summed to form the total expected number of deaths (E) for that group. The actual deaths in each group are also summed to form the observed number of deaths (O). Then the observed deaths are compared with the expected deaths in the following chi-square test on 1 degree of freedom:

$$\text{logrank } \chi^2 = \frac{(O_T - E_T)^2}{E_T} + \frac{(O_C - E_C)^2}{E_C}$$

where O_T and E_T are the observed and expected deaths in the treatment group and where O_C and E_C are the observed and expected deaths in the control group. Note that only two terms are needed, because the expected counts are not determined from row and column totals in a 2×2 table but instead are obtained by an independent method.

Proportional Hazard Models (Cox Models). The Kaplan-Meier approach has been made even more powerful by the development of statistical models

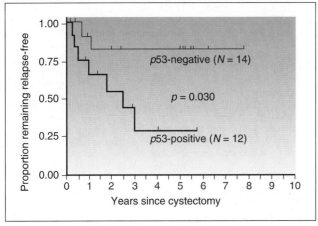

FIGURE 11–5. Graph showing a life table analysis using the Kaplan-Meier method in a study of the probability of remaining relapse-free over time for two groups of patients who had organ-confined transitional-cell cancer of the bladder with deep invasion into the muscularis propria (i.e., stage 3a disease) but without regional lymph node metastases. One group consisted of 14 patients with negative results in a test for p53 protein in the nuclei of tumor cells, and the other group consisted of 12 patients with positive results in the same test. (Adapted from Esrig, D., et al. Accumulation of nuclear p53 and tumor progression in bladder cancer. New England Journal of Medicine 331:1259–1264, 1994. Copyright 1994. Massachusetts Medical Society. All rights reserved.)

that enable dichotomous outcomes to be used as dependent variables in multiple logistic regression analyses, despite losses to follow-up and censorship of patients. Although a detailed discussion of these models is beyond the scope of this book, students should be aware that they are called proportional hazard models or Cox models and that their application is becoming increasingly common in medical studies. For more information, see Dawson-Saunders and Trapp (1994) or Tibshirani (1982).

SUMMARY

Bivariate analysis is the analysis of the relationship between one independent variable and one dependent variable. The statistical significance tests frequently used for this purpose are listed in Table 11–1.

The relationships between two variables that are both continuous should first be examined graphically. Then the data can be analyzed statistically to determine whether there is a real relationship between the variables, whether the relationship is linear or nonlinear, whether the correlation (r) is positive or negative, and whether the association is sufficiently strong that it is not likely to have occurred by chance alone. The strength of an association between two continuous variables can be determined by calculating the value of r^2, and the impact that variable x has on variable y can be determined by calculating the slope of the regression.

Both correlation and regression analysis indicate whether there is an association between two continuous variables, such as weight (y) and height (x). Correlation tells what proportion of the variation in y is explained by the variation in x. Linear regression estimates the value of y when the value of x is 0, and it also predicts the degree of expected change in y when x changes by one unit of measure.

There are numerous tests to determine the relationships between two ordinal variables. These include the Mann-Whitney U test (similar to the Student's t-test), the Wilcoxon test (similar to the paired t-test), the Kruskal-Wallis test (similar to the F-test), and the sign test. Of the tests that measure the correlation between two ordinal variables, the most important are the Spearman and the Kendall correlation coefficients, which are rho and tau, respectively. There are no linear regression tests for ordinal variables.

The bivariate analysis of dichotomous or nominal data may begin by placing the data for the two variables in a 2×2 contingency table. Then the null hypothesis of independence between the two variables is usually tested by using the chi-square test for unpaired data or the McNemar chi-square test for paired data. Less frequently, the Fisher exact probability test is used in the analysis of dichotomous unpaired data. For data in 2×2 tables, the phi coefficient can be used to test the strength of association, and methods are available to calculate standard errors and confidence intervals for proportions, risk ratios, or odds ratios.

Survival analysis employs various methods to study dichotomous outcome variables (e.g., death/survival) over time. Although the actuarial method of analysis is still used, the Kaplan-Meier (product-limit) method has become the most frequently used approach. Life table curves are constructed from the data, and two or more curves can be tested to see if they are significantly different. For actuarial curves, significance tests for proportions can be used. For Kaplan-Meier curves, the logrank test and proportional hazards (Cox) models are among the statistical tests available.

References Cited

Blalock, H. M., Jr. Social Statistics, 2nd ed. New York, McGraw-Hill Book Company, 1972.

Cohen, S. R. Mycosis fungoides: clinicopathologic relationships, survival, and therapy in 54 patients, with observation on occupation as a new prognostic factor. Master's thesis, Yale University School of Medicine, New Haven, Conn., 1977.

Currie, J., J. F. Jekel, and L. V. Klerman. Subsequent pregnancies among teenage mothers enrolled in a special program. American Journal of Public Health 62:1606–1611, 1972.

Cutler, S. J., and F. Ederer. Maximum utilization of the life table method in analyzing survival. Journal of Chronic Disease 8:699–713, 1958.

Dawson-Saunders, B., and R. G. Trapp. Basic and Clinical Biostatistics, 2nd ed. Norwalk, Conn., Appleton and Lange, 1994.

Dean, J., et al. EPIINFO, Version 5.01. Atlanta, Centers for Disease Control, Epidemiology Program Office, 1991.

Emerson, J. D., and G. A. Colditz. Use of statistical analysis. New England Journal of Medicine 309:709–713, 1983.

Esrig, D., et al. Accumulation of nuclear p53 and tumor progression in bladder cancer. New England Journal of Medicine 331:1259–1264, 1994.

Fleiss, J. L. Statistical Methods for Rates and Proportions, 2nd ed. New York, John Wiley and Sons, 1981.

Kaplan, E. L., and P. Meier. Nonparametric estimation from incomplete observations. Journal of the American Statistical Association 53:457–481, 1958.

Kleinbaum, D. G., and L. L. Kupper. Applied Regression Analysis and Other Multivariable Methods. North Scituate, Mass., Duxbury Press, 1978.

Phillips, D. S. Basic Statistics for Health Science Students. San Francisco, W. H. Freeman and Company, 1978.

Siegel, S. Nonparametric Statistics. New York, McGraw-Hill Book Company, 1956.

Snow, P. J. Effect of propranolol in myocardial infarction. Lancet 2:551–553, 1965.

Tibshirani, R. A plain man's guide to the proportional hazards model. Clinical and Investigative Medicine 5:63–68, 1982.

Veterans Administration Coronary Artery Bypass Surgery Cooperative Study Group. Eleven-year survival in the Veterans Administration randomized trial of coronary bypass surgery for stable angina. New England Journal of Medicine 311:1333–1339, 1984.

Selected Readings

Dawson-Saunders, B., and R. G. Trapp. Basic and Clinical Biostatistics, 2nd ed. Norwalk, Conn., Appleton and Lange, 1994.

Inglefinger, J. A., et al. Biostatistics in Clinical Medicine, 2nd ed. New York, Macmillan Publishing Company, 1987.

Kleinbaum, D. G., and L. L. Kupper. Applied Regression Analysis and Other Multivariable Methods. North Scituate, Mass., Duxbury Press, 1978.

Lee, E. T. Statistical Methods for Survival Data Analysis. Belmont, Calif., Lifetime Learning Publications, 1980.

CHAPTER TWELVE

SAMPLE SIZE,

RANDOMIZATION, AND

PROBABILITY THEORY

SAMPLE SIZE

Among the factors affecting the number of subjects required for a study are the following: whether the research design involves paired data (e.g., observations before treatment and after treatment in the same group of subjects) or unpaired data (e.g., observations in an experimental group and a control group); whether the investigator wishes to consider beta (type II or false-negative) errors in addition to alpha (type I or false-positive) errors; whether the investigator anticipates a large or small variance in the data sets; whether the investigator chooses the usual alpha level (p value of 0.05 in the two-tailed test and a confidence interval of 95%) or a smaller level; and whether the investigator wants to be able to detect a fairly small or extremely small difference between the means or proportions of the outcome variable.

Statisticians are probably consulted more often because an investigator wants to know the sample size needed for a study than for any other reason. Sample size calculations can be confusing even for many people who can do ordinary statistical analyses without trouble. As a test of intuition regarding sample size, try answering the following three questions:

(1) What size sample—large or small—would be needed if there was a very large variance?

(2) What size sample would be needed if the investigator wanted the answer to be very close to the true value (i.e., have very narrow confidence limits or a very small p value)?

(3) What size sample would be needed if the difference that the investigator wanted to be able to detect was extremely small?

If intuition suggested that all of the above requirements would create the need for a large sample size, that is correct. If intuition did not suggest the correct answers, review these questions again after reading the following information about how the basic formula for sample size is derived.

Derivation of the Basic Sample Size Formula

To derive the basic formula for calculating the sample size, it is easiest to start with the formula for the paired t-test:

$$t_\alpha = \frac{\bar{d}}{\dfrac{s_{\bar{d}}}{\sqrt{N}}}$$

where $\bar{d}$ is the mean difference that was observed, $s_{\bar{d}}$ is the standard error of that mean difference, and N is the sample size.

To solve for N, several rearrangements and substitutions of terms in the equation must be made. First, everything can be squared and the equation rearranged so that N is in the numerator:

$$t_\alpha^{\;2} = \frac{(\bar{d})^2}{(s_{\bar{d}}/\sqrt{N})^2} = \frac{(\bar{d})^2 \cdot N}{(s)^2}$$

Next, the terms can be rearranged so that the equation for N in a paired (before and after) study becomes:

$$N = \frac{t_\alpha^{\;2} \cdot (s)^2}{(\bar{d})^2}$$

Now the t in the formula must be replaced with z. This provides a solution to a circular problem: In order to know the value of t, the degrees of freedom (df) must be known. However, the df is dependent on N, which is what the investigator is trying to calculate in the first place. Because the value of z is not dependent on df and because z is equal to t when the sample size is large, z can be used instead of t. The formula therefore becomes:

$$N = \frac{z_\alpha^{\;2} \cdot (s)^2}{(\bar{d})^2}$$

In theory, using z instead of t might produce a slight underestimate of the sample size needed. In practice, however, using z seems to work well, and its use is customary.

Note that the above formula is for a study using the paired t-test, in which each subject serves as his or her own control. For a study using the Student's t-test, such as a randomized controlled trial with an experimental group and a control group, it would be necessary to calculate N for each group. Note also that the above formula only considers the problem of alpha error; to minimize the possibility of beta error, a z term for beta error must be introduced as well. Before these topics are discussed, however, the answers to the three questions posed earlier should be explored more fully in light of the information provided by the basic formula for N.

(1) The larger the variance is, the larger the sample size must be, because the variance is in the numerator of the above formula for N. It makes sense intuitively, because with a large variance (and therefore a large standard error), a bigger N is needed to compensate for the greater uncertainty of the estimate.

(2) To have considerable confidence that a mean difference shown in a study is real, the analysis must produce a small p value for the observed mean difference, which in turn implies that the value for t_α or z_α was large. Because z_α is in the numerator of the sample size formula, the larger z_α is, the larger the N (the sample size needed) will be. For example, for a two-tailed test, a p value of 0.05 (the alpha level chosen) would require a z_α of 1.96, which, when squared as in the formula, would equal 3.84. To be even more confident, the investigator might set alpha at 0.01. This would require a z_α of 2.58, which equals 6.66 when squared, 73% greater than when alpha is set at 0.05. To decrease the probability of being wrong from 5% to 1% would thus require the sample size to be almost doubled.

(3) If the investigator wanted to detect with confidence a very small difference between the mean values of two study groups, a very large N would be

needed, because the difference (squared) is in the denominator. The smaller the denominator is, the larger the ratio is and, hence, the larger the N must be. A precise estimate and therefore a large sample size is needed to detect a small difference.

The Problem of Beta Error

If a mean difference is examined with a t-test and it is statistically significant at the prestated level of alpha (e.g., 0.05), there is no need to worry about beta error (type II or false-negative error). If, however, an investigator observes a mean difference in the data that appears to be clinically important but the null hypothesis cannot be rejected at the desired level of confidence (e.g., alpha = 0.05), beta error may have occurred because the sample size was small. In planning a study, investigators want to avoid the likelihood of beta (false-negative) error as well as the likelihood of alpha (false-positive) error.

The need to be concerned about beta error was illustrated in a seminal article by Freiman et al. (1978). They found that in most of 71 "negative" randomized controlled trials of new therapies, the sample sizes were too small "to provide reasonable assurance that a clinically meaningful 'difference' (i.e., therapeutic effect) would not be missed." In their study, "reasonable assurance" was 90%. In fact, in 94% of these negative studies, the sample size was too small to detect a 25% improvement in outcome with reasonable (90%) assurance. In 75% of the studies, the sample size was too small to detect a 50% improvement in outcome with the same level of assurance.

A study with a large beta error has a low sensitivity for detecting a mean difference because, as discussed in Chapter 7:

$$\text{Sensitivity} + \text{False-negative (beta) error} = 1.00$$

When investigators speak of a study as opposed to a clinical test, however, they usually use the term "statistical power" instead of "sensitivity." With this substitution in terms,

$$\text{Statistical power} + \text{Beta error} = 1.00$$

which means that statistical power is equal to (1 − beta error). Therefore, in calculating a sample size, if the investigators accept a 20% possibility of missing a true finding (beta error = 0.2), the study should have a statistical power of 0.8, or 80%. That means the investigators are 80% confident that they will be able to detect a true mean difference of the size they specify with the sample size they determine.

The best way to incorporate beta error into a study is to include it beforehand in the determination of sample size. Incorporating beta in the sample size calculation is easy, but it is likely to increase the sample size considerably.

Steps in the Calculation of Sample Size

The first step in calculating sample size is to choose the appropriate formula to be used, based on

TABLE 12–1.   Formulas for the Calculation of Sample Size for Studies Commonly Pursued in Medical Research

Type of Study and Type of Errors to Be Considered	Appropriate Formula to Be Used*
Studies using the paired t-test (e.g., before and after studies) and considering alpha (type I) error only	$N = \dfrac{(z_\alpha)^2 \cdot (s)^2}{(\bar{d})^2}$
Studies using the Student's t-test (e.g., randomized controlled trials with one experimental group and one control group) and considering alpha error only	$N = \dfrac{(z_\alpha)^2 \cdot 2 \cdot (s)^2}{(\bar{d})^2}$
Studies using the Student's t-test and considering alpha (type I) and beta (type II) errors	$N = \dfrac{(z_\alpha + z_\beta)^2 \cdot 2 \cdot (s)^2}{(\bar{d})^2}$
Studies using a test of differences in proportions and considering alpha and beta errors	$N = \dfrac{(z_\alpha + z_\beta)^2 \cdot 2 \cdot \bar{p}(1-\bar{p})}{(\bar{d})^2}$

*The appropriate formula is based on the study design and the type of outcome data. In these formulas, N = sample size; z_α = value for alpha error; z_β = value for beta error; s^2 = variance; $\bar{p}$ = mean proportion of success; and $\bar{d}$ = difference to be detected. See Boxes 12–1, 12–2, 12–3, and 12–4 for examples of calculations using the formulas.

the type of study and the type of error to be considered. Four common formulas for calculating sample size are discussed in this chapter and listed in Table 12–1.

In the second step in calculating sample size, the investigators must specify the following values: the variance expected (s^2); the alpha desired (actually, z_α); the smallest clinically important difference $(\bar{d})$; and, usually, beta (actually, z_β). All but the variance must come from clinical and research judgment. The estimated variance, however, must be based on knowledge of data. If the outcome variable being studied is continuous, such as blood pressure, the estimate of variance can be obtained from the literature or from a small pilot study.

If the outcome is the proportion surviving for 5 years, for example, the variance is easier to estimate. The investigators need to estimate only the proportion that would survive 5 years with the new experimental treatment (which is p_1 and is, say, 60%) and the proportion expected to survive with the control group's treatment (which is p_2 and is, say, 40%). Assuming the two study groups are of approximately equal size, the investigators must determine the mean survival in the entire group (which would be $\bar{p} = 50\%$ in this example). The formula for the variance of a proportion is simply the following:

$$\text{Variance (proportion)} = \bar{p}\,(1 - \bar{p})$$

Once the investigators are armed with all of the above information, it is straightforward to compute the needed sample size, as shown in Boxes 12–1 through 12–4 and discussed below. Note that the N determined using the formulas in Boxes 12–2, 12–3, and 12–4 is only for the experimental group. This must be doubled to include the control group.

For some studies, investigators may find it easier to obtain control subjects than cases (or vice versa). In this situation, it is satisfactory to have more of one

---

BOX 12–1. Calculation of Sample Size for a Study Using the Paired *t*-Test and Considering Alpha Error Only

Part 1. Data on which the calculation will be based:

Study Characteristic	Assumptions Made by Investigator
Type of study	Before and after study of an antihypertensive drug
Data sets	Pretreatment and posttreatment observations in the same group of subjects
Variable	Systolic blood pressure
Standard deviation (s)	15 mm Hg
Variance (s^2)	225 mm Hg
Data for alpha (z_α)	$p = 0.05$; therefore, 95% confidence desired (two-tailed test); $z_\alpha = 1.96$
Difference to be detected $(\overline{d})$	10 mm Hg or larger difference between pretreatment and posttreatment blood pressure values

Part 2. Calculation of sample size (N):

$$N = \frac{(z_\alpha)^2 \cdot (s)^2}{(\overline{d})^2} = \frac{(1.96)^2 \cdot (15)^2}{(10)^2}$$

$$= \frac{(3.84)(225)}{100} = \frac{864}{100} = 8.64 = \textbf{9 subjects total}$$

Interpretation: Only 9 subjects would be needed in all, because each subject serves as his or her own control in a before and after study.

BOX 12–2. Calculation of Sample Size for a Study Using the Student's *t*-Test and Considering Alpha Error Only

Part 1. Data on which the calculation will be based:

Study Characteristic	Assumptions Made by Investigator
Type of study	Randomized controlled trial of an antihypertensive drug
Data sets	Observations in one experimental group and one control group of the same size
Variable	Systolic blood pressure
Standard deviation (s)	15 mm Hg
Variance (s^2)	225 mm Hg
Data for alpha (z_α)	$p = 0.05$; therefore, 95% confidence desired (two-tailed test); $z_\alpha = 1.96$
Difference to be detected $(\overline{d})$	10 mm Hg or larger difference between mean blood pressure values of the experimental group and control group

Part 2. Calculation of sample size (N):

$$N = \frac{(z_\alpha)^2 \cdot 2 \cdot (s)^2}{(\overline{d})^2} = \frac{(1.96)^2 \cdot 2 \cdot (15)^2}{(10)^2}$$

$$= \frac{(3.84)(2)(225)}{100} = \frac{1728}{100} = 17.28$$

$$= 18 \text{ subjects per group} \times 2 \text{ groups} = \textbf{36 subjects total}$$

Interpretation: Why is the total number of subjects needed in this box 4 times as large as the total number needed in Box 12–1, even though the values for $z_\alpha, s,$ and $\overline{d}$ are the same in both boxes? First, because two independent groups are being compared in this box, there are two sources of variance. This is why the variance estimate in the numerator of the formula is multiplied by 2. Second, for the type of study depicted in this box, 18 subjects will be needed in the experimental group and 18 in the control group, for a total of 36 study subjects.

---

group than the other, to maximize statistical power. The analysis will be somewhat more complicated, however, and the sample size formulas given in Boxes 12–2, 12–3, and 12–4 will need to be modified (see Kelsey, Thompson, and Evans 1986 for modified formulas).

Sample Size for Studies Using *t*-Tests

Box 12–1 shows the formula and the calculations for a before and after study of an antihypertensive drug—that is, a study for which a **paired *t*-test** will be used. Given the variance, alpha, and difference chosen by the investigator, only 9 subjects would be needed altogether. Clearly, this kind of study is efficient in terms of the sample size required. However, even most paired studies require far more than 9 subjects.

Box 12–2 shows the formula and the calculations for a randomized controlled trial of an antihyperten-

sive drug—that is, a study for which the **Student's *t*-test** will be used. This formula differs from the Box 12–1 formula only in that the variance estimate must be multiplied by 2. Given the same assumptions as in Box 12–1 concerning variance, alpha, and difference, it would be necessary to have a total of 36 study subjects for this randomized controlled trial, which is four times the number of subjects required for the before and after study described in Box 12–1. The larger sample size is needed for studies using the Student's *t*-test because there are two sources of variance instead of one and because a second person serves as the control for each experimental subject.

BOX 12–3.   Calculation of Sample Size for a Study Using the Student's *t*-Test and Considering Alpha and Beta Errors

---

Part 1. Data on which the calculation will be based:

Study Characteristic	Assumptions Made by Investigator
Type of study	Randomized controlled trial of an antihypertensive drug
Data sets	Observations in one experimental group and one control group of the same size
Variable	Systolic blood pressure
Standard deviation (s)	15 mm Hg
Variance (s^2)	225 mm Hg
Data for alpha (z_α)	$p = 0.05$; therefore, 95% confidence desired (two-tailed test); $z_\alpha = 1.96$
Data for beta (z_β)	20% beta error; therefore, 80% power desired (one-tailed test); $z_\beta = 0.84$
Difference to be detected $(\overline{d})$	10 mm Hg or larger difference between mean blood pressure values of the experimental group and control group

Part 2. Calculation of sample size (N):

$$N = \frac{(z_\alpha + z_\beta)^2 \cdot 2 \cdot (s)^2}{(\overline{d})^2}$$

$$= \frac{(1.96 + 0.84)^2 \cdot 2 \cdot (15)^2}{(10)^2}$$

$$= \frac{(7.84)(2)(225)}{100} = \frac{3528}{100} = 35.28$$

= 36 subjects per group × 2 groups = **72 subjects total**

Interpretation: Including z_β in the calculations doubled the sample size in this box, compared with the sample size in Box 12–2. If the investigators insisted on an even smaller beta error, the sample size would have increased even more.

The only difference between the formula shown in Box 12–2 and the one shown in Box 12–3 is that the latter considers **beta error** in addition to alpha error. Although there is no complete agreement on the level of beta error acceptable for most studies, usually a beta error of 20% (one-tailed test) is used; this corresponds to a *z* value of 0.84. When these beta estimates are used in Box 12–3, with the same z_α, variance, and mean difference as in Box 12–2, the calculations show that 72 study subjects are needed for the randomized controlled trial. In contrast, 36

subjects were needed if only alpha was considered, as shown in Box 12–2.

The issue of adequate versus excessive sample sizes continues to be debated. Some believe that the medical world may have overreacted to the beta error study by Freiman et al. (1978), with the result that investigators began using samples that were larger than necessary.

On the one hand, if the estimated variance used in the calculations was smaller than the observed variance (i.e., the estimate was too small), the sample size would be too small, and the study might miss showing statistical significance for a difference that was clinically important. Therefore, for safety, the actual sample size should be somewhat larger than that calculated from the formula in Box 12–2.

On the other hand, when z_α and z_β are added together before squaring (as shown in the formula in Box 12–3), the sample size may be excessive. Depending on the value of z_β used, this could as much as quadruple the *N* estimated, which would increase the cost of a study astronomically. The large sample sizes required are one of the reasons for the limited number of major studies that can now be funded nationally. Moreover, a needlessly large sample size introduces other problems for the investigators, who previously set the minimum difference they thought was worthwhile to detect. If the sample size is larger than necessary, when the analysis is done, differences smaller than those the investigators considered clinically important are now likely to become statistically significant, creating problems for the interpretation and possibly forcing the investigators to confront statistically significant differences that they did not consider clinically important. Here, it is important to focus on the original hypotheses.

Sample Size for a Test of Differences in Proportions

Often a dependent variable is measured as success/failure and is described as the proportion of outcomes that represent some form of success, such as improvement in health, remission of disease, or reduction in mortality. In this case, the formula for sample size must be expressed in terms of proportions, as shown in the formula in Box 12–4.

Box 12–4 provides an example of how to calculate the sample size for a randomized controlled trial of a drug to reduce the 5-year mortality in patients with a particular form of cancer. Before the calculations can be made, the investigators must decide which values they will use for z_α, z_β, variance, and the smallest difference to be detected. For alpha and beta, they decide to use a level of 95% confidence (two-tailed test, $p = 0.05$) and 80% power (one-tailed test), so that z_α equals 1.96 and z_β equals 0.84.

Initially, as shown in the first part of Box 12–4, the investigators decide they want to detect a 10% improvement in survival (i.e., a difference of 0.1 between the 5-year mortality of the experimental group and that of the control group). They also

BOX 12–4.   Initial and Subsequent Calculation of Sample Size for a Study Using a Test of Differences in Proportions and Considering Alpha and Beta Errors

Part 1A. Data on which the initial calculation is based:

Study Characteristic	Assumptions Made by Investigator
Type of study	Randomized controlled trial of a drug to reduce the 5-year mortality in patients with a particular form of cancer
Data sets	Observations in one experimental group (E) and one control group (C) of the same size
Variable	Success = 5-year survival after treatment; failure = death within 5 years of treatment
Variance, expressed as $\bar{p}(1-\bar{p})$	$\bar{p} = 0.55$; therefore, $(1-\bar{p}) = 0.45$
Data for alpha (z_α)	$p = 0.05$; therefore, 95% confidence desired (two-tailed test); $z_\alpha = 1.96$
Data for beta (z_β)	20% beta error; therefore, 80% power desired (one-tailed test); $z_\beta = 0.84$
Difference to be detected ($\bar{d}$)	0.1 or larger difference between the success (survival) of the experimental group and that of the control group (i.e., 10% difference—because $p_E = 0.6$, and $p_C = 0.5$)

Part 1B. Initial calculation of sample size (N):

$$N = \frac{(z_\alpha + z_\beta)^2 \cdot 2 \cdot \bar{p}(1-\bar{p})}{(\bar{d})^2} = \frac{(1.96 + 0.84)^2 \cdot 2 \cdot (0.55)(0.45)}{(0.1)^2}$$

$$= \frac{(7.84)(2)(0.2475)}{0.01} = \frac{3.88}{0.01} = 388$$

$$= 388 \text{ subjects per group} \times 2 \text{ groups} = \textbf{776 subjects total}$$

Part 2A. Changes in data on which the initial calculation was based:

Study Characteristic	Assumptions Made by Investigator
Variance, expressed as $\bar{p}(1-\bar{p})$	$\bar{p} = 0.60$; therefore, $(1-\bar{p}) = 0.40$
Difference to be detected ($\bar{d}$)	0.2 or larger difference between the success (survival) of the experimental group and that of the control group (i.e., 20% difference—because $p_E = 0.7$, and $p_C = 0.5$)

Part 2B. Subsequent (revised) calculation of sample size (N):

$$N = \frac{(z_\alpha + z_\beta)^2 \cdot 2 \cdot \bar{p}(1-\bar{p})}{(\bar{d})^2} = \frac{(1.96 + 0.84)^2 \cdot 2 \cdot (0.60)(0.40)}{(0.2)^2}$$

$$= \frac{(7.84)(2)(0.2400)}{0.04} = \frac{3.76}{0.04} = 94$$

$$= 94 \text{ subjects per group} \times 2 \text{ groups} = \textbf{188 subjects total}$$

Interpretation: As a result of changes in the data on which the initial calculation was based, the number of subjects needed was reduced from 776 to 188.

assume that the mean proportion of success $(\bar{p})$ for all subjects enrolled in the study will be 0.55. Based on these assumptions, the calculations show that they would need 388 subjects in the experimental group and 388 in the control group, for a total of 776 subjects. In all probability, this is an unreasonable number of patients to obtain. What can be done? Theoretically, any of the estimated values in the formula might be altered. However, the alpha and beta values that they chose are the ones customarily used, and the best estimate of variance should always be used. Therefore, the only place to rethink the sample size calculation is the requirement for the minimum difference to be detected. Perhaps a 10% improvement is not large enough to be very meaningful. What if it were changed to 20% (a difference of 0.2)? As shown in the second part of Box 12–4, changing the improvement requirement to 20% changes the variance estimate, so that $\bar{p}$ is equal to 0.6. Based on these revised assumptions, the calculations show that the investigators would need 94 subjects in the experimental group and 94 in the control group, for a total of 188 subjects. A study with this smaller sample size appears much more reasonable and more likely to be funded, but changing the difference the investigators want to detect after a sample size calculation is made may be trying to adjust truth to what is convenient. If the investigators really believe the small difference is clinically important, they should try to obtain funding for the large sample required.

In choosing the 10% difference initially, the investigators may have intuitively assumed (incorrectly) that it is easier to detect a small difference than a large one. Or they may just have had an interest in detecting a small difference, even though it would not be clinically important. In either case, the penalty in sample size may alert the investigators to the statistical realities of the situation and force them to think seriously about the smallest difference that would be clinically important. Once they have agreed on the minimal clinically important difference, they should retain it in their research, despite any sample size difficulties.

RANDOMIZATION

There is a distinction between **randomization,** which entails allocating the available subjects to one or another study group, and **random sampling,** which entails selecting a small group for study from a much larger group of potential study subjects. Randomization is usually used in clinical studies.

Goals of Randomization

An experimental design, of which the randomized clinical trial is the standard in clinical research, depends on an **unbiased allocation of study subjects** to the experimental and control groups. For most purposes, the only evidence of an unbiased allocation that will be accepted is randomization. Contrary to popular opinion, randomization does not guarantee that the two (or more) groups created by random allocation are identical in either size or subject characteristics. What randomization does guarantee, if properly done, is that the different groups will be free of selection bias and problems due to regression toward the mean.

Selection bias can occur if subjects are allowed to choose whether they will be in an intervention group or a control group, as occurred in the 1954 polio vaccine trials (see Chapter 4). Selection bias can also occur if investigators influence the assignment of subjects to one group or another. There may be considerable pressure from a patient and from his or her family members or other care givers to alter the randomization process and let the patient into the intervention group, especially in studies involving a community intervention (Lam, Hartwell, and Jekel 1994), but this pressure must be resisted.

Regression toward the mean, which is also known as the **statistical regression effect,** affects patients who were chosen to participate in a study precisely because they had an extreme measurement on some variable (e.g., a high number of throat infections during the past year). They are likely to have a measurement that is closer to average at a later time (e.g., during the subsequent year) for reasons unrelated to the type or efficacy of the treatment they are given. In a study comparing treatment methods in two groups of patients, both of which had extreme measurements at the beginning of the study, randomization cannot eliminate the tendency to regress toward the mean. However, randomization can equalize the tendency between the study groups, thereby preventing bias in the comparison. When Paradise et al. (1984), for example, undertook a randomized clinical trial of surgical treatment (tonsillectomy and adenoidectomy) versus medical treatment (antibiotics) of children with recurrent throat infections, they found that the children in both groups had fewer episodes of throat infection in the year following treatment than in the year before, although the surgically treated patients showed more improvement than the medically treated patients.

Methods of Randomization

When a study involving an experimental group and a control group is planned, the investigators must decide what method of randomization will be used to ensure that each subject has an equal probability of being assigned to the experimental group. As described below, some methods incorporate the use of a random number table such as that shown in the Appendix. Regardless of the method chosen, the best way to keep human preferences from creeping into the randomization process is to hide the results of randomization until they are needed for the analysis. If possible, the study subjects should not know which group they are in. This can be accomplished by "blinding" the study subjects (e.g., giving the control group a placebo that looks the same as the treatment for the experimental group) and blinding the persons who record the findings from the study subjects. If both of these are done, it is a **double-blind study.**

The methods described below all assume that an equal number of subjects is desired in the experimental and control groups. However, the methods can easily be modified to provide two control subjects for each experimental subject.

Simple Random Allocation

In this method, the investigators begin with a random number table (see the Appendix) and a stack of sequentially numbered envelopes (e.g., numbered from 1 to 100 in a study with 100 participants). They blindly put a pencil on a number in the random number table and proceed from that number in a predetermined direction (e.g., up the columns of the table). If the first number is even, they write "experimental group" on a slip of paper and put it in the first envelope. If the next number is odd, they write "control group" on a slip of paper and insert it in the second envelope. They continue until all of the envelopes contain a random group assignment.

The first patient enrolled in the study is assigned to whatever group is indicated in the first envelope. As each new eligible patient is enrolled, the investigators open the next sequentially numbered envelope to find out the patient's group assignment.

Randomization into Groups of Two

Patients can be randomized two at a time. Envelopes are numbered sequentially (e.g., from 1 to 100) and separated into groups of two. As in the above method, the investigators begin by blindly putting down a pencil on a number in the random number table and proceeding in a predetermined direction. If the first number is even, they write "experimental group" on a slip of paper and put it in the first envelope. For the paired envelope, they automatically write the alternative group—in this case, "control group." They use the random number table to determine the assignment of the first envelope in the second pair and continue in this manner for each pair of envelopes. Thus, any time an even number of patients have been admitted into the study, half will be in the experimental group and half in the control group.

Systematic Allocation

Systematic allocation in research studies is equivalent to the old military "Sound off!" The first patient is randomly assigned to a group, and the next patient is automatically assigned to the alternative group. Subsequent patients are given group assignments on an alternating basis. This will ensure that the experimental and control groups are of equal size if there is an even number of patients entered in the study.

There are advantages to this method beyond simplicity. Usually, the variance of the data from a systematic allocation is smaller than that from a simple random allocation, so the statistical power is improved. However, if there is any kind of "periodicity" in the way patients enter, there may be a bias. For example, suppose systematic sampling is used to allocate patients into two groups, and only two patients are admitted each day to the study (e.g., the first two new patients who enter the clinic each morning). If each intake day started so that the first patient was assigned to the experimental group and the second was assigned to the control group, all of the experimental group subjects would be the first patients to arrive at the clinic, perhaps very early in the morning. They might be systematically different (e.g., employed, eager, early risers) compared to those who come later in the day, in which case bias might be introduced into the study. This danger is easy to avoid, however, if the investigator reverses the sequence frequently, sometimes taking the first person each day into the control group. The convenience and statistical advantages of systematic sampling make it desirable to use whenever possible.

The systematic allocation method can also be used for allocating study subjects to three, four, or even more groups.

Stratified Allocation

In clinical research, stratified allocation is often called **prognostic stratification.** It is used when the investigators want to assign patients to different risk groups depending on such baseline variables as the severity of disease (e.g., stage of cancer) and age. When such risk groups have been created, each stratum can then be allocated randomly to the experimental group or the control group. This is usually done to ensure homogeneity of the study groups by severity of disease. If the experimental and control groups have been made prognostically similar, the analysis can be done both for the entire group and within the prognostic groups.

Special Issues Concerning Randomization

Randomization does not guarantee that two or more groups will be identical. Suppose an investigator, when checking how similar the experimental and control groups were after randomization, found that the two groups were of somewhat different size and that 1 out of 20 characteristics being compared showed a statistically significant difference between the groups. The fact that there are occasional differences which are statistically significant does not mean that the randomization was biased; some differences are expected by chance alone. However, there may be a legitimate concern that some of the observed differences between the randomized groups could confound the analysis. In that case, the variables of concern can be controlled for in the analysis.

Even though randomization is the fundamental technique of clinical trials, many other precautions must still be taken in clinical trials, including ensuring the accuracy of all of the data by blinding patients and observers, standardizing data collection instruments, and so forth.

One of the biggest problems of randomization has to do with the generalizability of findings of the study. Obviously, patients have the right to refuse to participate in a study. This means that a particular study is limited to patients who are willing to participate. Are these patients typical of patients who refused to participate, or are they an unusual subset of the entire population with the problem being studied? The results of a clinical trial can only be generalized to similar patients.

What happens if, following randomization, a patient is not doing well and the patient or physician wishes to switch from the experimental treatment to another medication? Ethically, the patient cannot be forced to continue a particular treatment. Once the switch occurs, it will be necessary to choose an alternative way of analyzing the data. There are several possible strategies, and the choice between them represents a philosophical position. Currently, the popular approach is to analyze the data as if the patient had remained in his or her original group, so that any negative outcomes are assigned to their original treatment. This strategy, called the **"intention to treat" approach,** is based on the belief that if the patient was doing so poorly as to want to switch, a negative outcome should be ascribed to that treatment. Other investigators prefer to analyze the data as if the patient had never participated in the study, but this could lead to a small, and probably biased, sample. Still others prefer to reassign the patient to a third group and analyze the data separately from the original groups. The problem with this approach is that the original groups are changed and it is not clear whom the remaining groups represent.

Another problem in randomized trials of treatment is deciding what to consider as the starting point for measuring the outcome. For example, if surgical treatment and medical treatment are being compared, should surgical mortality be included as part of the debit side for surgical treatment, or is the question "Given survival from initial surgical or medical therapy, does the other treatment do better?" (Sackett and Gent 1979). Most investigators recommend counting from the point of randomization.

DANGERS OF DATA DREDGING

In studies with large amounts of data, there is a temptation to use modern computer techniques to see which variables are associated with which other variables and to grind out hundreds of associations. This process is sometimes referred to as data dredging.

The search for associations can be appropriate as long as the investigator keeps two points in mind.

First, the scientific process requires that hypothesis development and hypothesis testing be based on different data sets. One data set is used to develop the hypothesis or model, which is used to make predictions, which are then tested on a new data set. Second, a correlational study (e.g., the Pearson correlation coefficient or the chi-square test) is useful only for developing hypotheses, not for testing them. Stated in slightly different terms, a correlational study is only a kind of screening method. Investigators who keep these points clearly in mind are unlikely to make the mistake of thinking every association found in a data set represents a true association.

One of the most celebrated examples of the problem of data dredging was seen in the report of an association between coffee consumption and pancreatic cancer (MacMahon et al. 1981), obtained by looking at many associations in a large data set, without repeating the analysis on another data set to see if it was consistent. This approach was severely criticized at the time (Feinstein et al. 1981), and several subsequent studies have failed to find a true association between coffee consumption and pancreatic cancer.

How does this problem arise? Suppose there were 10 variables in a descriptive study and the investigator wanted to try to associate each one with every other one. There would be 10×10 possible cells represented (Fig. 12–1). However, 10 of these would be each variable times itself, which is always a perfect correlation. That leaves 90 possible associations, but half of these would be "x times y" and the other half "y times x." Because the p values for bivariate tests are the same regardless of which is considered the independent variable and which is considered the dependent one, there are only half as many truly independent associations, or 45. If the $p = 0.05$ cutoff point is used for alpha, then out of 45 independent associations, slightly more than 2 "statistically significant" associations would be expected to occur by chance alone. In other words, chance would account for at least 1 out of 20 statistically significant associations (see Jekel 1977).

The problem with multiple hypotheses is similar to the problem with multiple associations: the greater the number of hypotheses that are tested, the more likely it is that at least one of them will be found "statistically significant" by chance alone. One possible way to handle this is to lower the p value required before rejecting the null hypothesis (e.g., make it less than 0.05). This was done in a study testing the same medical educational hypothesis at 5 different hospitals (Jekel et al. 1983). If the alpha level in the study had been set at 0.05, there would have been almost a 25% probability of finding a statistically significant difference by chance alone in at least 1 of the 5 hospitals. To keep the risk of a false-positive finding in the entire study to no more than 0.05, the alpha level chosen for rejecting the null hypothesis was made more stringent by divid-

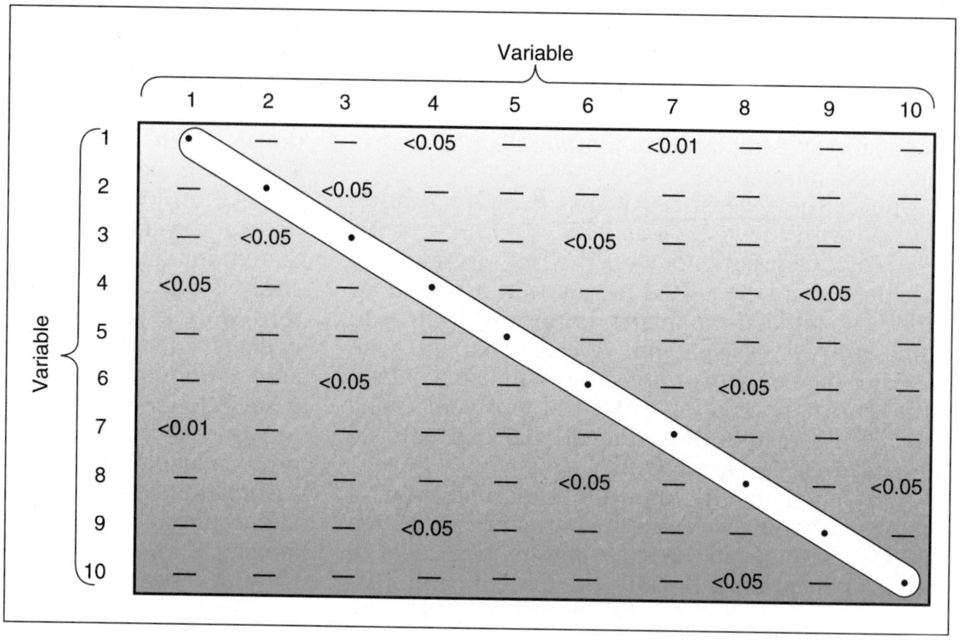

FIGURE 12–1. Matrix of possible statistical associations between 10 different variables from the same research study. Perfect correlations of one variable with itself are shown by dots; nonstatistically significant relationships are shown by dashes; and statistically significant associations are shown by the *p* values. (Redrawn from Jekel, J. F. Should we stop using the *p*-value in descriptive studies? Pediatrics 60:124–126, 1977. Reproduced by permission of Pediatrics, vol. 60, page 125, copyright 1977.)

ing alpha by 5 to make it 0.01. This method of adjusting for multiple hypotheses is called the **Bonferroni procedure.** There are other possible adjustments that are less stringent, but they are more complicated and are used in different situations. These include the Tukey procedure, the Scheffé procedure, and the Newman-Keuls procedure (see Dawson-Saunders and Trapp 1994).

ELEMENTARY PROBABILITY THEORY

A newsletter from a local insurance agent recently made the following argument:

Statistics indicate that if you are fortunate enough to reach age 65, the odds are . . . 50/50 you will spend time in a nursing home. . . . Ergo (our logic): If there are two of you, it would seem the odds are 100% that one of you will need . . . [nursing home] care.

Is this writer's logic correct when he states that if two married people reach the age of 65, there is essentially a 100% chance that at least one member of the couple will require nursing home care? Common sense would indicate that this is not true, because at least some couples are certain to escape. However, it is better to know where the fallacy in the writer's reasoning lies.

There are three basic rules of probability that should be kept in mind when considering arguments such as that used in the example: the independence rule, the product rule, and the addition rule.

The Independence Rule

If the insurance agent's statement that the husband and wife each have a 50% chance of

requiring care in a nursing home is true and if the probabilities are independent of each other, the correct probability that one of them will require nursing home care can be obtained by many trials of flipping an unbiased coin, twice in a row, repeated many times. Assume that the first flip of a trial is the probability that the husband would need nursing home care and that the second flip is the probability that the wife would. Two successive heads would mean both husband and wife would need such care (not necessarily at the same time); one head and one tail would mean that one partner would need care and one would not; and two tails would mean that neither would need care. Heads could be recorded as a plus sign (+), meaning that nursing home care is necessary; tails could be recorded as a minus sign (–), meaning that nursing home care is unnecessary; and the symbols H and W could be used for husband and wife.

Repeated trials of two flips would show the following: a 25% chance of getting two heads in a row (H+ and W+); a 25% chance of getting first a head and then a tail (H+ and W–); a 25% chance of getting first a tail and then a head (H– and W+); and a 25% chance of getting two tails (H– and W–). Therefore, if each member of a couple has a 50% probability of requiring nursing home care at some time and if these probabilities are independent, the chances that at least one member of the couple would require nursing home care at some time would be 75%, not 100%.

In this example, independence means that the overall probability of the husband's being confined to a nursing home is the same whether the wife is confined or not (and vice versa). In statistical terms, this statement can be expressed as follows: $p\{H+ \mid W+\} = p\{H+ \mid W-\}$. Here, p denotes probability, H+ denotes confinement of the husband, the vertical line means "given that" or "conditional upon" what immediately follows, W+ denotes confinement of the wife, and W− denotes no confinement of the wife.

The independence rule does not mean that the husband and wife must have an equal probability of being confined to a nursing home; it requires only that the probability of one partner (whatever that probability is) is not influenced by what happens to the other.

The Product Rule

The product rule is used to determine the probability of two things being true. The manner of calculation depends on whether the two things are independent.

In the example of the husband and wife, if independence is assumed, this simplifies the calculation. The probability that *both* the husband and wife will be confined to a nursing home is simply the product of their independent probabilities. Thus, $p\{H+ \text{ and } W+\} = p\{H+\} \times p\{W+\} = 0.5 \times 0.5 = 0.25$. The probability that *neither* will be confined to a nursing home is the product of the probabilities of not being in a nursing home. Thus, $p\{H− \text{ and } W−\} = p\{H−\} \times p\{W−\} = (1 − p\{H+\}) \times (1 − p\{W+\}) = (1 − 0.5) \times (1 − 0.5) = 0.25$. These answers are the same answers that were derived from flipping coins.

If independence cannot be assumed, a more general product rule must be used. In calculating the probability that *neither* would be confined to a nursing home, the general product rule says that $p\{H− \text{ and } W−\} = p\{H− \mid W−\} \times p\{W−\}$. The answer would be the same if the rule was expressed as $p\{H− \text{ and } W−\} = p\{W− \mid H−\} \times p\{H−\}$. In this example, the probability of the husband not being confined if the wife is not confined is 0.5, and the probability that the wife will not be confined is 0.5. Therefore, the $p\{H− \text{ and } W−\} = 0.5 \times 0.5 = 0.25$, again the same answer as derived from flipping coins.

Although the insurance agent assumed that the probabilities for the husband and wife were each 50%, a recent study by Kemper and Murtaugh (1991) estimated that the probability of confinement in a nursing home after age 65 is 33% for the husband and 52% for the wife. If independence between these probabilities is assumed, the probability that they both will be confined to a nursing home would be calculated as the product of the separate probabilities: $0.33 \times 0.52 = 0.17 = 17\%$.

The Addition Rule

One of the insurance agent's errors was adding the probabilities when he should have multiplied them. A quick way to know that adding the probabilities was incorrect would have been to say, "Suppose each partner had a 90% chance of being confined." If adding were the correct approach, the total probability would be 180%, which is impossible. According to the addition rule, all of the possible different prob-

abilities in a situation must add up to 1.0 (100%), no more and no less.

The addition rule is used to determine the probability of one thing being true under all possible conditions. For example, it may be used to determine the lifetime probability that the husband will be confined to a nursing home, taking into consideration that the wife may or may not be confined. In this case, the equation would be as follows: $p\{H+\} = p\{H+ \mid W+\} \times p\{W+\} + p\{H+ \mid W−\} \times p\{W−\}$. Box 12–5 shows the calculations for this formula, based on probabilities estimated from Kemper and Murtaugh (1991). Husbands have a lower probability of being in a nursing home than do wives, partly because wives are often younger and may take care of the husband at home, thus removing his need for a nursing home, and partly because women live longer and are more likely to reach the age at which many people require nursing home care.

Note that the numerator and the denominator of Bayes' theorem (see Chapter 8) are based on the general product rule and the addition rule, respectively.

SUMMARY

The most common reason biostatisticians are consulted is for help in calculating sample sizes needed for studies. Such help can be given only, however, if the investigator already has determined the basic numbers that will be used in the calculations: the level of alpha and beta to be used, the difference in outcome variables to be detected, and the variance expected. Determining the needed sample size is usually straightforward if these values are known. The equations commonly used are shown in Table 12–1.

Another process that is essential to much clinical research is random allocation. This is ordinarily not difficult to accomplish effectively if certain steps are followed carefully. It is especially important to keep the selection process secret until it is announced, and sealed envelopes are often a good way to achieve this. The basic methods of random allocation include simple random allocation, randomization into groups of two, systematic allocation, and stratified allocation.

In the analysis of data, investigators should be alert to the problem of multiple associations, which occurs when multiple hypotheses are tested. Without some statistical adjustment, testing multiple hypotheses increases the probability of false-positive statistical associations (alpha errors).

In the calculation of probabilities, three basic rules should be kept in mind: the independence rule, the product rule, and the addition rule. If the independence of two events can be assumed, then the probability of both events occurring jointly is the product of their separate probabilities. This is true whether the probability is that something will happen or that something will not happen.

BOX 12–5. Calculation of All Possible Probabilities of Husband and Wife Requiring or Not Requiring Care in a Nursing Home

Part 1. Definitions:

H+ = probability that the husband will require care in a nursing home at some time

H− = probability that the husband will not require care in a nursing home at some time

W+ = probability that the wife will require care in a nursing home at some time

W− = probability that the wife will not require care in a nursing home at some time

Part 2. Assumptions on which calculations are based:

(1) The following holds true if the wife does not require care in a nursing home: H+ = 0.3 and H− = 0.7

(2) The following holds true if the wife does require care in a nursing home: H+ = 0.4 and H− = 0.6

(3) The following holds true whether or not the husband requires care in a nursing home: W+ = 0.52 and W− = 0.48

Part 3. Calculations:

(1) Probability that neither the husband nor the wife will require care in a nursing home:

$$p\{\text{H}- \text{ and } \text{W}-\} = p\{\text{H}- \mid \text{W}-\} \times p\{\text{W}-\} = 0.7 \times 0.48 = \mathbf{0.336}$$

(2) Probability that both the husband and the wife will require care in a nursing home:

$$p\{\text{H}+ \text{ and } \text{W}+\} = p\{\text{H}+ \mid \text{W}+\} \times p\{\text{W}+\} = 0.4 \times 0.52 = \mathbf{0.208}$$

(3) Probability that the husband will require care and the wife will not require care in a nursing home:

$$p\{\text{H}+ \text{ and } \text{W}-\} = p\{\text{H}+ \mid \text{W}-\} \times p\{\text{W}-\} = 0.3 \times 0.48 = \mathbf{0.144}$$

(4) Probability that the husband will not require care and the wife will require care in a nursing home:

$$p\{\text{H}- \text{ and } \text{W}+\} = p\{\text{H}- \mid \text{W}+\} \times p\{\text{W}+\} = 0.6 \times 0.52 = \mathbf{0.312}$$

(5) Sum of the above probabilities (must always equal 1.00):

$$0.336 + 0.208 + 0.144 + 0.312 = \mathbf{1.00}$$

Note that, as it should, the sum of (1) and (3) equals the probability that the wife will not require care in a nursing home (0.336 + 0.144 = 0.48). Likewise, the sum of (2) and (4) equals the probability that the husband will not require care in a nursing home (0.208 + 0.312 = 0.52).

Source of data on which probability estimates are based: Kemper, P., and C. M. Murtaugh. Lifetime use of nursing home care. New England Journal of Medicine 324:595–560, 1991.

References Cited

Dawson-Saunders, B., and R. G. Trapp. Basic and Clinical Biostatistics, 2nd ed. Norwalk, Conn., Appleton and Lange, 1994.

Feinstein, A. R., et al. Coffee and pancreatic cancer: the problems of etiologic science and epidemiologic case-control research. Journal of the American Medical Association 246:957–961, 1981.

Freiman, J. A., et al. The importance of beta, the type II error, and sample size in the design and interpretation of the randomized control trial: a survey of 71 "negative" trials. New England Journal of Medicine 299:690–695, 1978.

Jekel, J. F. Should we stop using the p-value in descriptive studies? Pediatrics 60:124–126, 1977.

Jekel, J. F., et al. The regional educational impact of a renal stone center. Yale Journal of Biology and Medicine 56:97–108, 1983.

Kelsey, J. L., W. D. Thompson, and A. S. Evans. Methods in Observational Epidemiology. New York, Oxford University Press, 1986.

Kemper, P., and C. M. Murtaugh. Lifetime use of nursing home care. New England Journal of Medicine 324:595–600, 1991.

Lam, J. A., S. W. Hartwell, and J. F. Jekel. "I prayed real hard, so I know I'll get in": living with randomization. New Directions for Program Evaluation 63:55–66, 1994.

MacMahon, B., et al. Coffee and cancer of the pancreas. New England Journal of Medicine 304:630–633, 1981.

Paradise, J. L., et al. Efficacy of tonsillectomy for recurrent throat infection in severely affected children. New England Journal of Medicine 310:674–683, 1984.

Sackett, D. L., and M. Gent. Controversy in counting and attributing events in clinical trials. New England Journal of Medicine 301:1410–1412, 1979.

Selected Readings

Dawson-Saunders, B., and R. G. Trapp. Basic and Clinical Biostatistics, 2nd ed. Norwalk, Conn., Appleton and Lange, 1994.

Feinstein, A. R. The other side of "statistical significance": alpha, beta, delta, and the calculation of sample size. Clinical Pharmacology and Therapeutics 18:491–505, 1975.

Kelsey, J. L., W. D. Thompson, and A. S. Evans. Methods in Observational Epidemiology. New York, Oxford University Press, 1986.

CHAPTER THIRTEEN

MULTIVARIABLE ANALYSIS

AN OVERVIEW OF MULTIVARIABLE STATISTICS

However imperfect they may be, mathematical and statistical equations are attempts to model reality (Kac 1969). Statistical models often seek to represent only one dimension of reality, such as the effect of a change in one variable (e.g., a nutrient) on another variable (e.g., the growth rate of a rat). For such models to be meaningful, all factors other than the one being studied must be equalized in the research architecture, usually by randomization. Often, however, either the other influences cannot be adequately controlled by design or the investigator may actually wish to study the relative simultaneous influence of several independent (possibly causal) variables on a dependent (outcome) variable.

Statistical models that have one outcome variable but include more than one independent variable are generally called **multivariable models.** These models are intuitively attractive to investigators because they seem more true to life than the single-variable models. Multivariable analysis does not enable an investigator to ignore the basic principles of good research design and analysis, because multivariable analysis also has many limitations. The methodology and interpretation of findings in this type of analysis are difficult for most physicians, despite the fact that the methods and results of multivariable analysis are reported frequently in the medical literature and their use is increasing (Concato, Feinstein, and Holford 1993). Their conceptual attractiveness and the availability of high-speed computers contribute to making these methods popular. In order to be intelligent consumers of the medical literature, health care professionals should understand how to interpret the findings of multivariable analysis as they are presented in the literature.

A Conceptual Understanding of Equations

One of the reasons people "turn off" statistics is that the equations appear to be a jumble of meaningless symbols. That is especially true of multivariable techniques, but it is possible to understand conceptually, rather than mathematically, what is generally going on in multivariable analysis. For example, suppose that there is a study of the prognosis of patients at the time of diagnosis for a certain cancer for which there is not, as yet, an effective treatment. The physician might surmise that the length of survival for a patient would depend on at least four things: the patient's age, the anatomic stage of the disease at the time of diagnosis, the presence or absence of other diseases (comorbidity), and the degree of systemic symptoms such as weight loss. That relationship could be explained conceptually as follows:

$$\text{Cancer prognosis varies with Age and Stage and Comorbidity and Symptoms} \quad (13\text{--}1)$$

This statement could be made to look more mathematical simply by making a few slight changes:

$$\text{Cancer prognosis} \approx \text{Age} + \text{Stage} + \text{Comorbidity} + \text{Symptoms} \quad (13\text{--}2)$$

The four independent variables on the right side of the equation are not necessarily of equal importance. Expression 13–2 can be improved by giving each independent variable a **coefficient,** which is a **weighting factor** based on its relative importance in predicting prognosis. Thus, the equation becomes:

$$\text{Cancer prognosis} \approx (\text{Weight}_1)\,\text{Age} + (\text{Weight}_2)\,\text{Stage} + (\text{Weight}_3)\,\text{Comorbidity} + (\text{Weight}_4)\,\text{Symptoms} \quad (13\text{--}3)$$

Before equation 13–3 can become useful, two more things are needed. First, some sort of **anchor point** for the equation is needed. This anchor point must be something comparable to the a of the formula for simple regression ($y = a + bx$). Second, an **error term** is needed to make the equation true if the prediction is not perfect. By inserting the anchor point and the error term, the $\approx$ symbol (meaning "varies with") can be replaced by an equals sign. Abbreviating the weights with a W, the equation now becomes:

$$\text{Cancer prognosis} = \text{Anchor point} + W_1\text{Age} + W_2\text{Stage} + W_3\text{Comorbidity} + W_4\text{Symptoms} + \text{Error term} \quad (13\text{--}4)$$

In common statistical symbols, y is the dependent (outcome) variable (e.g., cancer prognosis) and is customarily placed on the left; $x_1 + x_2 + x_3 + x_4$ are the independent variables 1 (age) through 4 (symptoms), and they are lined up on the right; b_i is the statistical symbol for the weight of the ith independent variable; a is the estimated y-intercept (the anchor point); and e is the error term. Now, purely in statistical symbols, the equation can be expressed as follows:

$$y = a + b_1x_1 + b_2x_2 + b_3x_3 + b_4x_4 + e \quad (13\text{--}5)$$

Although equation 13–5 looks complex, it means exactly the same thing as equations 13–1 through 13–4.

Best Estimates

Equation 13–5 cannot be used to do any calculations, because the value for the error term (e) is not known until after the equation has been solved for a and all of the b's. Therefore, in multivariable statistics a further modification is made in the equation. Instead of y, the estimated value of y—namely, $\hat{y}$—is used, and there is no error term. (Because the estimate of y has a circumflex, or "hat," over it, it is usually called y-hat.) If the values of all of the observed y's and all of the x's are inserted, the following equation can be solved:

$$\hat{y} = a + b_1x_1 + b_2x_2 + b_3x_3 + b_4x_4 \quad (13\text{--}6)$$

When equation 13–6 is subtracted from equation 13–5, the following equation for the error term emerges:

$$(y - \hat{y}) = e \qquad (13\text{–}7)$$

The error term is the observed value of the outcome variable y for a given patient minus the predicted value of y for the same patient.

What happens to indicate when the best estimates of the values of a and b_i have been obtained? The best estimate has been achieved in this equation when the sum of the squared error term has been minimized. That sum is expressed as:

$$\sum(y_i - \hat{y})^2 = \sum(y_O - y_E)^2 = \sum e^2 \qquad (13\text{–}8)$$

This idea is not new, because as was noted in previous chapters, variation in statistics is measured as the sum of the squares of the observed value *(O)* minus the expected value *(E)*. In multivariable analysis, the error term e is often called a **residual.**

In straightforward language, the best estimates for the values of a and b_1 through b_4 are found when the total quantity of error (measured as the sum of squares of the error term, or, most simply, e^2) has been minimized. Those values of a and of the several b_i's which, taken together, give the smallest value for the squared error term are the best estimates that can be obtained from that set of data. Appropriately enough, this approach is called the **least-squares solution,** because the process is stopped when the sum of squares of the error term is the least.

The General Linear Model

The multivariable equation, with one dependent variable and one or more independent variables, as shown in equation 13–6, is usually called the general linear model. The model is "general" because there are many variations regarding the types of variables for y and x_i as well as the number of x variables that can be used. The model is "linear" because it is a linear combination of the x_i terms. For the x_i variables, a variety of transformations (e.g., square of x, cube of x, square root of x, or logarithm of x) could be used and the combination of terms would still be linear, so that the model would remain linear. What cannot happen if the model is to remain linear is for any of the coefficients (the b_i terms) to be a square, a square root, a logarithm, or another transformation.

Numerous procedures for multivariable analysis are based on the general linear model. These include methods with such imposing terms as analysis of variance (ANOVA), analysis of covariance (ANCOVA), multiple linear regression analysis, multiple logistic regression, the log-linear model, and discriminant function analysis. As discussed below, the choice of which procedure to use depends primarily on whether the dependent and independent variables are continuous, dichotomous, nominal, or ordinal. Knowing that the procedures are all variations of the same theme (the general linear model) helps to make them less confusing.

Uses of Multivariable Statistics

In some research, important findings can be presented more clearly in a contingency table (see Chapter 11) than by multivariable analysis. Sometimes, however, subtle findings and interactions could not have been discovered without multivariable analysis. One of the disadvantages of contingency tables compared to multivariable analysis is that unless the sample size is very large, the numbers in the cells of the final contingency tables might become very small. This is because controlling for other variables in contingency tables requires dividing the total sample size into many smaller tables containing subgroups. Multivariable analysis uses all of the observations in the analysis and therefore is often more efficient and robust than is contingency table analysis.

The usual purpose of multivariable analysis is to understand how important, both individually and when acting together, the independent variables are for explaining the variation in the dependent variable y. Often, there is considerable overlap in the ability of independent variables to explain the dependent variable. For example, both height and age predict body weight, but age and height are usually correlated; this is particularly true for the first two decades of life. During the growth years, height and weight both increase with age, so that age can be considered the underlying explanatory variable and height can be viewed as an intervening variable influencing weight. Children, however, grow at different rates, so that height would add explanatory power that age could not: those children who were tall for their age would, on the average, also be heavier than those children who were short for their age. Thus, each independent variable explains some of the variation in y beyond what any of the other variables explains.

Multivariable techniques also make it possible to determine whether there is an **interaction between variables.** Interaction is present when the value of one independent variable influences the way another independent variable explains y. In a large blood pressure survey in Connecticut, for example, Freeman et al. (1983) found that in black people under about 50 years of age, hypertension was more likely to occur in men than in women. After age 50, however, that trend was reversed, and hypertension was more likely to occur in women than in men. Thus, there was an interaction between age and gender in explaining the prevalence of hypertension.

In a clinical setting, such as an emergency room, it would be helpful to have some kind of scale or index that predicts whether or not a patient with chest pain is likely to have a myocardial infarction. One of several multivariable techniques can be used to develop such a **prediction model,** complete with coefficients for use in prediction. For example, Goldman et al. (1982) used a multivariable technique to develop a protocol to assist in the diagnosis of myocardial infarction in patients presenting to an emergency room with chest pain. Using various combinations of symptoms, signs, laboratory values, and electrocardiographic findings, the authors developed estimates for the probability of myocardial infarction. Multivariable analysis was also used by investigators in the Framingham Study to develop prediction equations for the 8-year risk of developing cardiovascular disease in people with various combinations of the following factors: smoking, elevated cholesterol levels, hypertension, glucose intolerance, and left ventricular hypertrophy (Breslow 1978). These prediction equations are now used in various health risk assessment programs.

If all goes well, the net effect of the complex calculations of multivariable analysis is that the investigators can determine which of the independent variables are the strongest predictors of *y* and which of the independent variables overlap with one another or interact in their ability to predict *y*.

PROCEDURES FOR MULTIVARIABLE ANALYSIS

As shown in Table 13–1, the choice of an appropriate statistical method for multivariable analysis depends on whether the dependent and independent variables are continuous, ordinal, dichotomous, or nominal. In cases in which more than one method could be used, the final choice will depend on the investigator's experience, personal preference, and comfort with the methods that are appropriate. Because there are many potential pitfalls in the use of multivariable techniques in medical research (see Concato, Feinstein, and Holford 1993), these techniques should not be used without experience or expert advice.

Analysis of Variance (ANOVA)

If the dependent variable is continuous and all of the independent variables are categorical (i.e., nominal, dichotomous, or ordinal), the correct multivariable technique is analysis of variance (ANOVA). One-way ANOVA and *N*-way ANOVA are discussed briefly below. Both techniques are based on the general linear model and can be used to analyze the results of an experimental design. If the design includes only one independent variable (e.g., treatment), the technique is called one-way analysis, regardless of how many different kinds of treatment (levels of analysis) are under consideration. If it includes more than one independent variable (e.g., treatment, age group, and gender), the technique is called *N*-way ANOVA.

One-Way ANOVA (The *F*-Test)

Suppose a team of investigators wanted to study the effects of drugs A and B on blood pressure. They might randomly allocate hypertensive patients into four treatment groups: those taking drug A alone,

TABLE 13–1. Choice of an Appropriate Procedure To Be Used in Multivariable Analysis (Analysis of One Dependent Variable and More Than One Independent Variable)

Characterization of Variables To Be Analyzed		Appropriate Procedure or Procedures
Dependent Variable	Independent Variables*	
Continuous	All are categorical.	Analysis of variance (ANOVA).
Continuous	Some are categorical and some are continuous.	Analysis of covariance (ANCOVA).
Continuous	All are continuous.	Multiple linear regression.
Ordinal	—	There is no formal multivariable procedure for ordinal dependent variables. Either treat the variables as if they were continuous (see above procedures) or perform log-linear analysis.
Dichotomous	All are categorical.	Logistic regression; log-linear analysis.
Dichotomous	Some are categorical and some are continuous.	Logistic regression.†
Dichotomous	All are continuous.	Logistic regression; discriminant function analysis.
Nominal	All are categorical.	Log-linear analysis.
Nominal	Some are categorical and some are continuous.	Group the continuous variables and perform log-linear analysis.
Nominal	All are continuous.	Discriminant function analysis; group the continuous variables and perform log-linear analysis.

*Categorical variables include ordinal, dichotomous, and nominal variables.
†If the outcome is a time-related dichotomous variable (such as live/die), then proportional-hazards (Cox) models are best.

those taking drug B alone, those taking drugs A and B in combination, and those taking a placebo. The investigators would measure systolic blood pressure before and after treatment in each patient and calculate a difference (posttreatment systolic pressure minus pretreatment systolic pressure). They would then calculate the mean difference for each group. The dependent (outcome) variable would therefore be the mean difference in systolic blood pressure.

The investigators would want to determine whether the difference in blood pressure found in one or more of the drug groups was large enough to be clinically important, assuming it was a drop. For example, a drop in mean systolic blood pressure from 150 mm Hg to 148 mm Hg would be too small to be clinically useful. If the results were not clinically useful, there would be little point in looking for an appropriate test of significance. If, however, one or more of the groups showed a clinically important drop in blood pressure, the investigators would want to determine whether the difference was likely to have occurred by chance alone. To do this, an appropriate statistical test of significance is needed.

The Student's t-test could be used to compare each pair of groups, but this would require six different t-tests: each of the three drug groups (A, B, and AB) versus the placebo group; drug A group versus drug B group; drug A group versus drug combination AB group; and drug B group versus drug combination AB group. This raises the problem of multiple hypotheses and multiple associations (see the discussion of alpha and p values under Dangers of Data Dredging in Chapter 12). Even if the investigators decided that the primary comparison should be each drug or drug combination with the placebo, this would still leave three hypotheses to test instead of just one. Moreover, if two or three groups did significantly better than the placebo group, it would be necessary to determine if one effective drug was significantly better than the others.

There are numerous complex ways of handling the problem of multiple associations (see Dawson-Saunders and Trapp 1994), but the best approach in cases such as this is to begin by performing an F-test, which is the first step of ANOVA. The F-test is a kind of "super t-test" that allows the investigators to compare more than two means simultaneously. The null hypothesis for the F-test is that the mean change in blood pressure $(\bar{d})$ will be the same for all four groups $(\bar{d}_1 = \bar{d}_2 = \bar{d}_3 = \bar{d}_4)$, indicating that all samples were from the same population and that any differences between the means are due to chance variation, rather than to true differences.

In creating the F-test (F is for Fisher), Sir Ronald Fisher reasoned that if two different methods could be found to estimate the variance and if all of the samples came from the same population, these two different estimates of variance should be similar. He therefore developed two measures of the variance of the observations. One is called **between-groups variance** and is based on the variation between (or among) the means. The other is called **within-groups variance** and is based on the variation within each group—i.e., variation around a single group mean. In ANOVA, these two measures of variance are also called the **between-groups mean square** and the **within-groups mean square.** (Mean square is simply another name for variance, which is defined as a sum of squares, or SS, divided by the appropriate number of degrees of freedom, or df.) The ratio of the two measures can therefore be expressed as follows:

$$F \text{ ratio} = \frac{\text{Between-groups variance}}{\text{Within-groups variance}} = \frac{\text{Between-groups mean square}}{\text{Within-groups mean square}}$$

If the F ratio is fairly close to 1.0, the two estimates of variance are similar, and the null hypothesis that all of the means came from the same underlying population is not rejected. If the ratio is much larger than 1.0, there must have been some force, attributable to group differences, pushing the means apart, and the null hypothesis of no difference is rejected.

The assumptions for the F-test are similar to those for the t-test. First, the dependent variable (in this case, blood pressure values) should be normally distributed, although with large samples this assumption can be relaxed because of the central limit theorem. Second, the several samples of the dependent variable should be independent random samples from populations with approximately equal variances. As with the t-test, the F-test requires that an alpha level be specified in advance. After the F statistic has been calculated, its p value can be looked up in a table of the F distribution to determine whether the results are statistically significant.

If the results of the F-test are not statistically significant, either the null hypothesis must be accepted or the study must be repeated using a larger sample. However, if the results are statistically significant, the investigators must take additional steps to determine which of the differences in means are the "true" differences. In the case of the example introduced earlier, involving four treatment groups (drug A alone, drug B alone, drugs A and B combined, and placebo), statistical significance could be found if any of the following were true: (1) the mean of one group differed greatly from that of the other three groups; (2) the means of two groups differed greatly from those of the remaining two groups; or (3) the means of the four groups were strung along a line representing values of the mean systolic blood pressures—for example, with drugs A and B combined showing the best results, drug A showing the second best, drug B showing the third best, and the placebo showing the worst.

Most advanced statistical computer packages include a program for ANOVA, allowing investigators to determine which of the differences are the "true" differences in cases such as this. While a detailed discussion of the various methods is beyond the scope of this book, it is important for readers to understand the logic behind this form of analysis and to recognize the circumstances under which one-way ANOVA is appropriate. As an example, Pearlman et al. (1992) performed a clinical trial in which asthma patients were randomized into three treatment groups: one that received 42 µg of salmeterol two times daily, one that received 180 µg of albuterol four times daily, and one that received a placebo. At the beginning and end of the study, the investigators measured the asthma patients' forced expiratory volume in 1 second (FEV_1), and they then used F-tests to compare the changes in FEV_1 values seen in the three different treatment groups. Based on the results of one-way ANOVA, they concluded that salmeterol was more effective than albuterol or placebo in increasing the morning peak expiratory flow rate.

N-Way ANOVA

The goal of ANOVA, stated in the simplest terms, is to explain (to "model") the total variation found in a study.

If only *one* independent variable is tested in a model and that variable happens to be gender, as shown in Box 13–1, the total amount of variation must be explained in terms of how much variation is due to gender and how much is not. Anything that is not due to gender is considered to be error (residual).

If *two* independent variables are tested in a model and those variables happen to be treatment and gender, the total amount of variation must be explained in terms of how much variation is due to each of the following: the independent effect of treatment, the independent effect of gender, the interaction between (joint effect of) treatment and gender, and error. If *more than two* independent variables are tested, the analysis becomes increasingly complicated, but the underlying logic remains the same. As long as the research design is balanced—that is, there are equal numbers of observations in all of the study groups—ANOVA can be used to analyze the individual and joint effects of the independent variables and to partition the total variation into the various component parts. Numerous computer programs are available to test significance using the *F*-test and to perform subsequent calculations of formulas based on the general linear model described earlier in this chapter.

An example in which *N*-way ANOVA procedures were used is the study performed by Finkelstein et al. (1994) to determine whether supplementing gonadotropin-releasing hormone (GnRH) with parathyroid hormone (PTH) would reduce the osteoporosis-causing effect of GnRH. In this study, the investigators used ANOVA to examine the effects of treatment and other independent variables on bone loss induced by estrogen deficiency.

Analysis of Covariance (ANCOVA)

As shown in Table 13–1, ANOVA and ANCOVA are methods for evaluating studies in which the dependent variable is continuous. If the independent variables are all of the categorical type (nominal or dichotomous), then ANOVA is used. If some of the independent variables are categorical and some are continuous, however, then ANCOVA is appropriate. ANCOVA would be used, for example, in a study in which the goal is to test the effects of antihypertensive drugs on systolic blood pressure (a continuous variable that is the dependent variable here). The independent variables are age (a continuous variable) and treatment (a categorical variable with four levels—i.e., those treated with drug A, those treated

---

BOX 13–1. The Analysis of Variance (ANOVA) Table

The goal of ANOVA, stated in the simplest terms, is to explain (i.e., to model) the total variation found in a study. Because the total variation is equal to the sum of squares (SS), the process of explaining total variation is a process that entails partitioning the SS into component parts. The logic behind this process was introduced in Chapter 10 (see Variation between Groups versus Variation within Groups), and the discussion there focused on the example of explaining the difference between the heights of men and women. In the example, the heights of 100 female and 100 male university students were measured, the total variation was found to be 10,000 cm^2, and 4,000 cm^2 of the variation was attributed to gender. Because that example is uncomplicated and involves round numbers, it is used here to illustrate the format for an ANOVA table.

Source of Variation	Sum of Squares (SS)	Degrees of Freedom *(df)*	Mean Square (MS)	*F* Ratio
TOTAL	10,000	199		
Model (gender)	4,000	1	4,000.0	132.0
Error	6,000	198	30.3	

The model in this example has only one independent variable—namely, gender, a dichotomous variable.

In the column labeled sum of the squares (SS), the figure of 4,000 represents the amount of variation due to gender (i.e., the between-groups variation noted in the ANOVA), while 6,000 represents the amount of variation due to error (i.e., the within-groups variation).

In the column labeled degrees of freedom *(df)*, the total *df* is listed as 199, reflecting the fact that there were 200 subjects and 1 *df* was lost in calculating the grand mean for all observations. The *df* for the model is calculated as the number of categories minus 1. Gender has only two categories (men and women), so 1 *df* is assigned to it. The *df* for error is calculated as the total *df* minus the number of *df* assigned to the model: 199 − 1 = 198.

The mean square (MS) is simply another name for variance and is equal to the SS divided by the appropriate *df*: 4,000/1 = 4,000.0, and 6,000/198 = 30.3.

The *F* ratio is calculated by dividing the model mean square by the error mean square: 4,000.0/30.3 = 132.0. Because the *F* ratio is so large, the *p* value would be extremely small ($p < 0.00001$), and the null hypothesis that there is no true difference between the mean heights of men and women would be rejected.

Note that if there was more than one independent variable in the model being analyzed, there would be more entries under the column labeled source of variation: TOTAL, model, interaction, and error. Interaction would refer to the portion of the variation that is due to interactions between the independent variables in the model. Error would then be defined as the variation not explained by any of the independent variables or their interactions.

with drug B, those treated with both A and B, and those treated with a placebo).

The ANCOVA procedure adjusts the dependent variable on the basis of the continuous independent variable or variables, and it then does an *N*-way ANOVA on the **adjusted dependent variable.** In the above example, the ANCOVA procedure would remove the effect of age from the analysis of the effect of the drugs on systolic blood pressure. Controlling for age means that (artificially) all of the study subjects are made the same age. Suppose that the mean systolic blood pressure in the study group is 150 mm Hg at an average age of 50 years. The first step (and this is all done by the computer packages that have ANCOVA) is to do a simple regression between age and blood pressure, which shows that the blood pressure increases, say, an average of 1 mm Hg for each year of age over 50 years and decreases an average of 1 mm Hg for each year of age under 50. Thus, if a subject's age is 59, then 9 mm Hg would be subtracted from that subject's current blood pressure to arrive at the adjusted blood pressure. If another subject's age is 35, then 15 mm Hg would be added to that subject's current blood pressure to arrive at the adjusted value. If a subject's age is 50, no adjustment is necessary, because that subject is already at the population mean age. ANCOVA can adjust the dependent variable for several continuous independent variables (called covariates) at the same time.

Stacpoole et al. (1992) used ANCOVA to evaluate the results of a controlled clinical trial of dichloroacetate for treatment of lactic acidosis in adults. ANCOVA adjusted the dependent variable for the pretreatment concentrations of arterial blood lactate in the study subjects, before the treatments were compared.

Multiple Linear Regression

If the dependent variable and all of the independent variables are continuous, the correct type of multivariable analysis is multiple linear regression. The formula looks like the general linear model formula as shown above in equation 13–6. Here, the intercept is really the mean of *y*, and each of the independent variables improves the prediction somewhat (depending on its strength of association).

There are several computerized methods of analyzing the data in a multiple linear regression. Probably the most common method is called stepwise linear regression. The investigator either chooses which variable to begin with (i.e., to enter first in the analysis) or else instructs the computer to start by entering the one variable that has the strongest association with the dependent variable. In either case, when only the first variable has entered, the result is a simple regression analysis. Next, the second variable is entered according to the investigator's instructions. The explanatory strength of the variable entered—that is, the r^2 (see Chapter 11)—changes as each new variable is entered. The "step-

ping" continues until none of the remaining independent variables meets the predetermined criterion for being entered (e.g., *p* is ≤ 0.1 or the increase in r^2 is ≥ 0.01) or until all of the variables have been entered. When the stepping stops, the analysis is complete.

In addition to watching for the statistical significance of the overall equation and of each variable entered, the investigator keeps a close watch on the overall r^2 for each step, which is the proportion of variation the model has explained so far. In multiple regression equations that are statistically significant, the r^2 indicates how much of the variation is being explained by the variable entered.

Multiple linear regression is not used very often in clinical medicine, but it is frequently used in health services research. For example, the dependent variable in such research may be the amount of profit (or loss) in dollars for a hospital over a time period such as a year. The independent variables are often such factors as the average length of stay, the bed occupancy rate, and the proportion of patients who require surgical care.

Other Procedures for Multivariable Analysis

Other major multivariable procedures include **logistic regression, log-linear analysis,** and **discriminant function analysis.** Like the procedures discussed above, these too are forms of the general linear model and function in an analogous manner. Their uses are outlined in Table 13–1.

If the dependent variable in a study is a dichotomous variable, logistic regression is the most powerful technique available. In medicine, the most commonly used form of logistic regression is the proportional-hazards (Cox) method. This is used to test for differences between Kaplan-Meier survival curves while controlling for other variables. It is also used to determine which variables are associated with better survival. Logistic regression was used, for example, by O'Connell et al. (1994) to compare the relapse-free survival of two groups of patients with rectal cancer: those treated with radiation plus a protracted infusion of fluorouracil and those given a bolus injection of fluorouracil. The patients treated with the combination of radiation and fluorouracil had a statistically lower rate of tumor recurrence, and the Cox analysis showed that increased age, greater lymph node involvement, and a higher tumor grade were associated with a shorter relapse-free time.

SUMMARY

Multivariable analysis is a statistical method of determining how well several independent (possibly causal) variables, both separately and together, explain the variation in a single dependent (outcome) variable.

In medical research, there are three common uses of multivariable analysis. The first is to improve the test of a hypothesis in a clinical trial by controlling for the joint effects of independent variables on the dependent variable. The second is to shed light on the etiology of a disease by estimating the relative impact that several independent variables have on the disease. The third is to develop weights for the different variables used in a diagnostic or prognostic scoring system.

As shown in Table 13–1, the choice of an appropriate procedure to be used in multivariable analysis depends on whether the dependent and independent variables are continuous, dichotomous, nominal, ordinal, or a combination of these. Because there are many potential problems and pitfalls in the use of multivariable techniques in clinical research, these procedures should be used with care.

References Cited

Breslow, L. Risk factor intervention for health maintenance. Science 200:908–912, 1978.

Concato, J., A. R. Feinstein, and T. Holford. The risk of determining risk with multivariable models. Annals of Internal Medicine 118:201–210, 1993.

Dawson-Saunders, B., and R. G. Trapp. Basic and Clinical Biostatistics, 2nd ed. Norwalk, Conn., Appleton and Lange, 1994.

Finkelstein, J. S., et al. Parathyroid hormone for the prevention of bone loss induced by estrogen deficiency. New England Journal of Medicine 331:1618–1623, 1994.

Freeman, D. H., Jr., et al. The prevalence distribution of hypertension: Connecticut adults, 1978–1979. Journal of Chronic Disease 36:171–181, 1983.

Goldman, L., et al. A computer-driven protocol to aid in the diagnosis of emergency room patients with acute chest pain. New England Journal of Medicine 307:588–596, 1982.

Kac, M. Some mathematical models in science. Science 166:695–699, 1969.

O'Connell, M. J., et al. Improving adjuvant therapy for rectal cancer by combining protracted-infusion fluorouracil with radiation therapy after curative surgery. New England Journal of Medicine 331:502–507, 1994.

Pearlman, D. S., et al. A comparison of salmeterol with albuterol in the treatment of mild-to-moderate asthma. New England Journal of Medicine 327:1420–1425, 1992.

Stacpoole, P. W., et al. A controlled clinical trial of dichloroacetate for treatment of lactic acidosis in adults. New England Journal of Medicine 327:1564–1569, 1992.

Selected Readings

Dawson-Saunders, B., and R. G. Trapp. Basic and Clinical Biostatistics, 2nd ed. Norwalk, Conn., Appleton and Lange, 1994. [Tests for multiple comparisons.]

Freeman, D. L., Jr. Applied Categorical Data Analysis. New York, Marcel Dekker, 1987. [Advanced text.]

Kleinbaum, D. G., and L. L. Kupper. Applied Regression Analysis and Other Multivariable Methods. North Scituate, Mass., Duxbury Press, 1978. [Moderately advanced text.]

SECTION III

PREVENTIVE MEDICINE AND PUBLIC HEALTH

CHAPTER FOURTEEN

INTRODUCTION TO PREVENTIVE

MEDICINE

BASIC CONCEPTS

The fields of preventive medicine and public health share the goals of preventing specific diseases, promoting health, and applying the concepts and techniques of epidemiology toward these goals. While preventive medicine seeks to enhance the lives of individuals by helping them enhance their own health, public health attempts to promote health in populations through the application of organized community efforts. Although preventive medicine and public health are discussed somewhat separately here, there should be a seamless continuum between the practice of preventive medicine by physicians and other health professionals, the attempts of individuals and families to promote their own and their neighbors' health, and the efforts of governments and voluntary agencies to achieve the same health goals.

By traditionally focusing on the diagnosis and treatment of disease, Western medical education and medical practice have tended to obscure the importance, scientific basis, and clinical process of promoting the overall health of individuals. Diagnosis and treatment of disease will always be important aspects of health care, but increasing emphasis now is also being placed on the preservation and enhancement of health. There are specialists who undertake research, teaching, and clinical practice in the field of preventive medicine, but prevention is no more the exclusive province of preventive medicine specialists than, for example, the care of older people is limited to geriatricians. On the contrary, prevention should be incorporated into the practice of all physicians and other health care providers.

Health

Health is more difficult to define than is disease. Perhaps the best-known definition of health comes from the preamble to the constitution of the World Health Organization: "Health is a state of complete physical, mental, and social well-being and not merely the absence of disease or infirmity." This definition has the strengths of recognizing that any meaningful concept of health must include all the dimensions of human life and that such a definition must be positive (i.e., "not merely the absence of disease or infirmity"). Nevertheless, the definition has been criticized for two weaknesses. It is too idealistic in its expectations for complete well-being, and it is too static in viewing health as a state rather than as a dynamic process that requires constant effort and activity to maintain.

Successful Adaptation

Decades ago, it was pointed out that "the states of health or disease are the expressions of the success or failure experienced by the organism in its efforts to respond adaptively to environmental challenges" (Dubos 1965:xvii). Those who developed many of the concepts of **stress** that are used today correctly understood that different stressors could induce helpful and harmful forms of stress ("eustress" and "dystress"). That is, good health requires the presence of eustress and also the limitation of dystress to a level to which the organism can adapt (Selye 1973). Even though the body may adapt successfully to environmental stressors in the short term, if continual major adaptation is required, it may exact a serious toll on the body, particularly the neural, neuroendocrine, and immune systems. The ongoing level of demand for adaptation in an individual is called the **allostatic load** on that person, and it may be an important contributor to many chronic diseases (McEwen and Stellar 1993).

Satisfactory Functioning

Often what matters most to people is how they function in their environment. The inability to function will bring many people to a doctor more quickly than the presence of discomfort per se: "Clearly, health and disease cannot be defined merely in terms of anatomical, physiological, or mental attributes. Their real measure is the ability of the individual to function in a manner acceptable to himself and to the group of which he is a part" (Dubos 1961:214).

However health is defined, it derives principally from forces other than medical care. Appropriate nutrition, adequate shelter, a nonthreatening environment, and a prudent life-style contribute far more to health and well-being than does the medical care system. Nevertheless, medicine contributes to health both directly through patient care and indirectly through the development and dissemination of knowledge.

MEASURES OF HEALTH STATUS

Historically, measures of health status have been based primarily on **mortality data** (see Chapter 2). Researchers assumed that a low age-adjusted death rate and a high life expectancy reflected good health in a population. Currently, a higher proportion of the population lives to old age than ever before, and this group accumulates various chronic and disabling illnesses. Consequently, health care investigators and practitioners have increasingly expressed dissatisfaction with using mortality data as the sole index for the overall level of health in a population and have also shown an increased concern with improving the **health-related quality of life.** Unfortunately, much more research needs to be done before quality of life can be adequately measured (Gill and Feinstein 1994). An appropriate societal goal is for people to age in a healthy manner, with minimal disability until shortly before death (Fries and Crapo 1981).

Considerable research effort now goes into the development of **health status indexes.** In their 1987 book, McDowell and Newell include many of the available scales and questionnaires for measuring the degree of functioning and the quality of life in individuals. Most of the indexes require that each subject complete some form of questionnaire, and most do not incorporate mortality data. Many health status measures seek to adjust life expectancy on the basis of morbidity, the perceived quality of life, or both. One example of the measures used is "quality-adjusted life years" (see Last 1988), and another example is "healthy life expectancy" or just "health expectancy" (see Barendregt et al. 1994).

Life expectancy is traditionally defined as the average number of years of life remaining at a given age. **Quality-adjusted life years** (QALY) incorporates both life expectancy and the perceived impact of illness and disability on the quality of life. People who have had a stroke and now suffer from hemiparesis, for example, may be asked to estimate how many years of life with their disability (limited years) would be equal to 1 year of life with good health (healthy years). If the answer is that 2 limited years is equivalent to 1 healthy year, a year of life following a stroke might be given a weight of 0.5. If 3 limited years were equivalent to 1 healthy year, each limited year would contribute 0.33 years to the QALY. Some people might consider being confined to a nursing home and unable to speak (as occurs with some strokes) to be as bad as or worse than no life at all, and, if so, the weighting factor would be 0.0 for such years.

Healthy life expectancy is a somewhat less subjective measure that attempts to combine both mortality and morbidity into one index. The index reflects the number of years of life remaining that are expected to be free of serious disease. The onset of a serious disease with permanent sequelae—for example, a stroke with serious permanent residual effects—reduces the index as much as if the person who has the sequelae had died from the disease.

Other indexes combine several measures of health status. For example, the **General Well-Being Adjustment Scale** is an index that measures "anxiety, depression, general health, positive well-being, self-control, and vitality" (Revicki et al. 1994). Another index is called the **Life Expectancy Free of Disability,** which is just what the name suggests. The US Centers for Disease Control and Prevention (CDC) developed an index called the **Health Related Quality of Life** (HR-QOL) based on data from the Behavioral Risk Factor Surveillance System (BRFSS) (see Centers for Disease Control and Prevention 1994). Using the BRFSS, investigators found that 86.6% of adults in the USA considered their health to be good to excellent. They also found that the mean number of good health days—i.e., the number of days free of both physical and mental health problems during the 30-day period preceding the interview—was 24.8 days in the adults surveyed (see Centers for Disease Control and Prevention 1995).

THE NATURAL HISTORY OF DISEASE

Rather than being viewed as static concepts, disease and illness should be viewed as dynamic concepts. According to Leavell and Clark (1965), variations are seen in the natural histories of different diseases, depending on whether the "disease-producing stimuli arise in the environment or within man." If the disease is an **infectious disease,** there are reasons why the causative organism was present in the patient's environment, why the patient was exposed to the organism, and why the patient was or was not resistant to the organism. If the disease is a **noninfectious disease,** such as atherosclerosis leading to myocardial infarction, there may be multiple **risk factors** present in the patient's genotype, nutrition, life-style, and environment. The risk factors may interact with one another to modify the risk that would be expected by simple addition of the contributions of individual risk factors (see Chapter 4).

In the case of myocardial infarction, risk factors include male gender, a family history of myocardial infarction or other illnesses (e.g., diabetes mellitus and hypertension), elevated serum lipid levels, a high-fat diet, cigarette smoking, sedentary life-style, and advancing age. Genotype is only one of many factors influencing the composition of serum lipids and the development of atherosclerosis. The speed with which coronary atherosclerosis develops in an individual will be modified not only by the diet but also by the pattern of physical activity over the course of a lifetime. Hypertension may accelerate the development of atherosclerosis, and it also may lead to increased myocardial oxygen demand, thus precipitating infarction earlier than it otherwise might have occurred and also making recovery more difficult.

LEVELS OF PREVENTION

A useful concept of prevention that was developed or at least popularized by Hugh Leavell (see Leavell and Clark 1965) has come to be known as **Leavell's levels.** Based on this concept, all of the activities of physicians and other health professionals have the goal of prevention. There are three levels of prevention, as shown in Table 14–1 and described below. What is to be prevented depends on the stage of health or disease in the individual receiving preventive care. **Primary prevention** keeps the disease process from becoming established by eliminating causes of disease or increasing resistance to disease (see Chapters 15 and 16). **Secondary prevention** interrupts the disease process before it becomes

TABLE 14–1. Modified Version of Leavell's Levels of Prevention*

Stage of Disease	Level of Prevention	Type of Response
Predisease	Primary prevention	Health promotion and specific protection.
Latent disease	Secondary prevention	Presymptomatic diagnosis and treatment.
Symptomatic disease	Tertiary prevention	Disability limitation for early symptomatic disease. Rehabilitation for late symptomatic disease.

*Modified from Leavell, H. R., and E. G. Clark. Preventive Medicine for the Doctor in His Community, 3rd ed. New York, McGraw-Hill Book Company, 1965. Although Leavell originally categorized disability limitation under secondary prevention, both in Europe and in the USA it has become customary to classify it as tertiary prevention because it involves the management of symptomatic disease.

symptomatic (see Chapter 17). **Tertiary prevention** limits the physical and social consequences of symptomatic disease (see Chapter 18).

Primary Prevention and Predisease

Most noninfectious diseases can be seen as having an early stage, during which the causal factors will start to produce physiologic abnormalities. In atherosclerosis, for example, there may be high levels of low-density lipoprotein (LDL) and very low density lipoprotein (VLDL) in the blood but no signs of atheroma during the predisease stage. The goal at this time is to modify risk factors in a favorable direction. Life-modifying activities, such as changing to a low-fat diet, pursuing a consistent program of aerobic exercise, and ceasing to smoke cigarettes, are considered to be methods of primary prevention because they are aimed at keeping the pathologic process from occurring.

Health Promotion

Health-promoting activities usually contribute to the prevention of a variety of diseases as well as enhancing a positive feeling of health and vigor. They consist of nonmedical changes, such as changes in life-style, nutrition, and the environment. Such activities may require structural changes in society to enable the majority of people to take part in them. Structural changes involve societal changes that make healthy choices easier. For example, dietary modification may be difficult unless a variety of low-fat, low-salt, low-sugar, yet tasty and nutrient-rich foods are available in stores. Exercise will be more difficult if bicycling or jogging is a risky activity because of automobile traffic or social violence. Even more basic to health promotion is the assurance of the basic necessities of life, including freedom from poverty, environmental pollution, and violence.

Health promotion applies both to noninfectious diseases and to infectious diseases. Infectious diseases are reduced in frequency and seriousness where the water is pure, liquid and solid wastes are disposed of in a sanitary manner, and arthropod and animal vectors of disease are controlled. Crowding promotes the spread of infectious diseases, whereas adequate housing and working environments tend to minimize the spread of disease. In the barracks of soldiers, for example, even a technique as simple as requiring some soldiers to sleep with their pillows at the head of the bed and others to sleep with their pillows at the foot of the bed, in an alternating pattern, can reduce the spread of respiratory diseases because it doubles the distance between noses during sleeping time.

Specific Protection

If health-promoting changes in environment, nutrition, and behavior are not fully effective, it may be necessary to employ what Leavell called specific protection. This form of primary prevention is targeted at a specific disease or type of injury. Examples include immunization against poliomyelitis; pharmacologic treatment of hypertension to limit end-organ damage; use of ear-protecting devices in loud working environments, such as around jet airplanes; and use of seat belts, air bags, and helmets to prevent bodily injuries in automobile and motorcycle crashes. Some measures provide specific protection while also contributing to the more general goal of health promotion. Fluoridation of water supplies, for example, not only prevents dental caries but is a nutritional intervention that promotes stronger bones and teeth.

Secondary Prevention and Latent Disease

Sooner or later, depending on the individual, a disease process such as coronary artery atherosclerosis will progress far enough to become detectable by medical tests, even though the individual is still asymptomatic. This may be thought of as the latent (hidden) stage of disease.

For many infectious and noninfectious diseases, the development of screening tests has made it possible to detect latent disease in individuals considered to be at high risk. Presymptomatic diagnosis and treatment through screening programs is referred to as secondary prevention because it is the secondary line of defense against disease. Although it does not prevent the cause from initiating the disease process, it may prevent permanent sequelae.

Tertiary Prevention and Symptomatic Disease

When disease has become symptomatic and medical assistance is sought, the goal of the clinician is to provide tertiary prevention in the form of disability limitation for patients with early symptomatic disease or in the form of rehabilitation for patients with late symptomatic disease.

Disability Limitation

Disability limitation is the term used by Leavell to describe medical and surgical measures aimed at correcting the anatomic and physiologic components of disease in symptomatic patients. The majority of care provided by physicians meets this description. It can be considered prevention because its goal is to halt the disease process and thereby prevent or limit the impairment (disability) caused by it. An example is the surgical removal of a tumor, which may prevent any further local invasion.

Rehabilitation

Rehabilitation is the last of Leavell's levels. Although many people are surprised to see rehabilitation considered a form of prevention, it is designed to mitigate the effects of disease and thereby prevent it from resulting in total social and functional disability. For example, a person who has been injured or who has suffered a stroke may be taught how to care for himself or herself in the **activities of daily living** (feeding, bathing, and so forth). This may enable him or her to avoid the adverse sequelae associated with prolonged inactivity (e.g., increasing muscle weakness and total disability).

Rehabilitation of a stroke patient begins with frequent mobilization of all joints during the period of maximum paralysis. This permits recovery of limb use, rather than the development of stiff joints and flexion contractures. Physical therapy helps the stroke patient to strengthen remaining muscle function and to use this remaining function to maximum effect in performing the activities of daily life. It is legitimate, therefore, to view rehabilitation as a form of prevention.

THE ECONOMICS OF PREVENTION

In an era of cost consciousness, there are increasing demands that health promotion and disease prevention be proven economically worthwhile either by means of **cost-benefit analysis** or by means of **cost-effectiveness analysis** (see Box 14–1). Although most people believe it makes sense to invest resources to maintain health and prevent disease, there are numerous factors that make it difficult to demonstrate that special programs devoted to these goals produce benefits that are greater than or equal to the associated costs (Russell 1986).

Demonstration of Benefits

Scientific proof of benefits may be difficult because it is often unpractical or unethical to undertake randomized trials using people as subjects. For example, it is not possible to randomly assign people to smoking and nonsmoking groups. Therefore, apart from some research done on animal models, investigators are limited to observational studies, which usually are not as convincing as experiments. Moreover, life is filled with risks for one disease or another, and many of these operate together to produce the levels of health observed in a population. These risks may be changing in frequency in different subpopulations, making it impossible to infer what proportion of the benefits observed over time in, say, the incidence of lung cancer is due to smoking reduction programs and what proportion is due to the elimination of smoking in workplaces and public areas, the increase in public awareness of (and action against) the presence of radon in homes, and other factors as yet poorly understood.

BOX 14–1.   Cost-Benefit and Cost-Effectiveness Analysis

Cost-benefit analysis measures the costs and the benefits of a proposed course of action in terms of the same units, usually monetary units such as dollars. For example, a cost-benefit analysis of a poliomyelitis immunization program would determine the number of dollars to be spent toward vaccines, equipment, personnel, and so forth, to immunize a particular population. It then would determine the number of dollars that would be saved by not having to pay for the hospitalizations, medical visits, and lost productivity that would occur if poliomyelitis were not prevented in that population.

It is difficult to incorporate ideas such as the dollar value of life, suffering, and the quality of life into such an analysis. However, cost-benefit analysis is useful if a particular budgetary entity (such as a government or business) is trying to determine whether the investment of resources in health would save money in the long run. It is also useful if a particular entity with a fixed budget is trying to make informed judgments concerning allocations in various sectors (health, transportation, education, and so forth) and to determine the sector in which an investment would produce the greatest economic benefit.

Cost-effectiveness analysis provides a way of comparing different proposed solutions in terms of the most appropriate measurement units. For example, by measuring hepatitis B cases prevented, deaths prevented, and life-years saved per 10,000 population, Bloom et al. (1993) were able to compare the effectiveness of four different strategies of dealing with the hepatitis B virus: (1) no vaccination; (2) universal vaccination; (3) screening followed by vaccination of unprotected individuals; and (4) a combination of the screening of pregnant women at delivery, the vaccination of the newborns of women found to be antibody-positive during screening, and the routine vaccination of all 10-year-old children.

After Bloom et al. estimated the numbers of persons involved in each step of each method, they determined the costs of screening, of purchasing and administering the vaccine, and of medical care for various forms and complications of hepatitis. They calculated that the fourth strategy would have an undiscounted cost of about $367 (or a discounted cost of $1205) per case of hepatitis B prevented, and they concluded that this was clearly the strategy with the lowest cost.

The concept of **discounting**, which is important in business and finance, must also be used in medical cost-benefit and cost-effectiveness analysis when the costs are incurred in the present but the benefits will occur some time in the future. Discounting is a reduction in the present value of delayed benefits (or an increase in their present costs) to account for the time value of money. If the administrators of a prevention program spend $1000 now to save $1000 of expenses in the future, they will take a net loss. This is because they will lose the use of $1000 in the interim and also because of the effects of inflation (the $1000 eventually saved will not be worth as much as the $1000 initially spent). Discounting attempts to adjust for these forces.

To discount a cost-benefit or cost-effectiveness analysis, the easiest way is to increase the present costs by a yearly factor, which can be thought of as the interest that would have to be paid in order to borrow the prevention money until the benefits occurred. For example, if it costs $1000 today to prevent a disease that would have occurred 20 years in the future, the present cost can be multiplied by $(1 + r)^n$, where r is the yearly interest rate for borrowing and n is the number of years until the benefit is realized. If the average yearly interest rate is 5% over 20 years, the formula becomes: $(1 + 0.05)^{20} = (1.05)^{20} = 2.653$. When this is multiplied by the present cost of $1000, the result is $2653. Thus, the expected savings 20 years in the future from a $1000 investment today would have to be greater than $2653 in order for the initial investment to be a financial gain.

Delay of Benefits

With most preventive programs, there is a long delay between the time that the preventive measures are instituted and the time that positive health changes become visible. For example, because the latent period (incubation period) for lung cancer caused by cigarette smoking is 20 years or more, investments made now in smoking reduction programs may not be clearly identified until 20 or more years have passed. There are similar delays between the time of smoking cessation and the demonstration of effect for other smoking-related cancers and for chronic obstructive pulmonary disease.

Accrual of Benefits

Even if a given program could be shown to produce meaningful economic benefit, it is critical to know where the benefits would accrue. For example, a financially stressed health insurance plan or health maintenance organization might cover a preventive measure if the financial benefit were fairly certain to be as great as or greater than the cost of the program and if most or all of this financial benefit would accrue to the insurance plan. If most of the financial benefit would go to the enrollees rather than to the insurance plan, the prevention program would be seen as only a financial cost by the insurance plan.

The same principle is true for even more financially strapped government budgets, such as local, state, and federal budgets. If the savings from prevention efforts would go directly to taxpayers, rather than to the government budget, the elected representatives might not support the prevention effort, even if the benefits clearly outweighed the costs. Moreover, elected representatives seek to show results before the next election campaign. Disease prevention often shows results only over an extended time period (e.g., 20 years) and therefore does not lend itself to political popularity.

Discounting

Discounting (see Box 14–1) is another reason that prevention may show a lower benefit-cost ratio than expected. If a preventive effort is made now by a government body, the costs are present costs, but the savings may not be evident until many years later. Even if the savings are expected to accrue to the same budgetary unit that provided the money for the preventive program, the delay in economic return means that the benefits are worth less to that unit now. In the jargon of economists, the present value of the benefits must be discounted, making it more difficult to demonstrate cost-effectiveness or a positive benefit-cost ratio.

Priorities

As the saying goes, the squeaky wheel is the one that gets greased. Current, obvious problems usually attract far more attention and concern than future, subtle problems. Emergency care for victims of motor vehicle crashes is easy to justify, regardless of costs. Even though prevention may be far more cost-effective, it is difficult to justify money for medical crises that have not yet appeared. The same dilemma applies to essentially every phase of life. It is difficult to get money for programs to prevent the loss of topsoil, to prevent illiteracy, and to prevent the decay of roads and bridges. Even on an individual level, many patients will not want to make changes in fundamental aspects of their lives, such as eating a healthier diet, exercising, and stopping smoking, because the risk of future problems does not speak to them urgently in the present.

SUMMARY

Preventive medicine seeks to enhance the lives of patients by helping them promote their own health and prevent specific diseases. Preventive medicine also tries to apply the concepts and techniques of health promotion and disease prevention to the organization and practice of medicine. Health is an elusive concept, but there is general agreement that it means much more than the absence of disease; it is a positive concept that includes the ability to adapt to stress and the ability to function in society.

The three levels of prevention define the various strategies that are available to practitioners to promote health and prevent disease, impairment, and disability at various stages of the natural history of disease. Primary prevention keeps a disease from becoming established by eliminating the causes of disease or increasing resistance to disease. Secondary prevention interrupts the disease process by detecting and treating it in the presymptomatic stage. Tertiary prevention limits the physical impairment and social consequences from symptomatic disease.

It is not easy for prevention programs to compete for funds in a tight fiscal climate because of the frequently long delays before the benefits of such investments are noted. One of the purposes of specialty training in preventive medicine is to prepare investigators who can demonstrate the cost-effectiveness of prevention.

References Cited

Barendregt, J. J., et al. Health expectancy: an indicator for change? Journal of Epidemiology and Community Health 48:482–487, 1994.

Bloom, B. S., et al. A reappraisal of hepatitis B virus vaccination strategies using cost-effectiveness analysis. Annals of Internal Medicine 118:298–306, 1993.

Centers for Disease Control and Prevention. Health-related quality of life measures: United States, 1993. Morbidity and Mortality Weekly Report 44:195–200, 1995.

Centers for Disease Control and Prevention. Quality of life as a new public health measure: Behavioral Risk Factor Surveillance System. Morbidity and Mortality Weekly Report 43:375–380, 1994.

Dubos, Rene. Man Adapting. New Haven, Conn., Yale University Press, 1965.

Dubos, Rene. Mirage of Health. New York, Doubleday and Company, 1961.

Fries, J. F., and L. M. Crapo. Vitality and Aging. San Francisco, W. H. Freeman and Company, 1981.

Gill, T. M., and A. R. Feinstein. A critical appraisal of the quality of quality-of-life measurements. Journal of the American Medical Association 272:619–626, 1994.

Last, J. M. A Dictionary of Epidemiology, 2nd ed. New York, Oxford University Press, 1988.

Leavell, H. R., and E. G. Clark. Preventive Medicine for the Doctor in His Community, 3rd ed. New York, McGraw-Hill Book Company, 1965.

McDowell, I., and C. Newell. Measuring Health: A Guide to Rating Scales and Questionnaires. New York, Oxford University Press, 1987.

McEwen, B. S., and E. Stellar. Stress and the individual. Archives of Internal Medicine 153:2093–2101, 1993.

Revicki, D. A., et al. Responsiveness and calibration of the General Well Being Adjustment Scale in patients with hypertension. Journal of Clinical Epidemiology 47:1333–1342, 1994.

Russell, L. B. Is Prevention Better than Cure? Washington, D. C., Brookings Institution, 1986.

Selye, H. The evolution of the stress concept. American Scientist 61:692–699, 1973.

Selected Readings

Dubos, Rene. Mirage of Health. New York, Doubleday and Company, 1961. [The concept of prevention.]

Evans, R. G. Manufacturing consensus, marketing truth: guidelines for economic evaluation. Annals of Internal Medicine 123:59–60, 1995. [Cost-effectiveness and cost-benefit analysis.]

Fries, J. F., and L. M. Crapo. Vitality and Aging. San Francisco, W. H. Freeman and Company, 1981. [The concept of prevention.]

Goldbloom, R. B., and R. S. Lawrence. Preventing Disease. New York, Springer-Verlag, 1990. [Techniques of prevention.]

Leavell, H. R., and E. G. Clark. Preventive Medicine for the Doctor in His Community, 3rd ed. New York, McGraw-Hill Book Company, 1965. [The concept of prevention.]

Russell, L. B. Is Prevention Better than Cure? Washington, D. C., Brookings Institution, 1986. [The concept of prevention.]

Task Force on Principles for Economic Analysis of Health Care Technology. Economic analysis of health care technology: a report on principles. Annals of Internal Medicine 123:61–70, 1995. [Cost-effectiveness and cost-benefit analysis.]

Udvarhelyi, S., et al. Cost-effectiveness and cost-benefit analyses in the medical literature: are the methods being used correctly? Annals of Internal Medicine 116:238–244, 1992. [Cost-effectiveness and cost-benefit analysis.]

US Preventive Services Task Force. Guide to Clinical Preventive Services. Baltimore, Williams and Wilkins, 1989. [Techniques of prevention.]

CHAPTER FIFTEEN

METHODS OF PRIMARY PREVENTION:

HEALTH PROMOTION

Methods of primary prevention have the goals of health promotion and specific protection (Leavell and Clark 1965). While health promotion is the focus of this chapter, specific protection is discussed in Chapter 16.

SOCIETY'S CONTRIBUTION TO HEALTH

In the absence of serious genetic disease, the most fundamental sources of health are adequate nutrition, a safe environment, and prudent behavior. Society provides the basic structure for these three sources of health, through the socioeconomic conditions, opportunities for safe employment, environmental systems (such as water supply and sewage disposal), and the regulation of the environment, commerce, and public safety. Society also helps to sustain social support systems such as families, neighborhoods, and churches, which are fundamental to health (Pratt 1976).

Because socioeconomic and other conditions vary greatly from country to country and from time to time, health problems and the success of health promotion efforts vary as well. For example, recent conditions in areas such as Somalia, Ethiopia, and Sudan precluded adequate nutrition, and even international relief efforts were hindered. Immediately following the chemical disaster in Bhopal, India, or the radiation disaster in Chernobyl, Ukraine, it was impossible for people in the immediate area to find a safe environment. And during wars, civil or otherwise, such as those in Chechnya and Rwanda in 1994 and 1995, ordinary standards of safe, civil behavior were abandoned.

Even in the presence of a reasonably ordered society, income must be sufficient to allow for adequate nutrition and a safe environment for individuals and families. Education is needed both to enhance employment opportunities and to provide sufficient understanding of the forces that promote good health.

In the United Kingdom, the relationship between socioeconomic status and health has been studied more than in most other nations. This is because for decades people in the UK have been assigned to one of the following five "social classes," based on their occupations and "general standing" in the community (Morris 1957): class I, consisting of professionals (e.g., company directors and physicians); class II, consisting of teachers, shopkeepers, and farm owners; class III, consisting of skilled workers (e.g., clerks and miners); class IV, consisting of partly skilled workers (including most agricultural and assembly line workers); and class V, consisting of laborers. Although this social classification system is controversial, studies using it have consistently shown that according to almost every measure, the best health is found in class I, with health measures declining steadily as one proceeds to class V. This trend applies not only to direct measures of health or lack of it (e.g., perinatal death rates) but also to nutrition, health behaviors, and fertility (Morris 1957).

The best known socioeconomic scale in the USA was developed by Hollingshead in the 1950s and is based on education, occupation, and residence. Using this scale to study the relationship between social class and mental illness, Hollingshead and Redlich (1958) showed a strong social class trend, with fewer cases of mental illness found in the upper classes than in the lower classes. It is difficult, however, to know whether the level of mental illness was the result of or the cause of the social class observed.

In the USA, as in the UK and elsewhere, there has been and continues to be much debate about what factors should be taken into account in defining socioeconomic groups. Some authors have suggested that other social classifications are more adequate for African-Americans in the USA (for example, see Billingsley 1968). In developing nations, social classifications also tend to show that the amount and types of illnesses are quite different among the middle and upper classes as opposed to those living in the rural areas and in poor urban areas. Even in poor nations, the wealthier persons tend to die of "Western" diseases, especially cardiovascular diseases and cancer, whereas the poor tend to die of infections and the sequelae of malnutrition. Current evidence indicates that socioeconomic differentials in mortality persist in the USA (Pappas et al. 1993).

NUTRITIONAL FACTORS IN HEALTH PROMOTION

Nutrition is a vast subject that can be covered only briefly here. In general, problems of undernutrition tend to be found more frequently in the poorer nations, whereas health problems from overnutrition tend to be more common in the industrialized nations and in the post-Communist nations. However, even in highly industrialized nations, such as the USA, both extremes of nutrition can be found. This point was emphasized in the 1968 televised documentary entitled "Hunger in America."

Undernutrition
Starvation, Marasmus, and Kwashiorkor

Most of the frank starvation in recent years has occurred as a result of war or civil unrest. Events in places such as Ethiopia, Sudan, Somalia, and Bosnia serve as reminders that adequate nutrition depends on a fragile chain of production, transportation, storage, processing, and marketing. Wars interfere with all of these steps.

In infants, severe malnutrition results in a severe wasting syndrome called marasmus. Marasmus causes almost total growth retardation and is the result of deficiencies in all nutrients, as occurs when the mother's milk fails and no substitute is available. Breast-feeding is absolutely essential for infant survival in most developing nations, because formula milk is often unavailable and because breast milk is nutritionally well-balanced, sterile, and contains antibodies that help infants fight off infection.

In slightly older children, nutritional deficiencies tend to develop during the weaning process, when the greatest deficiency is usually in vitamins and essential amino acids, while caloric intake may be closer to normal. In developing nations, gruel and other foods used to wean children tend to be starchy, are apt to be deficient in one or more essential amino acids, and are often prepared with polluted water. Under these circumstances, a condition called kwashiorkor (visceral protein malnutrition) can develop and lead to serious morbidity and mortality. The resulting infections and kwashiorkor produce liver damage and a reduction in serum proteins, both of which lead to ascites (fluid in the abdominal cavity). Because the abdominal ascites causes the stomach to swell, observers may think that affected children are fat, when actually they are severely undernourished.

The extent to which marasmus and kwashiorkor occur varies with many factors, including the type of staple food crops. In areas where the diet consists primarily of cassava, plantain, bananas, or a combination of these crops, the protein intake may be especially low (Hegsted 1978). But even in areas where the staple crops are relatively rich in amino acids, if the economy is based largely on a single staple crop, a deficiency of one or more amino acids may occur (King 1969). Corn, for example, is low in tryptophan, and beans are low in methionine. However, by mixing starchy crops that are deficient in different amino acids, it is possible to obtain a diet that is adequate in all of the essential amino acids. Successful programs based on this principle have been developed, making it possible to reduce the incidence of weaning malnutrition and child mortality resulting from amino acid deficits (King 1969).

Vitamins, in particular, may be deficient where nutrition is poor, and supplying vitamins alone may markedly reduce mortality from infectious disease. For example, Rahmathullah et al. (1990) showed that the mortality of preschool children in southern India could be reduced by more than half merely by giving the children vitamin A supplements.

Synergism of Malnutrition and Infection

In developing nations, there is a significant risk of both malnutrition and infection among children who are between their first and fifth birthday, particularly those in the process of being weaned from breast milk. Not only are malnutrition and infection frequently present together, but each makes the other worse (Scrimshaw, Taylor, and Gordon 1968; Hansen et al. 1968). This synergism between malnutrition and infection, which is discussed in Chapter 1 (see the section entitled Synergism of Factors Predisposing to Disease), is the underlying cause of a large proportion of deaths of young children in poor countries and is therefore the target of many programs designed to promote health.

Because the prevention of infection will improve the ratio of caloric intake to caloric need, programs that provide measles vaccinations and programs that make uncontaminated water supplies more accessible to the population will have a positive effect on the nutritional status of children in that population. Similarly, programs that provide improved nutrition, especially for young children, will help the children avoid death or permanent organ damage due to infections during the highest risk period of life. An important lesson of research on synergism, however, is that the approach to nutritional and infectious disease problems in regions of scarcity should be broad-based, attempting to improve all dimensions of life simultaneously.

Overnutrition

It is ironic that a major health problem in the USA and most of the other industrialized nations is overnutrition, while many people in the world suffer varying degrees of undernutrition.

Nutritional Excesses and Imbalances

Over the centuries, cooking has become an art form and eating a major source of pleasure for wealthier populations. In addition, now complicating the desire for special rich flavors is a pervasive time pressure for much of the population. Single persons, single-parent families, and families in which both husband and wife are employed outside the home may reduce the time of food preparation by buying partially or completely prepared foods. These "fast foods" may be adequate in proteins, calories, vitamins, and minerals, but they are likely to contain an excessive amount of fat, to be deficient in fiber, or to stimulate excessive insulin production from refined sugars.

High-Fat Diets. According to many sources, including the US Surgeon General's 1988 report concerning nutrition and health (see US Department of Health and Human Services 1988), excessive consumption of food, particularly foods high in fat, is an important threat to the health of the US population. The negative effect of a high-fat diet occurs through its role in the development of obesity and many chronic diseases, including coronary artery disease and breast cancer.

Cross-cultural studies have helped to document the impact of high-fat diets on the incidence of coronary artery disease. Among the earliest of these was a study performed by Keyes, Kimura, and Kusukawa (1958). The findings, as described by Diehl (1994), were as follows: "When Keyes and his colleagues studied Japanese men who had migrated to California, they found that these men had also left behind their very low-fat, low-cholesterol diets and their apparent immunity to heart disease. Their fat intake had moved from 10 to 40% of total calories, their serum cholesterol had climbed from . . . 150 mg% to . . . 238 mg%, and their CHD [coronary heart disease] death rate had increased tenfold, almost equaling that of American males."

Other studies and data have generally confirmed these findings, although, as discussed below, the level of fiber in the diet may also play a role. For example, disease statistics show that semistarvation in Nazi-occupied Europe during World War II led to a marked decrease in the coronary artery disease rate. Studies with laboratory animals have shown that reduction of food intake below normal levels lengthens the life expectancy considerably if micronutrient levels remain adequate.

The best sources of data on the dietary fat intake of US adults are probably the second National Health and Nutrition Examination Survey (NHANES) (see Carrol, Abraham, and Dresser 1983) and the first Continuing Survey of Food Intakes by Individuals (CSFII) (see US Department of Health and Human Services 1988). In these surveys, the average fat intake for US adults was found to be 37% of total calories. For the year 2000, the US national goal for all persons over 2 years of age is the reduction of total dietary fat intake to no more than 30% of total calories, with no more than 10% in saturated fat (see US Department of Health and Human Services 1990). Many authorities, however, argue that even the 30% fat intake standard is not low enough to have a major effect on heart disease. In particular, some experts now believe that the percentage of saturated fats and perhaps also the percentage of polyunsaturated fats should be less than 10% each and that a higher proportion of the fats should be monounsaturated fats, such as olive oil. Trans–fatty acids, which are produced when fats are "partially hydrogenated," should be avoided whenever possible.

The reasons for the human preference for a high intake of fats and calories are complex. It is probable that the human body is adapted to withstand frequent episodes of starvation, with intermittent periods of abundance (such as after a big kill or other harvest), rather than a steady abundance of food. The ability of the body to store calories as fat whenever an excess of food is available, the human preference for calorie-rich foods, and the increased metabolic efficiency observed in the use of energy during periods of caloric deficiency all may be biologic mechanisms that served *Homo sapiens* well in the distant past but are maladaptive under conditions of nutritional abundance, particularly when compounded by a sedentary life-style. These biologic mechanisms appear to be widespread throughout the animal kingdom. For example, when given a choice between low-fat and high-fat chow, laboratory rats usually select high-fat diets (Reed et al. 1991), and they may become obese.

Low-Fiber Diets.   While diets in industrialized nations tend to be high in fats, they are often deficient in fiber. Dietary fiber consists of a group of compounds, including cellulose, noncellulose polysaccharides, gums, mucilages, lignins, cutin, and suberin (Heaton 1994). The compounds can be divided into two types. The first type is soluble fiber, which tends to slow the absorption of lipids and glucose and to lower the lipid and glucose levels in the blood. The second type is insoluble fiber, which increases the bulk of the stool and provides benefits to the gastrointestinal tract. A mixed fiber diet slows the ingestion (the intake) of solid food; slows the digestion of starch and sugars; increases the absorption of short-chain fatty acids; changes the bacterial metabolism in the colon, thereby reducing the absorption of bacterial metabolites; and has a laxative effect that reduces straining upon evacuation of the bowels (Heaton 1994).

In his cross-cultural studies of nutrition and disease, Burkitt found that many common diseases in the industrialized nations are uncommon or even rare in Central Africa and in several other regions (see Chapter 1 and Table 1–3). Burkitt postulated that many of the differences in disease rates were due to the abundance of dietary fiber in Africa and the lack of it in industrialized nations (see Burkitt and Temple 1994). Although the precise roles of dietary fiber are not well understood, Heaton (1994) asserts that "bulky stools seem to protect against large bowel cancer and probably other diseases, and such stools are safely and reliably obtained by raising dietary fiber intake." He concludes that "by eating most of their plant food with its cellular structure intact, people can protect themselves from overnutrition and hyperinsulinemia and thereby lower their risk of diabetes, hypertension, coronary heart disease, and gallstones."

Obesity

Most people who are obese (120% or greater of ideal body weight) are unable to achieve sustainable weight loss, despite frequent attempts. According to self-reported heights and weights from people interviewed in the 1990 US National Health Interview Survey, 24% of males and 27% of females in the USA are at or above the obesity level (see US Department of Health and Human Services 1990).

Obesity is associated with coronary artery disease, hypertension, a variety of cancers, and increased mortality rates. It is not entirely clear whether obesity is directly causal, indirectly causal (e.g., by increasing blood pressure, which is a risk factor for coronary artery disease), or merely associated in a noncausal way. What is clear is that obesity has significant deleterious health effects for many individuals. Even in those for whom excess weight is not producing any discernible pathologic manifestations, there is often psychologic stress arising from dissatisfaction with body image and loss of self-esteem.

The solutions are more easily stated than achieved. People who are obese have a predisposition to accumulate calories as fat. Weight reduction requires sustainable decreases in caloric intake (often achieved by restricting dietary fat intake) along with sustainable increases in activity levels. Short-term dieting is ill-advised. The loss of weight from a brief diet is of no more value than is a short-term course of insulin for diabetes. In both cases, the underlying condition remains and lifelong management is necessary.

Nutritional Counseling

Despite the strong evidence that nutrition plays an important role in health promotion in general and the prevention of several diseases in particular, physicians are unlikely to counsel patients regarding nutrition during routine care. In the USA, only 20% of patients reported having had nutritional counseling from their physicians even "sometimes" during routine care, and only 12% reported having had it "often" (see US Department of Health and Human Services 1992).

Much of the reluctance of physicians to counsel patients may come from their lack of certainty as to what to recommend. Many nutrition studies appear contradictory, and experts often disagree with one another (Kolata 1995). Despite the lack of a final word in nutrition, there are many general principles that appear to be safe for recommending to patients, as emphasized by the US Preventive Services Task Force (1989). Table 15–1 lists some dependable general nutrition recommendations for persons who do not have a disease requiring specific dietary therapy. There is a growing consensus that similar recommendations—namely, recommendations for a diet that is varied and well-balanced, is low in fats (particularly saturated fats), and is high in fruits, vegetables, and whole grain foods—should be advocated for patients with obesity or diabetes mellitus and for prevention of atherosclerosis. A detailed discussion of the preventive approach to coronary artery disease can be found in Chapter 18.

ENVIRONMENTAL FACTORS IN HEALTH PROMOTION

Environmental conditions affecting health may be harmful (producing "dystress") or helpful (producing "eustress"). The environment should be understood in a broad sense to include not only microbiologic and chemical agents but also physical, social, and psychologic sources of dystress or eustress.

TABLE 15–1. Nutrition Recommendations on Which There Is General Agreement*

(1) The diet should be varied and well-balanced.
(2) Consumption of fruits and vegetables should be encouraged.
(3) Consumption of complex carbohydrates (e.g., whole grain breads) should be encouraged.
(4) The diet should include a significant amount of dietary fiber (e.g., raw fruits and vegetables, whole grain cereals, and whole grain breads).
(5) The fat content of meals should be kept low (less than 30% of all calories). However, monounsaturated fats (such as those found in olive oil) are still important.
(6) The intake of sodium (e.g., in table salt and many snack foods) and refined sugar (in many prepared cereals as well as sodas, candies, pastries, and donuts) should be limited.

*In cases in which a chronic illness is being managed and dietary compliance is essential, the patient should be referred to a trained nutritionist.

Public concern about the environment today tends to focus on hazards such as chemical toxins (e.g., dioxin), radiation (including electromagnetic, ionizing, and solar ultraviolet radiation), radon, "sick" buildings, and other relatively new and "high-tech" environmental hazards. In contrast, hazards related to crowding or loud noise from music or industrial exposure elicit little public concern or interest these days. Perhaps this is because in general people tend to be more fearful about risks over which they believe they have no control. People have control over some aspects of their environment (such as whether or not to smoke) but little control over other aspects of their environment (such as the quality of the air where they live).

Among the tasks of physicians in environmental health are the following: (1) helping patients interpret the dangers of environmental risks about which they are concerned, (2) exploring the possibility of environmental and occupational causes of acute and chronic disease in patients by performing histories and physical examinations that are environmentally sensitive, and (3) reporting diseases that might have an environmental source to public health agencies (see Chapter 19).

Routes and Effects of Exposure to Environmental Hazards

Chemical and biologic hazards ordinarily enter the body through one of its protective surfaces: the skin for external hazards, the gastrointestinal tract for ingested hazards, and the lung for inhaled hazards. Therefore, it is not surprising that all three of these organ systems are heavily affected by the environment. The environment also can damage the vision and hearing, which often happens in an occupational or recreational setting.

Knowledge of the probable **route of entry** of an environmental hazard is essential in devising adequate protection. The **skin** is damaged by microbial hazards, by chemicals (both direct damage and allergic reaction), and by heat and other energy sources, including ultraviolet radiation and kinetic energy that causes cuts or contusions. The **gastrointestinal tract** is particularly subject to microbial hazards, but it is also a portal of entry for ingested chemical toxins, including lead. The gastrointestinal tract also is sensitive to large doses of ionizing radiation. The **lung** is especially sensitive to airborne microbes, chemical aerosols, fumes, dusts, and allergens in the environment (including pollens, dust mites, animal danders, and molds).

Exposure to an environmental hazard can be classified as acute or chronic. The negative effects of **acute exposure** may result from short-term, high-level exposure to an infectious organism; to certain toxic substances, such as potassium cyanide or carbon monoxide; or to a source of high energy, such as heat (resulting in burns), noise (resulting in acute deafness), or a heavy blow (resulting in crushing or penetrating wounds). The negative effects of **chronic**

exposure may result from cumulative contact with or irritation of human tissues, as occurs, for example, with long-term exposure to asbestos, lead, mercury, and certain types of dust; with repetitive motion injuries (e.g., carpal tunnel syndrome); or with repeated exposure to loud noise of the type faced by airport ground crew and baggage handlers and by members or aficionados of rock bands.

Chronic exposures often show a **dose-response relationship** (see Chapter 4), such as that between the quantity of cigarette smoking and the risk of lung cancer. For cigarette smoking, a dose-response relationship has been found, whether the "dose" is estimated by duration of smoking, depth of inhalation, or pack-years (see US Department of Health and Human Services 1980). In research concerning a potential carcinogen, the dose-response relationship is measured beyond the usual **latent period** for the carcinogen (i.e., the period between the onset of exposure and the development of cancer). The latent period for lung cancer due to cigarette smoking is approximately 20 years, while the latent period for mesothelioma due to asbestos exposure is about 15–20 years.

Environmental exposures may or may not have a **threshold level** below which the body can adapt successfully and no harm will come. There is such a threshold level for most chemical and physical agents and even for most microbes. Usually, **nonthreshold exposures** are limited to those which alter genetic material, producing cancer or genetic mutations. Very low levels of exposure to a nonthreshold hazard, such as ionizing radiation, will produce some risk, such as for subsequent leukemia, even though the risk may be small. Generally, the more a person is exposed to a nonthreshold hazard, the greater is the risk of a disease.

Assessment of Environmental Risks

Table 15–2 lists five suggested steps in the assessment of an environmental risk. Many of these steps have been covered in detail in other chapters.

First, the environmental hazard must be identified. This step is qualitative, as in the investigation of an acute disease outbreak (see Chapter 3).

Second, the qualitative and quantitative aspects of exposure to the hazard must be determined (see above and Chapter 3): When did exposure occur? How many exposures were there? How long did each exposure last? How intense was each exposure?

Third, the nature of the disease or damage that results from the environmental exposure must be identified. This may be difficult to determine in the presence of multiple hazards, particularly because experimentation with human subjects is unethical and animal models of exposure to a toxin or other hazard must be used to estimate the type of damage. The Ames test is an example of a quick and frequently used test to estimate the mutagenic potential of a chemical substance. In the Ames test, *Salmonella typhimurium* bacteria are exposed to the suspected

TABLE 15–2. Suggested Steps in the Assessment of an Environmental Risk

(1) Identify the environmental hazard
(2) Characterize the exposure to the hazard in terms of the following:
    (a) Time of occurrence
    (b) Number of exposures
    (c) Duration of each exposure
    (d) Intensity (level) of each exposure
(3) Determine the nature of acute and chronic effects of exposure to the hazard
(4) Determine the relationship between the exposure level and the risk of each effect identified above
(5) Determine the risks for an exposed individual and the probable population impact (population attributable risk and population attributable risk percent)

toxin in the presence of mammalian enzymes and then observed for the mutation of a specific gene. Although the Ames test looks for mutations, not carcinogenesis, a high proportion of the chemicals that cause mutation in this test is also found to be carcinogenic in other, more complicated assays. A negative result in the Ames test, however, is not a guarantee that the tested chemical is not carcinogenic.

Fourth, the nature of the association between exposures and their presumed effects must be determined (see Chapter 4).

Fifth, the risks for an exposed individual and for the population must be assessed (see Chapter 6). This step is particularly difficult for many types of environmental hazards, because much of what is known about them is based on data concerning fairly high levels of exposure and the resulting risk of acute toxic effects. It is not clear to what extent such data can be extrapolated to low levels of exposure for a long period of time. Nevertheless, an estimate of risk for low levels of exposure can be obtained by plotting observed levels of exposure against associated known risks of death, disease, or damage and then calculating the regression line for this relationship.

Methods of Environmental Modification

The basic approach to environmental control is first to identify specific biologic, chemical, social, and physical factors that represent hazards to health or well-being and then to modify the environment in a manner that protects people from harmful exposures.

There are two basic methods for modifying the environment. The first method consists of eliminating or reducing the offending agent—for example, eradicating microorganisms such as the smallpox virus, discontinuing most production of chemicals such as the insecticide DDT in the USA, switching to lead-free gasoline, or controlling the level of heat in buildings. The second method consists of preventing contact between people and the environmental hazard. In some cases, this is accomplished by public measures, such as water sanitation, sewage disposal, restaurant sanitation, and control of disease vectors (e.g., mosquitoes and ticks). In other cases, it is accomplished by individual measures that are strongly encouraged (e.g., good hygiene, proper food handling practices in the home, and wearing of protective clothing and repellents in areas of ticks or mosquitoes) or legislatively mandated (e.g., requirements that motorcyclists wear helmets, that airport ground crew members wear devices for ear protection, and that septic tanks and private wells pass inspection).

Major Sources of Environmental Hazard

Air pollution, water pollution, solid wastes, contaminated food, and disease vectors represent major sources of environmental hazard.

Air Pollution

The air contains a variety of substances that not only affect the health, longevity, and quality of life for people and plants but also have positive and negative effects on nonliving aspects of the environment. In addition to playing a vital role in human respiration and metabolism, air is the source of entry for a variety of environmental hazards other than those normally considered under the term "air pollution." For example, because sound results from rapid variation in the air pressure on the eardrums, in a sense "noise pollution" is airborne. Moreover, many illnesses are caused by airborne microorganisms, with the rate of spread of the organisms influenced by the distance between people and their behavior (e.g., sneezing), by the degree of ventilation of indoor air spaces, and by the humidity of the ambient air.

Types of Air Pollutants. The lung is the most frequent site of serious contact with environmental hazards, not only because the lung tissue is extremely sensitive and absorptive but also because the volume of air inhaled and exhaled each day is so great—i.e., about 50 pounds per day (Moeller 1992). The lung is easily damaged by a variety of airborne pollutants, including particulate matter, metal fumes, gases, and dusts.

Particulate matter, whether from cigarette smoking or from fuel combustion, often contains carcinogenic substances, such as benzpyrene and other hydrocarbons and arsenic. The normal respiratory defense mechanisms are usually adequate against these unless they have been damaged by cigarette smoking or are overwhelmed during an episode of acute air pollution.

Metal fumes are gaseous metal oxides that come primarily from activities in occupational settings, such as welding without adequate ventilation. An acute syndrome called metal fume fever may occur a few hours following exposure and characteristically consists of flu-like symptoms, including fever, weakness, muscle aches, and headache, which subside within a day if exposure is stopped or within a few days if exposure is continued. Frequently, the syndrome is due to zinc oxide, copper oxide, or a combination of both, and these metals can be detected in the urine. Other metals responsible for air

pollution include arsenic, beryllium, cadmium, lead, and mercury. Lead in the air has been markedly reduced in most areas since the use of lead in gasoline has been restricted.

Gases of various types have negative effects on the lung. **Ozone,** a component of smog, is created by the action of sunlight on the reaction of nitrogen oxides and hydrocarbons. Inhalation of ozone produces acute and chronic changes in the respiratory tract, and these changes can predispose to respiratory infections. **Nitrogen dioxide** is produced from fuel combustion and automobile exhausts. Acute exposure may exacerbate bronchoconstriction, and chronic exposure may predispose to respiratory infections. **Sulfur dioxide** forms complexes with particulates. These complexes are toxic to the respiratory tract and can exacerbate respiratory infections and asthma. **Hydrocarbons** are emitted into the atmosphere in huge amounts (almost 30 million metric tons per year) from burning fossil fuels and from solvents and other chemicals. **Carbon monoxide** is an asphyxiant that is produced by sources of incomplete combustion, especially automobiles, poorly ventilated space heating devices, and cigarette smoking.

Dusts are an important cause of chronic lung disease. Inhalation of **coal dust** over a long period of time causes chronic bronchitis and fibrosis ("black lung" disease), which may result in death. Inhalation of **silica dust** is an occupational hazard for miners, stone masons, quarry workers, and foundry workers. The silica dust appears to stimulate varying degrees of pulmonary fibrosis and sometimes causes considerable interference with respiration. Occupational asthma (discussed in greater detail in Chapter 19) affects workers in a number of occupations and may be due to dusts from grain, wood, cotton, hemp, or flax, as well as to certain chemicals, especially isocyanates.

Outdoor versus Indoor Air Pollution. The importance of the distinction between outdoor and indoor air pollution has become clear only since World War II. The indoor environment protects people and objects from some types of air pollution (e.g., pollens) but concentrates other types (e.g., cigarette smoke). Among the factors that influence the relative concentration outdoors and indoors include where the pollutant is produced or released, the nature of the pollutant, the size of the air space available for dilution, and the rate of air exchange indoors.

Pollutants produced or released outdoors tend to be most concentrated outdoors. Examples include pollen, ozone, sulfur and nitrogen oxides, gasoline, and solvents. Industry is the greatest single source of particulate matter in the air. Most carbon monoxide comes from automobiles, whereas most sulfur and nitrogen oxides come from fuel combustion for power production and space heating.

Outdoor air is naturally mixed when there are lateral winds and when cooler air, which is usually above, sinks and the warmer air below rises. These diluting and cleansing mechanisms are usually fairly effective. Occasionally, however, **air inversions** occur, when the cooler air is found close to the earth and the warmer air is above, so that natural mixing does not occur. This allows a much greater than normal buildup of air pollutants in the outdoor environment. At such times, a large geographic area can become like a huge indoor environment, capable of concentrating all pollutants released in the area. In valleys protected from lateral winds, air inversions can be disastrous, as was the case with a fatal smog episode in Donora, Pennsylvania, in 1948, which killed 20 people (Roueché 1953) and with periodic smog episodes that have occurred in Mexico City.

Control of outdoor air pollution must come from a reduction in the release of pollutants, achieved either by altering the production process or by using filters, precipitators, or scrubbers before the pollutants are released into the ambient air.

Pollutants produced or released indoors almost always show higher concentrations indoors. Examples include microorganisms, allergens (such as those from pets and dust mites), allergenic molds, aerosols from products used indoors, cooking products, radon, tobacco smoke, and chemicals or fumes released by building or consumer products (such as urethane or formaldehyde from plywoods and carpets).

There have been cases in which significant numbers of people in a building complain of headaches, difficulty in concentrating or staying awake, wheezing or difficulty in breathing, watery eyes, and other such complaints whenever they enter a certain building. This is sometimes referred to as the **sick building syndrome.** Usually, it occurs in buildings that are tightly sealed for energy conservation, but increasing the ventilatory rate does not always ameliorate the symptoms (Menzies et al. 1993). Often, the sick building syndrome appears to be due to the joint action of many factors. Recently, for example, an older building was discovered to have elevated levels of carbon monoxide, and it appeared that a combination of heavy traffic outside and poor ventilation inside was responsible for the carbon monoxide buildup (Goldberg 1995).

Probably the most common and most serious indoor air pollutant is environmental tobacco smoke. According to the US Environmental Protection Agency (1992), environmental tobacco smoke causes lung cancer in nonsmoking adults; increases the risk of developing asthma and acute lower respiratory tract irritation and infections in children; and is associated with a higher risk of sudden infant death syndrome. The Council on Scientific Affairs of the American Medical Association concurred with these conclusions and recommended a number of steps that physicians should take, including (1) educating their patients about the risks associated with exposure to environmental tobacco smoke at home and at work; (2) encouraging parents to insist on smoke-free environments for children at day-care and preschool facilities; (3) supporting efforts to ban smoking from public places and workplaces; and (4) informing elected representatives about the dangers of environmental tobacco smoke (see American Medical Association 1994).

Control of other indoor pollutants also focuses on methods to reduce the production or release of the pollutants. Examples include improving stoves for better burning and changing behaviors that contribute to pollution (e.g., encouraging people to avoid the use of aerosols and poorly designed stoves). The next line of defense involves increasing the rate of air exchange (ventilation) at the source of the pollutant (e.g., by installing a hood over a cooking stove). The least effective approach is cleaning the air in a room or building by such methods as air filters or electrostatic precipitators.

Water Pollution

Water constitutes about two-thirds of the body weight in humans. Water contributes directly to health when ingested in liquids and as a constituent of food. It also contributes indirectly to health and well-being through its uses in agriculture, industry, power generation, waste disposal, recreation, and transportation.

Pollution of oceans, rivers, and lakes may cause human disease when toxins move through the food chain and enter into fish, which are subsequently caught and consumed by people. Perhaps the most striking example of this occurred in 1958 among the people who lived along Minamata Bay in Japan. Over 100 cases of central nervous system damage and some deaths occurred when the people ate fish contaminated by methylmercury from the dumping of toxic wastes by a vinyl chloride plant on the bay (Kurland et al. 1960). Pollution of sources of drinking water can also cause serious illnesses and deaths.

Sources of Potable Water. Potable water is water that does not contain harmful types or levels of chemical toxins, microorganisms, dissolved metals, or radioactivity and is therefore safe for human consumption. The provision of potable water has been one of the major methods of lowering the rates of death and disease throughout the world, and the decade from 1990 to 2000 was proclaimed the "Water Decade" by the World Health Organization. Surface water and ground water are the major sources of water for drinking.

Surface water includes protected surface reservoirs, lakes, and rivers. **Protected surface reservoirs** are usually the safest water sources. **Lakes** may be an excellent primary water source for a city if little or no pollution drains into the lakes from rivers or from cities and industries on the lake shores. However, many lakes are highly polluted. For example, the Great Lakes in the USA became seriously polluted after World War II, but environmental control efforts have helped them to recover considerably. The water from **rivers** may be polluted by a variety of sources and may therefore require considerable treatment to meet acceptable standards of potability. First, rivers are frequently used for the dumping of sewage by cities, often with only primary sewage treatment (i.e., letting the solids settle out first) or sometimes with no sewage treatment. Second, river water may contain industrial pollutants, such as chemical, biologic, or radioactive wastes. Third, rivers often are contaminated by runoff from farms, including biologic pollutants (animal waste) and chemical pollutants (fertilizers, pesticides, and fungicides).

Ground water exists in underground domes of water called **aquifers.** The rate of turnover of water in aquifers varies considerably, and when an aquifer becomes contaminated by chemical pollutants, such as gasoline from a leaking underground tank at a service station, it may be years or decades before the aquifer can cleanse itself to the point at which it is considered potable again. Therefore, protecting underground water sources is as important as protecting surface water sources.

Water Treatment. Although some surface and ground water supplies are safe for drinking without treatment, most states have laws requiring the treatment of any water supply going to more than one dwelling. The treatment of water involves removing some substances and adding others.

Filtration is the fundamental method for removing unwanted substances, including the cysts of *Giardia lamblia,* which are spread by beavers and other wild animals. Even if the water seems pure, as in the case of water from a mountain stream, there is a danger of giardiasis and other infectious diseases if the water has not been properly filtered.

The most common filtration methods are slow sand filtration and rapid sand filtration. **Slow sand filtration** requires the use of a large bed of packed sand, on which an organic layer forms and assists in the filtration process. The organic layer is called a *Schmutzdecke,* the German term for "dirt layer." When the *Schmutzdecke* becomes too thick, filtration is slowed and the layer must be shoveled off so water can get through and a new *Schmutzdecke* can form. In **rapid sand filtration,** a flocculent (usually aluminum sulfate, called alum) is added to the water before filtration. The flocculent coagulates and traps suspended materials, preventing them from passing through the sand with the filtered water. The flocculent is removed periodically by back flushing, and new flocculent is added to the next batch of water.

If the water contains chemicals that are hazardous or give the water a bad taste, they can be removed by **chemical filtration processes,** such as passing the water through activated carbon, but such techniques are expensive.

Additions are often made to drinking water. For example, chlorine is added to kill vegetative forms of microorganisms. Filtration of chlorinated water is necessary, however, because chlorination fails to kill many types of cysts and because even vegetative bacteria and viruses may be protected from the chlorine by the organic matter in unfiltered water. In many water systems, fluoride is added to help prevent dental caries. Despite considerable concern among some community groups that fluoride might be dangerous, no good evidence of danger from fluoridation (in the range of one part per million in tap water) has been found. There is now good evidence that there has been a considerable drop in the rate of decayed, missing, and filled teeth (called the DMF rate in dental epidemiology) in communities with fluoridated water.

Sewage Treatment. Human sewage poses a threat to more than just other human beings. Biologic wastes, rather than chemical toxins, are responsible for many, if not most, of the deaths occurring in fresh water fish. All living creatures in rivers and lakes, including fish at the top of the food chain, use dissolved oxygen in the water to sustain life. If the level of dissolved oxygen is too low, they will die. Sewage from humans and domestic animals contains aerobic bacteria (bacteria whose metabolism requires oxygen), and these bacteria lower the oxygen level in water. The quantity of oxygen that aerobic bacteria in a given amount of sewage will deplete from the water is called their **biologic oxygen demand.** Two goals of sewage treatment are to remove as much of the organic material as possible from the water (primary treatment) and then to reoxygenate the water (secondary treatment).

In the process of **primary sewage treatment,** water is held in a large basin until most of the solids have settled to the bottom. If the basin is long enough and the rate of water flow into the basin is slow enough, the water flowing out the top of the basin at the far end can be considered to have had primary treatment. Periodically, the basin is emptied and the sludge in the bottom is removed to dry either in sunlight or in a digester. If the sludge does not contain harmful metals, it can sometimes be used as a fertilizer. Otherwise, the treated sludge is buried or dumped at sea (this is not the same as dumping raw garbage at sea, a practice that is gradually being discontinued).

In the process of **secondary sewage treatment,** the water is aerated, usually by means of an activated sludge process or a trickling filter process. If the treated sewage water (called the effluent) must be essentially as clean as drinking water, it may be subjected to sand filtration and may even be chlorinated at the end of this process. Although secondary treatment usually destroys harmful bacteria, it does not always destroy viruses.

Solid Wastes

Each year, the average person in the USA generates about 1500 pounds of garbage and related solid wastes that must be disposed of by city governments and other governing bodies. The volume of solid waste produced by the industrial sector is even greater than that generated by the private sector. Both citizens and industry discard toxic waste, some of which is radioactive. Most of this waste goes to sanitary landfills, but it is becoming increasingly difficult to find locations for new landfills, and the existing landfills frequently leach toxic chemicals into the ground water. Recognizing that hazardous wastes are becoming an increasing problem, the US Congress passed the Superfund Act (Public Law 96-150) in 1980 and passed the Superfund Amendments and Re-authorization Act (Public Law 99-499) in 1986. It is clear more than a decade after the Superfund Act that the problem of toxic wastes is still enormous and probably getting worse.

Physicians may see patients who believe that their symptoms or even frank diseases, such as cancer, are due to their living in proximity to a facility that produces, releases, or disposes of toxic substances. Although such proximity has seldom been clearly established to cause disease in nearby residents (it is more likely to cause symptoms or disease in those working in the facility), such complaints by patients must be dealt with. Often, this will require communication with the local or state department of health.

Additional information concerning toxic agents and other potential health hazards is presented in Chapter 19.

Contaminated Food

Worldwide, foods contaminated with enteric bacteria, viruses, or parasites are a major source of reported morbidity. In the developing countries, they are also a source of mortality in infants who are not being breast-fed. In the USA, despite the fact that many outbreaks of food-borne illness are reported, it is believed that most individual cases go unreported.

To avoid contamination of food, a chain of safety procedures must be followed during production, transportation, storage, processing, marketing, and preparation. Contamination is possible at each stage. Examples of the ways in which hazards can be eliminated are adequate pasteurization of milk, ice cream, eggnog, and other milk products; proper sanitation in facilities handling food; and adequate refrigeration and cooking of foods.

Environmental Vectors

Until Lyme disease became a problem in the USA and was discovered to be a tick-borne illness, North Americans did not think much about the hazards of environmental vectors. Two serious types of mosquito-borne disease, malaria and dengue, were no longer spread indigenously, and various types of mosquito-borne encephalitis were rare. Tick-borne diseases, such as Rocky Mountain spotted fever, were not feared. However, the development of Lyme disease (and more recently, ehrlichiosis) called the attention of the public to potential tick hazards. Dengue may reemerge as a threat in the southern part of the USA, and malaria and tick-borne diseases continue to be leading killers in other parts of the world.

Prevention of vector-borne diseases usually consists of a variety of health promotion and specific protection methods, such as identifying and controlling mosquito-breeding swamps and encouraging travelers to take personal precautions (e.g., wear appropriate clothing, sleep under mosquito netting, use mosquito repellent, and take prophylactic anti-microbial agents) when visiting areas where the risk of malaria is high.

BEHAVIORAL FACTORS IN HEALTH PROMOTION

Human behavior is difficult to separate from nutrition and the environment, because human choices and behaviors have a profound influence on both. This is true, for example, of decisions regarding the types, quantities, and methods of preparation of the foodstuffs that are available to an individual or family.

Similarly, people make choices from the range of possible environments in which they live, work, and play. For example, the choice of a rural or semirural home environment means that the water supply and sewage disposal are likely to be individual responsibilities; the control of vectors (such as the ticks that carry Lyme disease) is a greater problem than in urban residential areas; there is a reduced threat of gang-related violence but probably more time is spent traveling in automobiles; and loneliness and isolation may cause social or psychologic problems. Choices regarding substances that are released into the indoor air space, such as cigarette smoking and aerosols, will influence the indoor ambient environment.

Because the level of education influences the types of jobs available to an individual, it also influences the environment in which he or she will work (office, factory, mine, and so forth) and thereby determines the types of occupational risks that will be faced. Like occupational pursuits, recreational pursuits also have an effect on the level of risk faced by individuals. Although mountain climbing, hang gliding, sky diving, and scuba diving are known to involve high risks, almost any sport has some risk involved, including jogging, even though jogging is touted to have a net benefit of extending life.

Physicians may not be aware of many of the individual behavioral choices made by their patients and may not feel comfortable in trying to influence them anyway. Rather, physicians are more likely to counsel a patient in a special situation or concerning a special topic, such as family planning, nutrition and behavior during pregnancy, and care of a newborn infant. Physicians may also decide to counsel a patient when they discover definite risk factors for disease, such as obesity, hypertension, elevated cholesterol levels, or unprotected sexual activity. Another window of opportunity for counseling occurs following the development of symptomatic disease, such as coronary artery disease, when the patients' motivation to modify diet and to exercise may be at its peak (see Chapter 18).

Counseling of Women before and during Pregnancy

Family planning and the counseling of pregnant women are generally discussed in textbooks of obstetrics and gynecology. However, recent research has emphasized the importance of certain items that will be discussed here.

A woman who might become pregnant should seriously consider taking supplements of folic acid to reduce the risk of neural tube defects in the fetus (see Centers for Disease Control and Prevention 1992). If this supplementation is to be of benefit, it must be present in the first days following conception. Even early prenatal visits are too late to provide the benefit of folic acid supplements, so public health officials in the USA and other nations are considering the possibility of adding folic acid to flour. An excellent natural source of folic acid is leafy green vegetables.

Currently, cigarette smoking is one of the most frequent factors contributing to premature delivery and the delivery of infants with low birth weight or intrauterine growth retardation. Maternal alcohol consumption, even in small quantities, can have serious negative effects on the developing fetus, and consumption in large quantities can cause fetal alcohol syndrome in the newborn. The intake of illegal drugs, particularly opiates and cocaine, can have negative effects on the infant. The exact nature and magnitude of these effects are difficult to predict, however, and the impact of illegal drugs is difficult to separate from the impact of medical, psychosocial, and economic problems that often accompany illegal drug use.

Because the ingestion of alcohol and illegal drugs and cigarette smoking are personal choices that involve habituation or addiction, solutions are not easy for the patient or physician. Nevertheless, identification of problems, counseling, and appropriate referrals are necessary steps, even if they are not always successful.

Counseling of Parents

Topics to be discussed with parents of infants and toddlers include nutrition (breast-feeding and other forms); safety (e.g., use of car seats, placement of barriers at the tops of stairs to prevent falls, and proper storage of harmful substances that might be ingested); immunizations (see Chapter 16); and the scheduling of routine medical examinations. The counseling of parents becomes more difficult and specialized when their offspring reach adolescence, a time during which behavioral problems may develop or become more pronounced. Most pediatric and adolescent medicine books offer guidelines concerning the types of health and safety topics that become pertinent as children reach specific ages.

Counseling of Patients with Risk Factors

Patients in whom a physician discovers risk factors often need and want counseling. If there are medications that could be prescribed, it is tempting for the physician to give them as the first line of attack for obesity, smoking, hypertension, and elevated cholesterol levels. Nevertheless, unless the problem is severe when the patient is first seen, generally the best approach is to try first to modify diet, exercise, or other aspects of life-style, such as eliminating smoking. If these approaches to reducing risk factors are refused or are not successful within a reasonable time, medications should be introduced.

Even if a physician is not comfortable with risk factor counseling, either because of perceived lack of

---

BOX 15–1. The Approach to Smoking Cessation that the National Heart, Lung, and Blood Institute and the American Lung Association Recommend for Use by Physicians in Counseling Their Patients

Step 1. Act as a role model by not smoking. Measures include adopting a no-smoking policy in the physician's office, posting no-smoking signs, and making pamphlets about smoking cessation available in the office.

Step 2. Provide the patient with information on the risks associated with smoking and the reduction of risks if smoking is stopped. In addition to outlining the patient's risks for specific diseases, the information should outline the risks faced by members of the patient's household, particularly children.

Step 3. Encourage abstinence by direct advice and suggestions. The patient is more likely to stop smoking if the physician recommends it clearly and forcefully. The approach should be brief, direct, unambiguous, and informative. Instead of using a "scare tactic," which is likely to arouse defense mechanisms, the physician should emphasize the benefits that will result from cessation of smoking. The reasons for smoking should be taken into account, and the advice should be tailored to individual needs. For example, an emphasis on the health benefits that will result may be most effective for an individual who has symptoms of heart or lung disease, whereas an emphasis on sports performance or how

one smells to others may be more effective for an adolescent. If the patient is willing to try smoking cessation, it is important to set a quit-smoking date. If the patient is unwilling to do this, it may be possible to persuade him or her to take some other positive action, such as contacting a smoking-cessation program, by a defined time. Most successful quitters have tried and failed several times before they finally succeed, and knowing this may help the patient.

Step 4. Refer the patient to a smoking-cessation program. Local hospitals or offices of the American Lung Association or American Cancer Society are good sources to find smoking-cessation programs.

Step 5. Follow up on the use of specific cessation and maintenance strategies. The patient must know that the physician is not abandoning him or her by referral but only enlisting specialized assistance. The physician should schedule specific follow-up visits for physical checkups and for emotional support both during and after the smoking-cessation process. Continual emotional support may be helpful in preventing the patient from smoking again or in encouraging the patient to cease smoking if relapse does occur.

Source of data: National Heart, Lung, and Blood Institute. Clinical Opportunities for Smoking Intervention: A Guide for Busy Physicians. NIH Publication No. 92-2178. Washington, D. C., Government Printing Office, June 1992.

counseling skills or shortage of time, he or she does have the responsibility to identify the problem, state firmly that it affects the patient's health and therefore requires attention, and offer recommendations to the patient concerning how to proceed (e.g., refer the patient to a specialist, such as a dietitian or nutritionist, or to a smoking-cessation program).

Perhaps the single most important behavior change for improving health is smoking cessation. Each year about 3.3 million smokers quit smoking, because they want to and because they are concerned about their health (see National Heart, Lung, and Blood Institute 1992). Signs of tobacco dependence include the continuous use of tobacco for at least 1 month plus at least one of the following: a history of unsuccessful attempts to stop smoking on a permanent basis, withdrawal symptoms after an attempt to stop smoking, or continuing use of tobacco despite a serious physical disorder the patient knows is made worse by tobacco use, such as lung or heart disease (see American Psychiatric Association 1980). Box 15–1 summarizes the approach that the National Heart, Lung, and Blood Institute and the American Lung Association recommend for use by physicians in counseling their patients.

Regardless of the extent of the physician's activity in behavior change, the physician has the responsibility for monitoring the progress of the patient on a regular basis and for changing the approach if sufficient progress is not being made. If necessary, the physician can assist the process of risk factor modification by careful prescription of medications, such as nicotine patches or nicotine inhalers for cessation of smoking (see Tonnesen et al. 1993) or acetyl-CoA reductase inhibitors for reduction of cholesterol levels. Patients using these medications require close monitoring for potential side effects.

In patients with hypertension (see Chapter 18), antihypertensive medications are indicated immediately if at the time of diagnosis the patient has a severely elevated blood pressure with evidence of end-organ damage. If the patient has a moderately elevated blood pressure with no evidence of end-organ damage, dietary change and exercise should be tried first. Only if these measures do not reduce blood pressure to satisfactory levels in an acceptable period of time should medication be started.

SUMMARY

Primary prevention begins with health promotion, which is working to improve the nutritional, environmental, social, and behavioral conditions in which people are conceived, born, raised, and live out their lives.

Proper nutrition is fundamental to good health and requires the intake of adequate amounts of proteins, carbohydrates, fats, vitamins, and minerals. In the developing nations, undernutrition is frequently a problem and usually takes the form of starvation, marasmus, or kwashiorkor. In industrialized nations, nutritional excesses and imbalances (high-fat and low-fiber diets) can lead to malnutrition and obesity.

The physical, biologic, and social environment has an impact on health and safety, with environmental threats taking the form of air pollution, water pollution, improper disposal of solid wastes, ingestion of contaminated food, contact with environmental disease vectors, and problems associated with crowded living conditions.

Many behavioral factors contribute to good or poor health. Negative factors include dangerous personal habits (such as smoking, use of illegal drugs, excessive intake of alcohol, and excessive intake of saturated fats), risk taking (such as risky driving or recreational activities), and failure to use available preventive measures (such as failure to be immunized). The physician's role in counseling patients regarding personal habits is underutilized. In particular, many physicians do not counsel patients until after a health problem is detected or an adverse event occurs.

References Cited

American Medical Association, Council on Scientific Affairs. Environmental tobacco smoke: health effects and prevention policies. Archives of Family Medicine 3:865–871, 1994.

American Psychiatric Association. Diagnostic and Statistical Manual of Mental Disorders, 3rd ed. Washington, D. C., American Psychiatric Association, 1980.

Billingsley, A. Black Families in White America. Englewood Cliffs, N. J., Prentice-Hall, 1968.

Burkitt, D. P., and N. J. Temple, eds. Western Diseases: Their Dietary Prevention and Reversibility. Totowa, N. J., Humana Press, 1994.

Carrol, M. D., S. Abraham, and C. M. Dresser. Dietary Intake Source Data: United States, 1976–1980. DHHS Publication No. (PHS)83-1681. Washington, D. C., Government Printing Office, March 1983.

Centers for Disease Control and Prevention. Recommendations for the use of folic acid to reduce the number of cases of spina bifida and other neural tube defects. Morbidity and Mortality Weekly Report 41:1–7, 1992.

Diehl, H. Reversing coronary heart disease. In Burkitt, D. P., and N. J. Temple, eds. Western Diseases: Their Dietary Prevention and Reversibility. Totowa, N. J., Humana Press, 1994.

Goldberg, C. When office air is hazardous. The New York Times, June 14, 1995.

Hansen, J. D., et al. Evaluating the synergism of infection and nutrition in the field. In Scrimshaw, N. S., and J. E. Gordon, eds. Malnutrition, Learning, and Behavior. Cambridge, Mass., MIT Press, 1968.

Heaton, K. W. Dietary fiber. In Burkitt, D. P., and N. J. Temple, eds. Western Diseases: Their Dietary Prevention and Reversibility. Totowa, N. J., Humana Press, 1994.

Hegsted, D. M. Protein-calorie malnutrition. American Scientist 66:61–65, 1978.

Hollingshead, A. B., and F. C. Redlich. Social Class and Mental Illness: Appendix 2. New York, John Wiley and Sons, 1958.

Keyes, A., N. Kimura, and A. Kusukawa. Lessons from serum cholesterol studies in Japan, Hawaii, and Los Angeles. Annals of Internal Medicine 48:83–94, 1958.

King, K. W. The world food crisis: a partial answer. Research/Development, September, pp. 22–25, 1969.

Kolata, G. Benefit of standard low-fat diet is doubted. The New York Times, April 15, 1995.

Kurland, L. T., et al. Minamata disease. World Neurology 1:370, 1960.

Leavell, H. R., and E. G. Clark. Preventive Medicine for the Doctor in His Community, 3rd ed. New York, McGraw-Hill Book Company, 1965.

Menzies, R., et al. The effect of varying levels of outdoor air supply on the symptoms of sick building syndrome. New England Journal of Medicine 328:821–827, 1993.

Moeller, D. W. Environmental Health. Cambridge, Mass., Harvard University Press, 1992.

Morris, J. N. The Uses of Epidemiology. Edinburgh, E. and S. Livingstone, Ltd., 1957.

National Heart, Lung, and Blood Institute. Clinical Opportunities for Smoking Intervention: A Guide for Busy Physicians. NIH Publication No. 92-2178. Washington, D. C., Government Printing Office, June 1992.

Pappas, G., et al. The increasing disparity in mortality between socioeconomic groups in the United States, 1960 and 1986. New England Journal of Medicine 329:103–109, 1993.

Pratt, L. Changes in health care ideology in relation to self-care by families. Paper presented at the annual meeting of the American Public Health Association, Miami Beach, Fla., 1976.

Rahmathullah, L., et al. Reduced mortality among children in southern India receiving a small weekly dose of vitamin A. New England Journal of Medicine 323:929–935, 1990.

Reed, D. R., et al. Enhanced acceptance and metabolism of fats by rats fed a high-fat diet. American Journal of Physiology 261:1084–1088, 1991.

Roueché, B. Eleven Blue Men. New York, Berkeley Publishing Corporation, 1953.

Scrimshaw, N. S., C. E. Taylor, and J. E. Gordon. Interactions of Nutrition and Infection. Geneva, World Health Organization, 1968.

Tonnesen, P., et al. A double-blind trial of a nicotine inhaler for smoking cessation. Journal of the American Medical Association 269:1268–1271, 1993.

US Department of Health and Human Services. Health, United States, 1991, and Prevention Profile. DHHS Publication No. (PHS)92-12320. Hyattsville, Md., US National Center for Health Statistics, 1992.

US Department of Health and Human Services. Healthy People 2000: National Health Promotion and Disease Prevention Objectives. DHHS Publication No. (PHS)91-50212. Washington, D. C., Government Printing Office, 1990.

US Department of Health and Human Services. The Surgeon General's Report on the Health Consequences of Smoking for Women. Washington, D. C., Government Printing Office, 1980.

US Department of Health and Human Services. The Surgeon General's Report on Nutrition and Health. DHHS Publication No. (PHS)88-50210. Washington, D. C., Government Printing Office, 1988.

US Environmental Protection Agency, Indoor Air Division, Office of Air and Radiation. Respiratory Health Effects of Passive Smoking: Lung Cancer and Other Disorders. Washington, D. C., Government Printing Office, 1992.

US Preventive Services Task Force. Guide to Clinical Preventive Services. Baltimore, Williams and Wilkins, 1989.

Selected Readings

Burkitt, D. P., and N. J. Temple, eds. Western Diseases: Their Dietary Prevention and Reversibility. Totowa, N. J., Humana Press, 1994.

Cassens, B. J., ed. Preventive Medicine and Public Health, 2nd ed. Malvern, Pa., Harwal Publishing Company, 1992.

Institute of Medicine. Environmental Health: Integrating a Missing Element into Medical Education. Washington, D. C., National Academy Press, 1995.

Last, J. M., and R. B. Wallace. Public Health and Preventive Medicine, 13th ed. Norwalk, Conn., Appleton and Lange, 1992.

Moeller, D. W. Environmental Health. Cambridge, Mass., Harvard University Press, 1992.

CHAPTER SIXTEEN

METHODS OF PRIMARY PREVENTION:

SPECIFIC PROTECTION

Three major goals of primary prevention are (1) prevention of **specific diseases** (e.g., by using vaccines and antimicrobial prophylaxis); (2) prevention of **specific deficiency states** (e.g., by using iodized salt to prevent iodine deficiency goiter and by using fluoride to prevent dental caries and osteoporosis); and (3) prevention of **specific injuries and toxic exposures** (e.g., by using helmets to prevent head injuries in construction workers, goggles to prevent eye injuries in machine tool operators, and ventilation systems to control dusts). Vaccines will be discussed as the prototype of a scientifically developed specific method of protection.

PREVENTION OF DISEASES BY USE OF VACCINES

An intact immune system in a well-nourished and otherwise healthy person provides basic protection against infectious diseases. **Intact immunity** implies that the immune system has not suffered damage from a disease such as infection with type 1 human immunodeficiency virus (HIV-1) or damage from medications such as certain anticancer drugs or long-term steroid use. Besides infections and medications, there is some evidence that depression and loneliness can suppress normal functioning of the immune system (Roitt 1991). There are also reports that experimental animals are more resistant to infections when in the presence of other animals of the same species (Cassel 1974).

Types of Immunity

Passive immunity is protection against an infectious disease provided by circulating antibodies made in another organism. Newborn infants are protected, for example, by **maternal antibodies** transferred through the placenta before birth and through breast milk after birth. If a person has recently been exposed to hepatitis B virus and has not been immunized with hepatitis B vaccine, he or she can be given **human immune globulin,** which confers passive immunity and protects against infection with this virus. In an emergency, a specific type of **antitoxin,** if available, can be used to confer passive immunity. For example, diphtheria antitoxin is used in the presence of clinical diphtheria, and trivalent botulinum antitoxin is used in the presence of botulism. Passive immunity provides incomplete protection and usually is of short duration.

Vaccines confer **active immunity.** Some types of vaccines, such as the inactivated polio vaccine (see Chapter 1), do this by stimulating the production of **humoral (blood) antibody** to the antigen in the vaccine. Other types, such as the live attenuated polio vaccine, not only elicit this humoral antibody response but also stimulate the body to develop **cell-mediated immunity.** This tissue-based cellular response to foreign antigens involves mobilization of killer T cells. Active immunity is far superior to passive immunity, because active immunity lasts longer (a lifetime in some cases) and is rapidly

stimulated to high levels by a reexposure to the same or closely related antigens.

All types of vaccines provide the immunized person with some level of **individual immunity** to a specific disease. Some vaccines also reduce or prevent the shedding (spread) of infectious organisms from an immunized person to others, and this contributes to **herd immunity,** a phenomenon discussed in Chapter 1 and illustrated in Fig. 1–3.

Types of Vaccines

As shown in Table 16–1, some vaccines are **inactivated** (killed), some are **live,** some are **attenuated** (altered), and others are referred to as **toxoids** (inactivated or altered bacterial exotoxins).

The older pertussis and typhoid vaccines are examples of **inactivated bacterial vaccines,** while influenza vaccine and the inactivated poliomyelitis vaccine are examples of **inactivated viral vaccines.** The bacillus Calmette-Guérin (BCG) vaccine against tuberculosis is an example of a **live attenuated bacterial vaccine,** and the measles and oral poliomyelitis vaccines are examples of **live attenuated viral vaccines.** Live attenuated vaccines are created by altering the organisms so that they are no longer pathogenic but still have antigenicity.

Diphtheria vaccine and tetanus vaccine are the primary examples of **toxoids.** *Corynebacterium diphtheriae,* the organism that causes diphtheria, produces a potent toxin when it is in the lysogenic state with corynebacteriophage. *Clostridium tetani,* an organism that is part of the normal flora of many animals and is frequently found in the soil, can cause tetanus in unimmunized people with infected wounds. This is because *C. tetani* produces a potent toxin when it grows under anaerobic conditions, such as those found in wounds with necrotic tissue. Tetanus is almost nonexistent in populations with high immunization levels.

Immunization Recommendations and Schedules
Active Immunization of Children

The American Academy of Pediatrics (AAP) publishes periodically updated versions of the *Report of the Committee on Infectious Diseases,* a comprehensive book commonly called the "Red Book" because it invariably comes in a bright red cover. In its extensive discussion of the use of active and passive immunization in children, the book includes an immunization schedule for healthy infants and children whose immunizations start early in life, another immunization schedule for children whose immunizations did not begin during the first year of life, and a discussion of immunization in special clinical circumstances (e.g., in the presence of HIV infection). This publication is essential for physicians providing care to children.

The Advisory Committee on Immunization Practices (ACIP) of the Centers for Disease Control and Prevention (CDC) also publishes immunization

TABLE 16–1. Prevention of Infectious Diseases by Vaccines Available in the USA

Disease	Vaccine
Anthrax	Anthrax vaccine contains inactivated bacteria and is administered subcutaneously.
Cholera	Cholera vaccine contains inactivated bacteria and is administered subcutaneously or intradermally.
Diphtheria	Several combination vaccines are available: DTP is a combined diphtheria, tetanus, and pertussis vaccine; DTaP is a combined diphtheria, tetanus, and acellular pertussis vaccine; DT is a combined diphtheria and tetanus vaccine; Td is like DT but with a reduced amount of diphtheria antigen; and Tetramune is the trade name for a new tetravalent vaccine combining DTP and *Haemophilus* b conjugate vaccine. In all cases, the diphtheria component is a toxoid and the intramuscular route of administration is used.
Haemophilus influenzae infection	The *H. influenzae* type b conjugate vaccine (Hib) contains bacterial polysaccharide conjugated to protein. It is administered intramuscularly. A tetravalent vaccine against diphtheria, tetanus, pertussis, and *H. influenzae* type b is also available and is marketed under the trade name Tetramune.
Hepatitis B	Hepatitis B conjugate vaccine (HBV) contains inactivated viral antigen and is administered intramuscularly.
Influenza	Influenza vaccine contains inactivated virus or viral components and is administered intramuscularly.
Japanese encephalitis	Encephalitis vaccine contains inactivated virus and is administered subcutaneously.
Measles	A vaccine against measles, mumps, and rubella (MMR) is available and contains live viruses. The vaccine is administered subcutaneously.
Meningococcal disease	Meningococcal vaccine contains bacterial polysaccharides of serotypes A, C, Y, and W-135 and is administered subcutaneously.
Mumps	A vaccine against measles, mumps, and rubella (MMR) is available and contains live viruses. A vaccine against mumps alone is also available. The vaccines are administered subcutaneously.
Pertussis	Three combination vaccines are available: DTP, DTaP, and Tetramune (see discussion under diphtheria, above). A vaccine against pertussis alone is also available. In all cases, the pertussis component consists of inactivated bacteria and the intramuscular route of administration is used.
Plague	Plague vaccine contains inactivated bacteria and is administered intramuscularly.
Pneumococcal disease	Pneumococcal vaccine contains bacterial polysaccharides from 23 strains of *Streptococcus pneumoniae*. It is administered intramuscularly or subcutaneously.
Poliomyelitis	Two vaccines are available. The oral polio vaccine (OPV) contains live polioviruses of all three types. The inactivated polio vaccine (IPV) contains inactivated polioviruses of all three types. The OPV, which is administered orally, is also referred to as the Sabin vaccine. The IPV, which is administered subcutaneously, is also referred to as the Salk vaccine.
Rabies	Human diploid cell vaccine (HDCV) contains inactivated virus and can be administered subcutaneously or intramuscularly. The subcutaneous dose is lower than the intramuscular dose and is used only for preexposure vaccination.
Rubella	A vaccine against measles, mumps, and rubella (MMR) is available and contains live viruses. A vaccine against rubella alone is also available and contains live attenuated virus. The vaccines are administered subcutaneously.
Tetanus	Several combination vaccines are available: DTP, DTaP, DT, Td, and Tetramune (see discussion under diphtheria, above). A vaccine against tetanus alone is also available. In all cases, the tetanus component is a toxoid and the intramuscular route of administration is used.
Tuberculosis	The bacillus Calmette-Guérin (BCG) vaccine contains live attenuated mycobacteria and is administered intradermally or subcutaneously.
Typhoid	The older typhoid vaccine contains inactivated bacteria and is administered subcutaneously. Two newer vaccines appear to be as antigenic as the older vaccine and to have fewer side effects. One is called the Ty21A oral vaccine and contains live attenuated bacteria. The other contains capsular polysaccharide and is administered intramuscularly.
Varicella	Varicella (chickenpox) vaccine contains live virus and is administered subcutaneously.
Yellow fever	Yellow fever vaccine contains live virus and is administered subcutaneously.

Sources of data: (1) Centers for Disease Control and Prevention (CDC). Advisory Committee on Immunization Practices (ACIP): general recommendations on immunization. Morbidity and Mortality Weekly Report 43(RR-1), 1994. (2) American Academy of Pediatrics (AAP). Report of the Committee on Infectious Diseases, 22nd ed. Elk Grove Village, Ill., AAP, 1991. (3) CDC. ACIP: recommendations for use of *Haemophilus* b conjugate vaccines and a combined diphtheria, tetanus, pertussis, and *Haemophilus* b vaccine. Morbidity and Mortality Weekly Report 42(RR-13), 1993. (4) CDC. ACIP: typhoid immunization. Morbidity and Mortality Weekly Report 43(RR-14), 1994. (5) CDC. ACIP: diphtheria, tetanus, and pertussis—recommendations for vaccine use and other preventive measures. Morbidity and Mortality Weekly Report 40(RR-10), 1991. (6) CDC. Varicella vaccination. Morbidity and Mortality Weekly Report 44:264, 1995.

schedules and other information in the Recommendations and Reports (RR) supplements to the *Morbidity and Mortality Weekly Report.* The recommendations of the AAP and the ACIP are similar, but because the latter are more frequently updated, they are discussed here and form the basis for Table 16–2.

Table 16–2 shows the recommended immunization schedule for healthy children without specific contraindications (such as immunodeficiency). The recommendations for immunizing children who did not start immunizations as infants have similar intervals between vaccine doses, and the most important difference is that the measles, mumps, and rubella (MMR) vaccine should be started immediately in older children.

Children with altered immunocompetence, whether due to HIV-1 infection or another reason, should not be given live attenuated virus vaccines, including oral polio vaccine; measles, mumps, and rubella vaccine; and yellow fever vaccine. Killed vaccines may be given according to clinical judgment. A tetravalent vaccine combining diphtheria, tetanus, and pertussis (DTP) with Hib has been produced under the trade name of Tetramune (see Centers for Disease Control and Prevention 1993).

Active Immunization of Adults

The need for adequate immunization levels in adults was shown by the dramatic epidemic of diphtheria that occurred in the new independent states of the former Soviet Union, where over 50,000 cases were reported between 1990 and 1994. In 70% of the cases, diphtheria occurred in persons 15 years or older. Almost 2000 deaths resulted (see Centers for Disease Control and Prevention 1995).

The immunization of adults builds on the foundation of vaccines given during childhood. If an adult

TABLE 16–2. Recommended Schedule for Active Immunization of Healthy Infants and Children

Recommended Age	Vaccine and Dose Number*	Comments
Birth	HBV #1	HBV #1 must be given to infant at birth if mother is HBsAg-positive. HBV #1 can be given to infant at birth or at 1 or 2 months if mother is HBsAg-negative.
2 months	DTP #1 OPV #1 Hib #1 HBV #1 or #2	DTP #1 and Hib #1 can be given earlier in areas of high endemicity. HBV #2 is given at 2 months if HBV #1 was given earlier.
4 months	DTP #2 OPV #2 Hib #2 HBV #2	An interval of 6–8 weeks between OPV doses is necessary. HBV #2 is given at 4 months if it was not given sooner.
6 months	DTP #3 OPV #3 Hib #3	DTP #3 should be given at 6 months in areas of high endemicity; otherwise, it can be given at 6 months or any time up to 18 months.
15 months	MMR #1 DTP #4 Hib #4	DTaP may be substituted for DTP.
6–18 months	HBV #3	
4–6 years	DTP #5 OPV #4 MMR #2	DTP #5 is given at or before school entry. DTP #5 and MMR #2 are boosters. DTaP may be substituted for DTP.
14–16 years	Td	Td is given as a booster at 14–16 years of age and every 10 years thereafter.

*Abbreviations are as follows: DTP = diphtheria, tetanus, and pertussis vaccine; DTaP = diphtheria, tetanus, and acellular pertussis vaccine; HBV = hepatitis B conjugate vaccine; Hib = *Haemophilus influenzae* type b conjugate vaccine; MMR = measles, mumps, and rubella vaccine; OPV = oral polio vaccine; Td = tetanus and diphtheria vaccine with a reduced amount of diphtheria antigen. A tetravalent vaccine combining DTP and *H. influenzae* type b conjugate vaccine is now available under the trade name of Tetramune.

Sources of data: (1) Centers for Disease Control and Prevention (CDC). Advisory Committee on Immunization Practices (ACIP): general recommendations on immunization. Morbidity and Mortality Weekly Report 43(RR-1), 1994. (2) ACIP, American Academy of Pediatrics, and American Academy of Family Physicians. Recommended childhood immunization schedule: United States, January 1995. Journal of the American Medical Association 273:693, 1995. (3) CDC. Recommended childhood immunization schedule: United States, 1995. Morbidity and Mortality Weekly Report 44(RR-5), 1995.

is missing polio, diphtheria, and tetanus vaccines, these should be started immediately. Many adults need boosters because they were immunized as children and their immunity levels have declined since they were immunized. For adults, it is better to use the oral polio vaccine (OPV) and to use the combined tetanus and diphtheria (Td) vaccine, which has reduced diphtheria antigen to decrease the number of reactions. In addition, some now recommend that adults be immunized with acellular pertussis vaccine because it may provide some herd immunity against pertussis to children.

The measles, mumps, and rubella (MMR) vaccine should be administered to most adults who were born after 1956 and lack evidence of immunity to measles (a definite history of measles or measles immunization after age 12 months). The exceptions are pregnant women and immunocompromised patients.

Hepatitis B vaccine should be given to susceptible persons who are at high risk for hepatitis B because of their professions (health care workers, persons with jobs in certain countries overseas, etc.); homosexual activity or intravenous drug use; or frequent exposure to blood or blood products.

Pneumococcal polysaccharide vaccine should be given at least once to persons 65 years and older and to those persons with chronic diseases that increase their risk of mortality or serious morbidity from pneumococcal infection, such as chronic pulmonary or cardiac disease, cancer, renal or hepatic disease, asplenia, and immunosuppression. Experts recommend that influenza vaccine be given annually in the late autumn to the same risk groups, and some believe that the influenza vaccine should be given to the general population, although this is not a national recommendation.

See Box 16–1 for information on vaccines for international travelers.

Passive Immunization

The medical indications for passive immunization are far more limited than those for active immunization. Table 16–3 provides information about the biologic agents available in the USA and the indications for their use in immunocompetent persons (those with normal immune systems) and immunocompromised persons (those with impaired immune systems).

For immunocompetent persons who are at high risk for exposure to hepatitis A, usually because of travel to a country where it is common, hepatitis A vaccine can be administered if there is time (see Medical Letter on Drugs and Therapeutics 1995a), or immune globulin can be administered prior to the travel as a method of **preexposure prophylaxis.** For those who were recently exposed to hepatitis B or rabies, a specific immune globulin can be used as a method of **postexposure prophylaxis.** For those who lack active immunity to exotoxin-producing bacteria already causing symptoms (such as *Clostridium botulinum*, the organism responsible for botulism), the injection of a specific antitoxin is recommended after tests are performed to rule out hypersensitivity to the antitoxin (see American Academy of Pediatrics 1991 and Benenson 1990).

For immunocompromised persons who have been exposed to a common but potentially life-threatening infection such as chickenpox, immune globulin can be lifesaving if given intravenously soon after exposure.

Vaccine Surveillance and Testing

As discussed in Chapter 3, the rates and patterns of reportable diseases are monitored, and any cases that are thought to be vaccine-associated are investigated. The goals are to monitor the effectiveness of vaccines and to detect vaccine failures or adverse effects.

Randomized Field Trials

The standard way to measure the effectiveness of a new vaccine is through a randomized field trial (the public health equivalent of a randomized controlled trial, although the level of "control" usually is somewhat less). In this type of trial, susceptible persons are randomized into two groups and are then given the vaccine or a placebo, usually at the

---

BOX 16–1. Information on Vaccines and Other Protective Measures for International Travelers

Basic immunity

Several vaccine-preventable diseases that have been largely eliminated from the USA and other highly industrialized countries can still be found in many of the lesser developed countries throughout the world. Plans for international travel to lesser developed regions should therefore serve as a stimulus for updating immunizations. In general, all children and adults who plan to travel to these regions should have had recent boosters for **tetanus, diphtheria, and poliomyelitis.** Because exposure to **measles** is a real possibility in many areas of the world, measles vaccination or revaccination is also indicated for those who have never had the disease and have not received measles vaccine at 15 months of age or later. In addition, female travelers of childbearing age should have immunity against **rubella.** Children should also be immunized against **pertussis** and *Haemophilus influenzae* **type b.** The 23-valent vaccine against **pneumococcal disease** should be given to persons 65 years or older and to persons with chronic illness.

Required or recommended vaccines

Proof of recent administration of **yellow fever** vaccine may be required for entry into some countries if the traveler has come from areas in South America or Africa where the disease is found. Yellow fever was reported in 14 countries in late 1994. Most countries allow travelers to enter from areas where **cholera** is endemic, but a traveler to an area with cholera may wish to obtain the vaccine for self-protection. In late 1994, cholera was reported in 50 countries, most of which were located in Central and South America, central Africa, and the Indian subcontinent.

Diphtheria vaccine is recommended for travel to Russia and the other former states of the Soviet Union. **Typhoid fever** might be a threat for a traveler to the Indian subcontinent or Peru, for example, and **meningococcal disease** may be a threat to those visiting the Indian subcontinent, the Arabian peninsula, and sub-Saharan Africa.

It is wise for travelers to have been immunized against **hepatitis B,** which is a problem not only in developing countries but also in many of the rapidly industrializing countries of the Pacific rim. If there is any question of sanitation being inadequate, particularly in rural areas, the traveler should receive passive immunization (human immune globulin) against **hepatitis A.** Any immune globulin should be given at least 2 weeks after the last dose of all active vaccines has been given. This schedule will prevent neutralization of the antigen.

Ordinary travel does not justify being immunized against diseases such as tuberculosis, Japanese encephalitis, and rabies.

Additional information

International travelers should contact a state-licensed official vaccination center in their state. Information about the nearest official center can be obtained from the local or state health department.

Physicians who care for patients before and after they travel internationally may wish to consult special guides for international health travel, such as Jong's *Travel and Tropical Medicine Manual* (1987) and Hill's "Immunizations for Foreign Travel" (1992). Hill's article discusses indications and precautions concerning special groups of travelers, such as pregnant women.

TABLE 16–3. Indications for Use of Immune Globulins and Antitoxins Available in the USA

Biologic Agent	Type	Indication
Botulinum antitoxin	Specific equine antibody	Treatment of botulism.
Cytomegalovirus immune globulin	Specific human antibody	Prophylaxis for bone marrow and renal transplant recipients.
Diphtheria antitoxin	Specific equine antibody	Treatment of respiratory diphtheria.
Immune globulin (intramuscular)	Pooled human antibody	Hepatitis A preexposure and postexposure prophylaxis.
Immune globulin (intravenous)	Pooled human antibody	Replacement therapy for antibody deficiency disorders.
Hepatitis B immune globulin	Specific human antibody	Hepatitis B postexposure prophylaxis.
Rabies immune globulin	Specific human antibody	Rabies postexposure management of persons not previously immunized with rabies vaccine.
Tetanus immune globulin	Specific human antibody	Treatment of tetanus; postexposure management of persons not previously immunized wth tetanus vaccine.
Vaccinia immune globulin	Specific human antibody	Postexposure prophylaxis for susceptible immunocompromised persons and for perinatally exposed newborns.

Source of data: Centers for Disease Control and Prevention (CDC). Advisory Committee on Immunization Practices (ACIP): general recommendations on immunization. Morbidity and Mortality Weekly Report 43(RR-1), 1994.

beginning of the high-risk season of the year. The vaccinated subjects and unvaccinated controls are followed through the high-risk season to determine the **attack rate** (AR) in each group:

$$AR = \frac{\text{Number of persons ill}}{\text{Number of persons exposed to the disease}}$$

Next, the **vaccine effectiveness** (VE) is calculated:

$$VE = \frac{AR_{(unvaccinated)} - AR_{(vaccinated)}}{AR_{(unvaccinated)}} \times 100$$

In the VE equation, the numerator is the observed reduction in AR due to the vaccination, and the denominator represents the total amount of risk that could be reduced by the vaccine.

Testing the efficacy of vaccines by randomized field trials is very costly, but it may be required the first time a new vaccine is introduced. Field trials were used to evaluate inactivated polio vaccine (see Chapter 1 and Francis et al. 1955), oral polio vaccine, and measles and influenza vaccines.

Retrospective Cohort Studies

The antigenic variability of influenza virus (see Chapter 1) necessitates frequent (often yearly) changes in the constituents of influenza vaccines to keep them up to date with new strains of the virus. This in turn requires constant surveillance of the disease and of the protective efficacy of the vaccine. Because there are insufficient resources and time to perform a randomized controlled trial of each new influenza vaccine, retrospective cohort studies are sometimes done during the influenza season to evaluate the protective efficacy of the vaccines.

In these studies, because there is no randomization, investigators cannot be sure that there was no selection bias on the part of the physicians who recommended the vaccine or the individuals who agreed to be immunized. If selection bias were present, those who were immunized might be either sicker or more interested in their health than those who were not immunized. Studies of influenza vaccine effectiveness in nursing homes have indicated that rates vary from near 0% to about 40% (for example, see Cartter et al. 1990). The low protection rates may be due to inadequate antibody production by older people and to the delay from the time vaccine is given until an outbreak appears.

Case-Control Studies

Because randomized field trials require large sample sizes (often over 100,000), they are almost impossible to perform for uncommon diseases, such as *Haemophilus influenzae* infections or pneumococcal pneumonia. To overcome this problem, many investigators have recommended using case-control studies (see, for example, Clemens and Shapiro 1984; Shapiro et al. 1991). Their recommendation is based on the fact that when the risk of disease in the

population is low, the vaccine efficacy (VE) formula above may be rewritten as follows:

$$VE = 1 - \left[\frac{AR_{(vaccinated)}}{AR_{(unvaccinated)}} \right] = (1 - RR) \cong (1 - OR)$$

The risk ratio (RR) is closely approximated by the odds ratio (OR) when the disease is uncommon, as in the cases of *H. influenzae* infections in children and pneumococcal infections in adults.

When Shapiro et al. (1991) performed a case-control study of pneumococcal vaccine, which is a polyvalent vaccine containing capsular polysaccharide antigens of 23 strains of *Streptococcus pneumoniae,* they found that the vaccine showed fairly good efficacy against the strains contained in the vaccine and no efficacy against other *S. pneumoniae* strains. The fact that the risks from strains not in the vaccine were comparable in the case and control groups suggests that the differences in protective efficacy for strains that were in the vaccine were not due to any selection bias.

Incidence Density Measures

Among the questions that vaccine research and surveillance are designed to answer are the following: When should a new vaccine be given? What is the duration of the immunity produced?

In the case of measles vaccine, surveillance studies suggested that when the vaccine was given to infants before 12 months of age, often it was not effective, presumably because the vaccine antigen was neutralized by residual maternal antibody. To determine the answers to both of the questions above, Marks, Halpin, and Orenstein (1978) performed a study in which they monitored the incidence density of measles cases in Ohio over an extended period of time. In order to adjust for the duration of exposure to measles, which varied between individuals, they used incidence density (see Chapter 2) as their measure of measles incidence. The formula for incidence density (ID) is as follows:

$$ID = \frac{\text{Number of new cases of a disease}}{\text{Person-time of exposure}}$$

The denominator (person-time) can be expressed in terms of the number of person-days, person-weeks, person-months, or even person-years of exposure to the risk.

Marks, Halpin, and Orenstein obtained the results shown in Box 16–2, which, along with other studies, suggested that measles vaccine should be postponed until children reach approximately 15 months of age. One concern in delaying the vaccine is the fact that measles is more severe in newborns than in older infants. Partly to reduce the likelihood of exposure of newborns to measles, experts have recommended that all children be revaccinated with measles vaccine before they enter school, at age 5 or 6 years. Another concern has been the duration of immunity. As shown in the second part of Box 16–2,

---

BOX 16–2.   Data Showing Why Measles Vaccine Is Now Postponed until Children Reach the Age of 15 Months

---

Part 1. Correlation of age at vaccination with data on measles incidence (rate of disease per 1000 person-weeks) and data on measles risk (relative risk of those vaccinated at the age shown in comparison with those vaccinated at 15 months of age):

Age at Vaccination	Measles Incidence per 1000 Person-Weeks	Relative Risk Compared to Risk in Children Vaccinated at 15 Months
Never	155.3	33.0
< 11 months	39.6	8.5
11 months	15.0	3.2
12 months	7.1	1.5
13 months	5.2	1.1
14 months	4.7	1.0

Part 2. Correlation of time since vaccination with data on measles incidence (rate of disease per 1000 person-weeks) and data on measles risk (relative risk):

Time Since Vaccination	Measles Incidence per 1000 Person-Weeks	Relative Risk
0–3 years	4.0	1.0
4–6 years	4.2	1.1
7–9 years	5.4	1.4
10–12 years	11.7	2.9

Source of data: Marks, J., T. J. Halpin, and W. A. Orenstein. Measles vaccine efficacy in children previously vaccinated at 12 months of age. Pediatrics 62:955–960, 1978.

---

the measles vaccine lost its protective ability slowly during the first 6 years, but the relative risk of acquiring measles had almost tripled by 10–12 years after immunization. This is another line of evidence that led to the recommendation that children be revaccinated at the age of 5 or 6 years.

Immunization Goals

The strategy of developing disease control programs through the use of vaccines depends upon the objectives of the vaccine campaign. The goal may be **eradication of disease** (as has been achieved for smallpox), **regional elimination of disease** (as has been achieved for poliomyelitis in the Western hemisphere), or **control of disease** to reduce morbidity and mortality.

Disease eradication by immunization is feasible only for diseases in which human beings are the sole reservoir of the infectious organism. Although vaccines are available to prevent some diseases with reservoirs in other animals (e.g., rabies, plague, and encephalitis) and some diseases with reservoirs in the environment (e.g., typhoid fever), they are not candidates for eradication programs. The surveil-

lance systems to achieve eradication or regional elimination must be excellent, and any eradication or elimination program would require considerably more resources and time, as well as general political and popular support, than would a disease control program. For these reasons, immunization strategies are frequently the subject of much scrutiny and debate.

For years, immunization experts in the USA have been debating whether or not to recommend total population coverage with a new varicella (chickenpox) vaccine. On the one hand, the live virus vaccine performed well in controlled trials (Weibel et al. 1984), and administering it during childhood could reduce disease-related morbidity, children's loss of time from school, and parents' loss of time from work to care for the children with chickenpox. In addition, it might prevent herpes zoster in later life. On the other hand, if the varicella immunization program did not immunize enough people to eliminate the virus, many could reach adulthood without adequate immunity to it. Varicella infection in adults can be quite serious, particularly when skin lesions are accompanied by pneumonia. Moreover, because the vaccine is a live herpesvirus vaccine, some people have expressed concerns that the virus may become reactivated or that a new kind of herpes zoster may arise and not be detected for decades. Those who are worried about general use of the new vaccine claim that for the relatively low price the population pays in terms of morbidity and lost productivity due to chickenpox, it gets "automatic" immunization from the wild virus infection without any direct financial cost. Recently, the Food and Drug Administration approved the vaccine for general use (see Medical Letter on Drugs and Therapeutics 1995b).

The Expanded Program on Immunization

In May of 1974, the World Health Assembly adopted a global Expanded Program on Immunization (EPI), with the goal of cooperation between the World Health Organization and the member governments in establishing or expanding existing national immunization programs. A particular emphasis of the EPI has been the surveillance of vaccine-preventable illnesses and the monitoring of immunization levels in the member countries (see Centers for Disease Control and Prevention 1994a and 1994b).

The Vaccines for Children Program

In the USA, because of requirements for complete immunization before children enter school at the age of approximately 5 years, the rate of vaccine-preventable diseases has generally been falling and levels of adequate immunization have been high in school-age children. In 2-year-old children, however, the immunization rates have remained disappointing. **Adequate immunization** is defined as receiving the recommended number of doses of vaccines by the ages shown in Table 16–2. In 1993, the percentages of 2-year-olds who had received adequate immunization were as follows: 72% for diphtheria, tetanus, and pertussis vaccine (4+ doses of DTP); 79% for oral polio vaccine (3+ doses of OPV); 84% for measles-containing vaccines (1 dose, usually of MMR, the combined measles, mumps, and rubella vaccine); 55% for *H. influenzae* vaccine; and 16% for hepatitis B vaccine. When the basic combination of 4 DTP doses plus 3 OPV doses plus 1 MMR dose is considered, only 67% of children were adequately immunized (see Centers for Disease Control and Prevention 1994c).

The generally poor immunization levels for preschool children led to the establishment of the Vaccines for Children Program (see Centers for Disease Control and Prevention 1994d). This program is designed to provide free vaccines to children at participating private and public health care provider sites. The eligible groups include American Indians, Alaskan Natives, children on Medicaid, children who lack health insurance, and children whose health insurance does not cover immunizations.

Explanations for Inadequate Immunization Levels

Why are immunization levels so low? This question has been studied extensively, without definitive answers. The process of obtaining vaccines is complex, and attitudes toward immunization are diverse. Beliefs about personal risks of acquiring a disease, concerns about vaccine-related lawsuits, and traditions are among the explanations for inadequate immunization levels.

Health Beliefs

Research concerning why people may not seek immunizations or other preventive measures for themselves or their children led to the development of what is often called the **health belief model** (see Rosenstock 1974). According to the model, before seeking preventive measures, people generally must believe (1) that the disease at issue is serious, if acquired; (2) that they or their children are personally at risk for the disease; (3) that the preventive measure is effective in warding off the disease; and (4) that there are no serious risks or barriers involved in obtaining the preventive measure. In addition, there need to be cues to action, consisting of information regarding how and when to obtain the preventive measure, as well as the encouragement from or support of other people.

The health belief model is useful in guiding the educational aspect of an immunization program. The "swine flu" (H1N1 viral influenza) vaccine campaign in 1976 had major difficulties, partly because the public was not convinced of any of the four items above. First, the public was not sure whether the disease would be a pandemic (as in 1918–1919) or just another outbreak which, while annoying and dangerous for a few, was not cause for alarm. Second, people were not sure if they were personally at risk. A few people had been found to harbor the H1N1 virus, but it was not clear that it would spread to large numbers of people. Third, experts were involved in debates about how effective the vaccine would be in preventing influenza if the H1N1 virus did establish a widespread infection. Fourth, there were conflicting stories about possible side effects from the vaccine.

Ironically, one of the reasons for inadequate immunization levels in the USA today is the very success of immunization programs in the past (Jekel 1972). People who do not remember how widespread or serious a disease was in the past tend to be less concerned with preventing it in the future.

In the case of pertussis vaccine, debates and continued concerns about the potential for serious side effects caused the British population largely to abandon its use of the vaccine and to suffer epidemics of pertussis as a consequence (Johnstone 1983). These concerns have also been present in the USA, although not to the extent they were in Great Britain. Evidence reported recently (see Medical Letter on Drugs and Therapeutics 1992) suggests that the new acellular pertussis vaccine has a much lower risk of negative effects, and this may eliminate most of the population's concerns about pertussis vaccine.

Vaccine-Related Lawsuits

In the USA, the number of lawsuits related to vaccine use increased from 1 lawsuit in 1978 to 219 lawsuits in 1985, and the damages claimed (but not necessarily awarded) increased from $10 million to over $3 billion (Herwaldt 1993). As a consequence of naming vaccine manufacturers in many of these lawsuits, there has been a decrease in the number of companies making vaccines.

In response to the problem, the federal government instituted the National Vaccine Injury Compensation Program. This program covers diphtheria, tetanus, pertussis, measles, mumps, rubella, and both oral and inactivated polio vaccines. It is limited to claims for injuries or deaths that are attributable to vaccines given after October 1, 1988. Claims concerning injury must be filed within 3 years of the first symptoms (e.g., anaphylactic shock, paralytic poliomyelitis, seizure disorders, or encephalopathy). Claims concerning death must be filed within 4 years of the first symptoms and 2 years of death. The program essentially protects vaccine manufacturers from liability lawsuits, unless it can be shown that their vaccines differed from the federal requirements. It also simplifies the process and reduces the costs for those people making a claim, and almost all of the costs are borne by the federal government.

Missed Opportunities

In the USA, the immunization levels are consistently lower in the poorer population groups. It is not clear whether this is due to less education among these groups, inadequate medical care, or inability to put such things as immunization high on a struggling family's list of priorities. One of the problems is that both the medical care system and the physicians have largely failed to adapt immunization practices to accommodate the special needs of the poor and, hence, have missed many opportunities for immunizing poor children. The new Vaccines for Children Program is one response to this problem, but it is far from clear that it will accomplish much in the absence of major changes in the way that medical care is organized and financed.

Studies have been undertaken to determine how many and what kind of missed opportunities for immunization occur in the context of medical care, especially during sick child visits (see Centers for Disease Control and Prevention 1994d). Often, physicians do not vaccinate children who have a mild upper respiratory infection without complications, even though part of the reason for their office visit may have been to receive a vaccination. More recent guidelines have emphasized that such children should receive the appropriate vaccines. Frequently, the siblings of a child who is being seen by the physician or nurse will be brought along by the parent, and these siblings should receive vaccinations if their immunization record is not up to date, although this is seldom done. These two scenarios are especially common in emergency departments, but opportunities are often missed here because providers lack records, time, and a relationship with the patients.

Hospitalized children whose immunization records are not up to date should be given the appropriate vaccines unless there are clear contraindications. Unfortunately, clinicians are often ill-informed about contraindications. As discussed in some detail in the pediatric "Red Book" (see American Academy of Pediatrics 1991), the following are *not* contraindications to immunizing children: a mild reaction to a previous DTP dose, consisting of redness and swelling at the injection site, a temperature under 40.5°C (105°F), or both; the presence of nonspecific allergies; the presence of a mild illness or diarrhea with low-grade fever in an otherwise healthy child who is scheduled for vaccination; current therapy with an antimicrobial drug in a child who is convalescing well; breast-feeding of an infant scheduled for immunization; and pregnancy of someone else in the household. False contraindications account for part of the reason that US physicians have not adequately immunized children.

PREVENTION OF DISEASES BY USE OF ANTIMICROBIAL DRUGS

Another form of specific protection, which can be used for varying lengths of time, is **antimicrobial prophylaxis.**

For travelers to countries where malaria is endemic, antimicrobial protection against the causative organism, *Plasmodium,* may be desirable. Oral chemoprophylaxis for adults may consist of the use of chloroquine phosphate before and during travel, followed by the use of primaquine for a few weeks after returning home. However, if chloroquine-resistant strains of *Plasmodium* have been reported in the area to be visited, an alternative drug, such as mefloquine, may be given instead (Bia 1992).

The chemoprophylaxis of tuberculosis is discussed in detail in Chapter 19. The usual prophylaxis is isoniazid (INH), given daily for 6 months, beginning from the time of the recognition of a recent exposure or the diagnosis of skin test conversion. This chemoprophylaxis reduces the probability of active tuberculosis.

In patients who have had rheumatic fever with valvular disease, a short-term course of bactericidal antibiotics is recommended before dental or other manipulative medical procedures are performed.

People who have been exposed to virulent meningococcal disease, either meningitis or meningococcal sepsis, should be given prophylactic antibiotics. The most common antibiotic used for this purpose is rifampin.

A high dose of ceftriaxone is sometimes given to prevent syphilis or gonorrhea in people who are known to have had sexual contact with an infected person during the period in which the disease was communicable.

PREVENTION OF DEFICIENCY STATES

When specific vitamin and mineral deficiencies were identified in the past, it was possible to fortify food or water to ensure that most people would obtain sufficient amounts of nutrients of a specific type. The most well-known examples are iodine in salt, which has essentially eliminated goiter; vitamin D in milk, which has largely eliminated rickets; and fluoride ion in water, which has markedly reduced the incidence of dental caries in children who grow up in areas with fluoridated water.

The frequent use of vitamin and mineral supplements and the fortification of most breakfast cereals with a number of vitamins and minerals have largely eliminated vitamin B deficiencies in populations with reasonably normal nutrition. Nevertheless, vitamin B deficiencies are still found in some elderly persons.

PREVENTION OF INJURIES AND TOXIC EXPOSURES

In the USA today, there is intense activity, often mandated through government regulations or carried out by government agencies, to protect the population from specific injuries and exposure to harmful environmental agents. These activities are so broad in scope that just a few can be mentioned.

The activities of the Department of Agriculture are designed to protect the food sold in the USA. They include supervision of meat packing and milk production in the country, as well as inspection of imported food products. The regulations of the Food and Drug Administration are designed to ensure that prescription and over-the-counter drugs are safe and effective and that foods are safe and properly labeled. Major new food labeling is now required to enable shoppers to determine the fat and salt content of foods.

Continual efforts are made to protect the public through federal or state laws governing land, sea, and air transportation and equipment, ranging from regulations for those who construct highways and automobiles to regulations for those who use them (e.g., laws about seat belts, air bags, speed limits, maximum lengths of air time or driving time in a day or a week for pilots or truck drivers, and penalties for operating equipment under the influence of drugs or alcohol).

Local regulations regarding building codes are largely for home and workplace safety and include requirements for hard-wired smoke alarms in new houses and hotels, as well as for properly lighted safety exits and automatic sprinklers in public buildings. Workplace protection regulations are enforced by the Occupational Safety and Health Administration (OSHA). These consist of regulations in **chemical**

safety (e.g., publication of all chemicals used in a manufacturing or research setting); **biologic safety** (e.g., protection for laboratory technicians working with hazardous microorganisms and proper immunizations for health care workers); and **physical safety** (e.g., protection against repetitive motion injuries and against harmful levels of exposure to noise, heat, and cold). Some common specific protection devices include helmets for construction workers, ear protection for those working around jet aircraft, and masks for those removing asbestos from old buildings or working in dusty areas.

PREVENTION OF IATROGENIC DISEASES AND INJURIES

Among the most preventable of health problems are those generated during the process of treatment—i.e., diseases and injuries that are iatrogenic (from the Greek *iatros,* which means physician, and *gennao,* which means to produce). Examples include infections, falls, medication errors, unnecessary surgery, and surgical and medical errors (see, for example, Bates et al. 1995; Inlander et al. 1988; and Leape et al. 1991).

Nosocomial infections (hospital-acquired infections) are more common than often supposed. Based on a review of the literature, Inlander et al. (1988) concluded that there were at least 100,000 nosocomial infection–related deaths each year in the USA. Ensuring that all health care workers wash their hands before going from one patient to another is the single most important method of reducing the spread of infections in hospitals. Proper sterile techniques, appropriate isolation techniques, and proper disposal of needles and other sharp objects are also critical.

Falls in hospitals and other institutions may result from improper supervision of patients whose illness or medication causes them to become confused or lose their footing. Falls can be prevented by careful monitoring of patients.

Medication errors include incorrect dosages, incorrect medications, and drug interactions. Medication errors can be reduced if careful ward procedures are followed, pharmacists are well informed, and pharmacy information systems that check dosages and drug interactions are used.

Unnecessary surgery is being reduced by increasing requirements for second opinions concerning elective surgical procedures.

Surgical and medical errors will always occur, but their frequency can be limited by the proper training and evaluation of surgeons and physicians, by the surveillance of complications, and by medical care studies of morbidity and mortality in patients undergoing surgical or medical procedures. A classic example of a health problem produced by medical error was the epidemic of retrolental fibroplasia that occurred when 100% oxygen was delivered to preterm infants. This caused vasoconstriction and destruction of small blood vessels, followed by an overgrowth of capillaries and fibrous tissue in the eye. Usually, keeping the oxygen tension in the infant's air at 40% or less, for as short a time as possible, will prevent retrolental fibroplasia.

SUMMARY

Many primary prevention strategies focus on the use of specific biologic, nutritional, or environmental interventions to protect individuals against specific diseases, deficiency states, injuries, or toxic exposures. The prototype of specific protection is the vaccine, which is directed against one specific disease and prevents the disease by increasing host resistance. Host resistance can be temporarily increased by passive immunization or even by prophylactic antibiotic therapy.

Specific nutritional deficiencies can be eliminated by adding nutrients (such as iodine) to commonly used foods (such as salt) to prevent a particular disease (in this case, goiter). Among construction workers, the incidence of head injury and eye injury can be reduced by the use of helmets and goggles, two examples of specific protection against environmental hazards.

Both specific protection and health promotion may be used together. In the case of noise produced by jet aircraft, for example, the ear protection devices worn by aircraft mechanics and airport personnel who cannot avoid exposure to the noise would be considered specific protection against hearing loss. Engineering changes designed to reduce the general level of noise produced by jets could be considered health promotion.

References Cited

American Academy of Pediatrics. Report of the Committee on Infectious Diseases, 22nd ed. Elk Grove Village, Ill., American Academy of Pediatrics, 1991.

Bates, D. W., et al. Incidence of adverse drug events and potential adverse drug events. Journal of the American Medical Association 274:29–43, 1995.

Benenson, A. S. (editor). Control of Communicable Diseases in Man, 15th ed. Washington, D.C., American Public Health Association, 1990.

Bia, F. J. Malaria prophylaxis: taking aim at constantly moving targets. Yale Journal of Biology and Medicine 65:329–336, 1992.

Cartter, M. L., et al. Influenza outbreaks in nursing homes: how effective is influenza vaccine in the institutionalized elderly? Infection Control and Hospital Epidemiology 11:473–478, 1990.

Cassel, J. Psychological processes and stress: theoretical formulation. International Journal of Health Services 4:471–482, 1974.

Centers for Disease Control and Prevention. Advisory Committee on Immunization Practices: general recommendations on immunization. Morbidity and Mortality Weekly Report 43(RR-1), 1994a.

Centers for Disease Control and Prevention. Advisory Committee on Immunization Practices: recommendations for use of Haemophilus b conjugate vaccines and a combined diphtheria, tetanus, pertussis, and Haemophilus b vaccine. Morbidity and Mortality Weekly Report 42(RR-13), 1993.

Centers for Disease Control and Prevention. Diphtheria epidemic: new independent states of the former Soviet Union, 1990–1994. Morbidity and Mortality Weekly Report 44:177–181, 1995.

Centers for Disease Control and Prevention. Update: childhood vaccine—United States, 1994. Morbidity and Mortality Weekly Report 43:718–720, 1994b.

Centers for Disease Control and Prevention. Vaccination coverage of 2-year-old children: United States, 1993. Morbidity and Mortality Weekly Report 43:705–709, 1994c.

Centers for Disease Control and Prevention. The Vaccines for Children Program, 1994. Morbidity and Mortality Weekly Report 43:705, 1994d.

Clemens, J. D., and E. D. Shapiro. Resolving the pneumococcal vaccine controversy: are there alternatives to randomized clinical trials? Reviews of Infectious Diseases 6:589–600, 1984.

Francis, T., Jr., et al. An evaluation of the 1954 poliomyelitis vaccine trials. American Journal of Public Health, April supplement, 1955.

Herwaldt, L. A. Pertussis and pertussis vaccines in adults. Journal of the American Medical Association 269:93–94, 1993.

Hill, D. R. Immunizations for foreign travel. Yale Journal of Biology and Medicine 65:293–315, 1992.

Inlander, C. B., et al. Medicine on Trial. New Jersey, Prentice-Hall Press, 1988.

Jekel, J. F. Communicable disease control in the 1970s: hot war, cold war, or peaceful coexistence? American Journal of Public Health 62:1578–1585, 1972.

Johnstone, T. Whooping cough in the United States and Britain (letter). New England Journal of Medicine 309:108–109, 1983.

Jong, E. C. The Travel and Tropical Medicine Manual. Philadelphia, W. B. Saunders Company, 1987.

Leape, L. L., et al. Adverse events and negligence in hospitalized patients. Iatrogenics 1:17–21, 1991.

Marks, J., T. J. Halpin, and W. A. Orenstein. Measles vaccine efficacy in children previously vaccinated at 12 months of age. Pediatrics 62:955–960, 1978.

Medical Letter on Drugs and Therapeutics. Hepatitis A vaccine. Medical Letter on Drugs and Therapeutics 37:51–52, 1995a.

Medical Letter on Drugs and Therapeutics. New recommendations for immunization against pertussis and hepatitis B. Medical Letter on Drugs and Therapeutics 34:69–70, 1992.

Medical Letter on Drugs and Therapeutics. Varicella vaccine. Medical Letter on Drugs and Therapeutics 37:55–57, 1995b.

Roitt, I. M. Essential Immunology, 7th ed. Oxford, Blackwell Scientific Publications, 1991.

Rosenstock, I. M. Historical origins of the health belief model. Health Education Monographs 2:328–335, 1974.

Shapiro, E. D., et al. The protective efficacy of polyvalent pneumococcal polysaccharide vaccine. New England Journal of Medicine 325:1453–1460, 1991.

Weibel, R. E., et al. Live attenuated varicella virus vaccine: efficacy trial in healthy children. New England Journal of Medicine 310:1409–1415, 1984.

Selected Readings

American Academy of Pediatrics. Report of the Committee on Infectious Diseases, 22nd ed. Elk Grove Village, Ill., American Academy of Pediatrics, 1991. [Immunization and infectious diseases.]

Benenson, A. S. (editor). Control of Communicable Diseases in Man, 16th ed. Washington, D.C., American Public Health Association, 1995. [Immunization and infectious diseases.]

Centers for Disease Control and Prevention. Advisory Committee on Immunization Practices: general recommendations on immunization. Morbidity and Mortality Weekly Report 43(RR-1), 1994. [Immunization and infectious diseases.]

Hill, D. R. Immunizations for foreign travel. Yale Journal of Biology and Medicine 65:293–315, 1992. [International travel.]

Jong, E. C. The Travel and Tropical Medicine Manual. Philadelphia, W. B. Saunders Company, 1987. [International travel.]

CHAPTER SEVENTEEN

METHODS OF SECONDARY

PREVENTION

Secondary prevention is aimed at early detection of disease, either through screening or case finding, followed by treatment.

Screening is the process of identifying a subgroup of people who are at high risk for having asymptomatic disease or who have a risk factor that puts them at high risk for developing a disease or becoming injured. Unlike case finding, which is defined below, screening takes place in a **community setting** and is applied to a community population, such as students in a school or workers in an industry. A positive screening test result in an individual is not diagnostic of a disease. It merely identifies a person as being at high risk for having that disease. As shown in Fig. 17–1, the process of screening is complex and involves a cascade of actions that should follow if each step along the way yields positive results. In this regard, initiating a screening program is like getting on a roller coaster, and those involved must continue until the end of the process is reached.

Screening is usually distinguished from **case finding,** which is the process of searching for asymptomatic diseases or risk factors among people while they are in a **clinical setting** (i.e., among people who are under medical care). If a patient is being seen for the first time in a medical care setting, whether it is

in a private or group practice or a health maintenance organization (HMO), physicians and other health care workers will usually take a thorough medical history and perform a careful physical examination and any indicated laboratory tests. Establishing baseline values in this way may produce case finding (if problems are discovered) and is considered by many to be good medicine, but it is not screening.

A program to take annual blood pressures of the people employed in a business or industry would be considered "screening," whereas performing a chest x-ray and measuring the blood pressure of a patient who was just admitted to a hospital for elective surgery would be called "case finding." Unfortunately, the distinction between screening and case finding is frequently ignored in the literature and in practice. The distinction is important because many of the criteria for community screening do not need to be met during the process of case finding. Because the purposes and criteria for community screening differ considerably from those for case finding, the discussion of these will be separated below.

In Chapter 7, some of the quantitative issues involved in screening were considered, including sensitivity, specificity, and predictive value of tests. In this chapter, it is assumed that the reader is comfort-

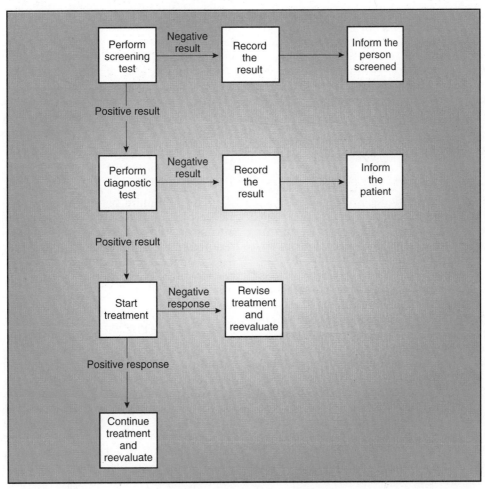

FIGURE 17–1. The process of screening.

TABLE 17-1.   Different Possible Objectives of Screening Programs

Target	Objective	Example
Disease	Treatment to cure patients	Cancer
Disease	Treatment to prevent complications	Hypertension
Disease	Measures to eradicate infection and prevent its spread	Gonorrhea, syphilis, or tuberculosis
Disease	Change in diet and lifestyle	Coronary artery disease or type II diabetes mellitus
Behavioral risk factor	Change in life-style or occupation	Cigarette smoking or unsafe sexual practices
Environmental risk factor	Change in occupation	Chronic obstructive pulmonary disease from work in a dusty trade
Metabolic risk factor	Treatment or change in diet and life-style	Coronary artery disease or elevated serum cholesterol levels

able with these concepts. The purpose here is to discuss broader issues concerning screening and case finding.

COMMUNITY SCREENING
Objectives of Screening

Community screening programs seek to test large numbers of persons for one or more diseases or risk factors in a community setting (e.g., in an educational, employment, or recreational setting), on a voluntary basis, usually with little or no direct financial outlay by the persons being screened. Table 17–1 lists various objectives of community screening and provides examples.

Ethical and Practical Concerns about Community Screening

If a patient comes to see a physician because of a medical problem, the practitioner is ethically and legally obligated to provide the best of medical care but is not obligated to guarantee the success of an appropriate and standard treatment. However, when an apparently well population of individuals who have not sought medical care is screened, the professionals involved in the screening program have a greater obligation to show that the benefits of being screened outweigh the costs. The methods used in performing any public screening program, therefore, should be safe, with minimal side effects.

Test errors are a major concern in screening. **False-positive test results** lead to extra time and costs and can also cause anxiety and discomfort to those whose results were in error. **False-negative test results** are, in some ways, even worse. One implied promise made to people is that if they are screened for a particular disease and found to have negative results, they do not have to worry about that disease. False-negative test results may lead people with early symptoms to be less concerned and therefore to delay medical visits that they might otherwise have made promptly. Thus, false-negative test results can be detrimental to the health of the people whose results were in error, and if the results delay the diagnosis in people who have an infectious disease, such as tuberculosis, they can be dangerous to the health of others as well.

It is not easy to establish the value of a community screening effort unless a randomized controlled trial is conducted. One of the scientific reasons that this type of trial is needed is that an association between having been screened and longer survival does not necessarily prove a cause-and-effect relationship, since two problems could have occurred: lead-time bias and length bias (Bailar 1976).

Lead-time bias occurs when screening detects disease earlier in its natural history than would otherwise have happened, so that the length of time from diagnosis to death is lengthened. Having additional lead time may not alter the natural history of the disease and, therefore, may not extend the length of life. This lead-time bias tends to operate in screening for cancers, no matter how aggressive the tumors are. **Length bias** occurs when the full spectrum of a particular tumor, such as prostate cancer, is composed of cancers that range from very aggressive to quite indolent. Persons discovered by screening programs are more likely to have a less aggressive tumor (because such persons survive longer to be detected) and therefore are likely to survive longer after detection, regardless of the treatment given. It should be noted that both lead-time bias and length bias apply to case finding as well as to community screening.

Given all of the potential problems in demonstrating the true effectiveness of screening, a great deal of care must be exercised to make sure a community screening program is worthwhile.

Minimum Requirements for Community Screening Programs

The minimum requirements for establishing a safe, ethical, and cost-effective screening program fall into three areas: disease requirements, screening test requirements, and health care system requirements. If any of the requirements are not at least partially met, population-wide screening may be inappropriate.

Disease Requirements

(1) The disease must be serious (i.e., produce significant morbidity or mortality), or there is no reason to screen in the first place.

(2) Even if a disease is serious, there must be an effective therapy for the disease if it is detected. Screening is of no value unless there is a good chance that detecting the disease in the presymptomatic stage will result in effective therapy. At the present time, there is no value in screening for pancreatic cancer, because the chance of cure by standard medical and surgical methods is so small.

(3) The natural history of a disease must be understood clearly enough to know that there is a significant window of time during which the disease is detectable and to believe that detection would probably lead to a cure or at least to effective treatment. For example, early detection and surgical removal of a malignant tumor in the colon could prevent intestinal obstruction and considerable morbidity, and it might be curative if all of the tumor were removed.

(4) The disease or condition must not be too rare or too common. Screening for a rare disease usually means that many false-positive test results would be expected (see Chapter 7). This increases the cost and difficulties of discovering those who truly are ill or at high risk, and it also causes anxiety and inconvenience for those who must undergo retesting because of erroneous test results. Unless the benefits from discovering one case are very high (such as in the case of treating a newborn child who has phenylketonuria or congenital hypothyroidism), it will seldom be cost-effective to screen general populations for a rare disease.

There is also no reason to do community screening for extremely common conditions, such as dental caries, because most of the screened population will need to return for further diagnosis or treatment. However, screening for some common conditions, such as elevated cholesterol levels, may provide opportunities for education and motivation, if it occurs in the context of medical care.

Screening Test Requirements

(1) The screening test must be reasonably quick, easy, and inexpensive, or the costs of large-scale screening in terms of time, effort, and money will be prohibitive.

(2) The screening test must be safe and acceptable both to the persons being screened and to their physicians. If the persons to be screened object to a procedure (as frequently occurs with colonoscopies), they are unlikely to participate.

(3) The sensitivity, specificity, positive predictive value, and other operating characteristics of a screening test must be known and be acceptable. As discussed above, both false-positive and false-negative test results are serious.

Health Care System Requirements

(1) There must be adequate follow-up for all persons who have positive results in the screening test. Because screening only sets apart a high-risk group, persons who have positive results must receive further diagnostic testing to rule in or rule out actual disease, even though the follow-up testing may be expensive, time-consuming, painful, and even entail some risk. With some screening programs, the majority of effort and costs are in the follow-up phase, not in the initial screening.

(2) Before a screening program for a particular disease is undertaken, there should already be adequate and accessible treatment for people known to have that disease. If there are limited resources, it does not make sense, either ethically or in terms of cost-effectiveness, to allow persons with symptoms of the disease to go untreated and yet look for the same disease in persons without symptoms.

(3) Those who are screened and diagnosed as having the disease in question must have access to treatment, or the process is ethically flawed. In addition to being unethical, it makes no medical sense to bring the persons screened to the point of informing them of a positive test result and then abandoning them. This is a major problem for community screening efforts, because many people who come for screening will have little or no medical care coverage, and the cost for their treatment will need to be borne by a local hospital or other institution.

(4) The treatment should be acceptable to those being screened. Otherwise, those who require treatment will not undertake it and the screening will have accomplished nothing. For example, some men will not want surgery for prostate cancer, because of possible interference with sexual functioning.

(5) The population to be screened should be clearly defined, so that the resulting data will be epidemiologically useful. Although screening at "health fairs" and in shopping centers provides the opportunity to educate the public about health matters, the data obtained are seldom useful because the screening population is not well-defined and tends to be self-selected and highly biased in favor of those concerned about their health (Berwick 1985).

(6) It should be clear who is responsible for the screening, what the cutoff points are for calling a test result positive, and how the findings will become part of a participant's medical record at his or her usual place of care.

Application of the Criteria to Examples

Table 17–2 applies the above criteria to four conditions for which community screening has commonly been undertaken: (1) hypertension, tested by a sphygmomanometer reading of blood pressure; (2) elevated cholesterol levels, with total cholesterol measurement based on a rapid screening of blood; (3) breast cancer, tested by mammography; and (4) lung cancer, tested by chest x-ray.

Investigators have agreed that a screening program using chest x-rays to detect lung cancer fails at some critical points, particularly in respect to treatment. Specifically, numerous studies have shown that only a small proportion of cancers detected by chest x-rays can be cured by the time they are visible (see, for example, Greenberg 1956; Brett 1968; Boucot and Weiss 1973). Because of the problems reported in early studies, community screening for lung cancer by chest x-rays is no longer recommended.

TABLE 17–2.   Requirements for Screening Programs and Ratings of Example Methods to Detect Hypertension, Elevated Cholesterol Levels, Breast Cancer, and Lung Cancer

Requirements	Screening Method and Rating*			
	Sphygmomanometer Reading	Serum Cholesterol Test	Mammogram	Chest X-Ray
Disease requirements				
(1) The disease is serious.	++	++	++	++
(2) Effective treatment exists.	++	+	+	+/–
(3) The natural history of the disease is understood.	++	+	+	+
(4) The disease occurs frequently.	++	++	++	++
(5) Other diseases or conditions may be detected.	–	–	–	+
Screening test requirements				
(1) The test is quick to perform.	++	+	+	++
(2) The test is easy to administer.	++	+	+	+
(3) The test is inexpensive.	++	+	+	+
(4) The test is safe.	++	++	+	+
(5) The test is acceptable to participants.	++	+	+	++
(6) The sensitivity, specificity, and other operating characteristics of the test are acceptable.	++	+	+	–
Health care system requirements				
(1) The method meets the requirements for screening in a community setting.	++	++	+	–
(2) The method meets the requirements for case finding in a medical care setting.	++	++	++	+

*Ratings are applied to four conditions for which community screening has commonly been undertaken: hypertension, tested by a sphygmomanometer reading of blood pressure; elevated cholesterol levels, with total cholesterol measurement based on a rapid screening of blood; breast cancer, tested by mammography; and lung cancer, tested by chest x-ray. Ratings are as follows: ++ means good, + means satisfactory, and – means unsatisfactory.

Although the other screening methods indicated in Table 17–2 are now generally accepted, as is cervical cancer screening by Papanicolaou test, there is still considerable debate about issues such as what age to start the screening, how often to repeat it, and whether the methods yield accurate results (Elmore et al. 1994).

Newer screening methods are being debated even more sharply. For example, investigators are questioning whether active treatment of prostate cancer detected by prostate-specific antigen (PSA) testing really changes the natural history of the disease. Recent evidence suggests that aggressive treatment of prostate cancers detected through PSA screening may actually decrease the quality of life without adding compensatory benefits (Krahn et al. 1994; Litwin et al. 1995; Potosky et al. 1995).

Repetition of Screening Programs

Deciding how frequently a screening program will be repeated in the future must be based on knowledge of the following: (1) whether resources are available for screening and whether their use for this purpose would be cost-effective in comparison to their use for other purposes; (2) how well previous similar screening programs worked in the same community, including the effectiveness of follow-up diagnosis and treatment and the benefits obtained by those who were diagnosed and treated in this way; (3) what percentage of the community was involved in the previous screening efforts and how much time has elapsed since screening was undertaken; and (4) what the incidence and natural history are for the disease being screened.

There are dangers in not giving careful thought to the details of repeat screening efforts. Strangely enough, this is particularly true if an initial major screening effort is considered a great success, in which case enthusiasm may lead the organizers to repeat the screening too soon (e.g., a year later). Almost inevitably, unless the population screened the second time is very different from the one screened the first time, a screening effort repeated after a short interval will be quite disappointing. This is because the initial screening will have detected prevalent cases (cases accumulated over many years), whereas the repeated screening will detect only incident cases (new cases since the last screening), making the number of detected cases smaller (Christopherson, Parker, and Drye 1962).

Multiphasic Screening

Multiphasic screening programs are those which involve screening for a variety of diseases in the same individual. Some investigators have argued that multiphasic screening makes community efforts more efficient. Once a sample of blood is drawn, for example, it is easy to perform a variety of tests, using modern, automated laboratory equipment. The yield of multiphasic screening, however, has come under serious question (Bates and Yellin 1972).

One problem is that multiphasic screening in an elderly population will often detect diseases or abnormal conditions that have been found earlier and are already being treated, in which case funds are being used for unnecessary testing. Another problem is that multiphasic screening results in a relatively high frequency of false-positive results, and this requires many participants to return for more expensive follow-up tests.

For each disease-free person screened, the probability that at least one of the screening tests will yield a false-positive finding can be expressed as $[1 - (1 - \text{alpha})^n]$, where alpha is the false-positive error rate (see Chapter 7) and n is the number of screening tests done. If two screening tests are performed and alpha is 5% (making the test specificity 95%), the probability of a disease-free person being recalled for further testing is $[1 - (0.95)^2] = [1 - (0.9025)] = $ almost 10%. If four tests are performed, the probability is $[1 - (0.95)^4] = [1 - (0.8145)] = 18.5\%$. As Table 17–3 shows, if 25 tests are performed, over 70% of disease-free individuals would be brought back for unnecessary but often costly follow-up testing.

Persons with one or more diseases or conditions that would be detected by multiphasic screening would have a slightly smaller probability of having one or more false-positive findings, only because the number of tests eligible to be falsely called positive would be reduced by the number of truly positive tests.

When Olsen, Kane, and Proctor (1976) undertook a controlled trial of multiphasic screening, they subjected one group of individuals to a battery of special screening tests that included hearing and vision tests, ocular pressure measurements, blood pressure measurements, spirometry, electrocardiography, mammography and breast examination, Papanicolaou smear, chest x-ray, urinalysis, complete blood count, and 12 blood chemistry tests. When they compared the findings in this group with the findings in a control group that was not subjected to the battery of special tests, they found that there were no major differences in the health knowledge or the mortality and morbidity rates of the two groups. However, the group that underwent multiphasic screening did spend more nights in the hospital.

INDIVIDUAL CASE FINDING
The Periodic Health Examination

Historically, the most common method of prevention in clinical medicine, especially in adults, has

been the annual physical checkup, which has come to be known as the periodic health examination.

After World War II, the number of available treatments for chronic illnesses increased greatly, and more people began to have an annual checkup, usually consisting of a medical history, physical examination, complete blood count, urinalysis, chest x-ray, and electrocardiogram. Despite the popularity of these checkups, the number of people who received them was limited by the fact that many insurance plans would not cover their costs, although some corporations provided them as a perquisite for high-level managers. In fact, most research on the periodic health examination prior to the 1960s concerned examinations that were sponsored by businesses or industries or were conducted by the few large health plans existing at the time.

An annotated bibliography of 152 early studies of periodic health examinations (Siegel 1963) shows that reports published prior to 1940 were mostly anecdotal and were enthusiastic about the examinations. Reports published between 1940 and 1962 were more likely to include quantitative data and, although still supportive, increasingly raised serious questions about "routine" use of examinations. With the subsequent increase in the number of health maintenance organizations (HMOs) came an increase in the use of periodic examinations, and even though most investigators agreed that examinations in children were beneficial, more and more studies began to cast doubts about the cost-effectiveness of examinations in adults (for example, see Schor et al. 1964; Roberts et al. 1969; Spitzer and Brown 1975; Spark 1976).

During the 1970s, investigators began moving toward the idea of modifying the periodic examination to focus only on those conditions and diseases that would be most likely to be found in a person of a given age, gender, and family history. This approach was given the term "lifetime health monitoring" by Breslow and Somers (1977). The biggest support for a new approach came in 1979, when the Canadian Task Force on the Periodic Physical Examination recommended that the traditional form of periodic checkup be replaced by the use of **health protection packages** that included sex-appropriate and age-appropriate immunizations, screening, and counseling of patients on a periodic basis. Specifically, the task force recommended that "with certain exceptions, the procedures be carried out as case finding rather than screening techniques; that is, they should be performed when the patient is attending for unrelated symptoms rather than for a specific preventive purpose." Among the "certain exceptions" noted by the task force were pregnant women, the very young, and the very old, for whom they recommended regular visits specifically for preventive purposes.

US Preventive Services Task Force

In an effort to clarify many of the issues concerning screening and case finding and to make well-studied recommendations, the US Department of

TABLE 17–3. Correlation between Number of Screening Tests Performed and Percentage of Persons with at Least One False-Positive Test Result

Number of Screening Tests Performed	Percentage of Persons with at Least One False-Positive Test Result*
1	5.0
2	9.8
4	18.5
5	22.6
10	40.1
20	64.2
25	72.3

Source of data: Schoenberg, B. S. The "abnormal" laboratory result. Postgraduate Medicine 47:151–155, 1970.

*Percentages are based on tests that each have a 5% false-positive error rate.

Health and Human Services created the US Preventive Services Task Force (USPSTF). In its investigations, the USPSTF reviewed data concerning the efficacy of a variety of interventions, including the following: (1) immunizations in children and adults; (2) postexposure prophylaxis of certain infectious diseases, such as *Haemophilus influenzae* type b disease, meningococcal infections, hepatitis A and B, tuberculosis, and rabies; (3) estrogen and aspirin use to prevent myocardial infarction; (4) counseling to prevent dental disease, tobacco use, motor vehicle injuries, household and environmental injuries, unintended pregnancy, and type 1 human immunodeficiency virus (HIV-1) infection and other sexually transmitted diseases; and (5) counseling to increase exercise and improve nutrition.

The first report of the USPSTF was issued in 1989 and consisted of an assessment of the effectiveness of a total of 169 interventions considered to be preventive in nature. This report, which is summarized in Box 17–1, has become a standard reference for investigators and health care workers in the field of preventive medicine.

In the area of screening tests and programs, the USPSTF recommendations are based not only on the efficacy of screening tests in detecting disease and adverse conditions but also on the extent to which early detection actually improves health. In this regard, the US task force borrowed much of the methodology developed by the Canadian task force and applied it more broadly. For example, using the latter's idea of "health protection packages," the USPSTF listed the following for each age group: (1) conditions to be the subject of screening efforts using the medical history, physical examination, and laboratory or other diagnostic procedures; (2) items for counseling regarding diet, exercise, substance use, sexual practices, injury prevention, dental health, and other matters; (3) immunizations and chemoprophylaxis; and (4) problems or concerns about which physicians should be particularly alert, such as those listed in Box 17–2.

Health Risk Assessments

Health risk assessments (HRAs) use questionnaires or computer programs to elicit and evaluate information concerning individuals in a clinical or industrial medical practice. Each assessed person receives information concerning his or her life expectancy and the types of interventions that are likely to have a positive impact on health or longevity.

For more than 25 years, the idea of HRAs has been promoted by physicians who are enthusiastic about detecting disease and risk factors in individuals. Based on the original work of Robbins and Hall (1970), a professional organization called the Society for Prospective Medicine has been formed. Its members seek to improve the construction and use of HRAs and the practice of preventive ("prospective") medicine in the context of a clinical or industrial medical practice (see Society for Prospective Medi-

cine 1995). Toward this end, they promote the use of HRAs for (1) assessing the needs of individual patients as they enter a medical care system or of employees in an industrial setting, (2) developing health education information for those who complete the assessment, and (3) developing cost-containment strategies based on better acquisition of health risk information from individuals.

Most HRAs use questionnaires or interactive computer programs to gather data concerning each person being assessed. In addition to data such as height, weight, blood pressure, cholesterol level, and previous and present diseases, the information usually includes details concerning the person's life-style and his or her family history. A computer then calculates the person's "risk age" on the basis of the data and an algorithm. Most HRAs use an algorithm based on findings of the Framingham Study. The **risk age** is defined as the age at which the average individual would have the same risk of dying as the person being assessed. If the assessed person's risk age is older than his or her chronologic age, that means that he or she has a higher risk of dying than the average individual of the same chronologic age. Likewise, if the assessed person's risk age is younger than the chronologic age, the person has a lower risk of dying than the average individual of the same chronologic age.

The HRAs usually provide a printed report about the assessed person's relative risk of dying or risk age, combined with some sort of educational message regarding the types of interventions that would have the most positive effect on the person's life expectancy if they were instituted. The printed reports have become more sophisticated in recent years and are sometimes supplemented with video cassettes providing tailor-made educational messages.

At least 27 currently available HRAs are listed and discussed in a major publication by the Society for Prospective Medicine (see Peterson and Hilles 1992). Some, such as the popular version from the Carter Center, are in the public domain and are self-contained. Others are proprietary programs for which the developer gets a fee for each person assessed.

HRAs have been extensively evaluated, with mixed results (see, for example, Foxman and Edington 1987; Kirscht 1989; Schoenbach 1987; Smith, McKinlay, and McKinlay 1989; Smith, McKinlay, and Thorington 1987). So far, criticisms have focused on errors or lack of information by the persons entering the data; difficulties in validating the predictions; uncertainties concerning the correct reference population for baseline risks; limitations related to the fact that the instruments focus mainly or exclusively on mortality and not on morbidity or the quality of life; and limitations associated with the middle-class orientation of all of the instruments developed to date. The greatest strength of HRAs may be their ability to clarify how nutritional and life-style factors affect an assessed person's risk of death and to motivate that person to make changes in a positive direction.

BOX 17–1. US Preventive Services Task Force Recommendations Regarding Screening for Specific Diseases, Conditions, and Risk Factors in Asymptomatic Persons*

Disease, Condition, or Risk Factor	Recommendation
Cancers	
Breast cancer	Annual clinical breast examination is recommended for women 40 years or older. Mammography every 1–2 years is recommended for women between 50 and 75 years of age.
Cervical cancer	Papanicolaou testing every 1–3 years is recommended for all women who are or have been sexually active.
Colorectal cancer	There is insufficient evidence to recommend for or against fecal occult blood testing and sigmoidoscopy; these may be of value in persons who are 50 years or older and have a positive family history. Periodic colonoscopy is recommended for persons with a family history of polyposis.
Lung cancer	Routine screening by chest x-ray or sputum cytology is not recommended.
Oral cancer	Routine screening is not recommended, although it may be of value in those with risk factors such as smoking or chewing tobacco. Examination should be incorporated into regular dental visits.
Ovarian cancer	Routine screening is not recommended.
Pancreatic cancer	Routine screening is not recommended.
Prostate cancer	There is insufficient evidence to recommend for or against routine digital rectal examination in asymptomatic men. Transrectal ultrasound and serum tests for tumor markers, such as prostate-specific antigen, are not recommended for routine screening.
Skin cancer	Routine screening is recommended for persons at high risk, such as those with light skin, easy burning, and major sun exposure. Primary prevention by avoiding excessive sunlight and by use of sunscreens is also recommended.
Testicular cancer	Periodic screening is recommended for men with a history of cryptorchidism, orchiopexy, or testicular atrophy. There is insufficient evidence to recommend for or against testicular self-examination or routine screening of other men.
Congenital and perinatal conditions	
Birth defects	Amniocentesis for karyotyping should be offered to any pregnant woman who is 35 years or older. Unless the pregnant woman does not have access to counseling and follow-up services, her serum alpha-fetoprotein level should be measured between week 16 and week 18 of gestation. In normal pregnancies, routine ultrasound examination is not recommended as a screening measure for birth defects.
Fetal distress	In pregnant women, the fetal heart rate should be monitored by auscultation during labor. Electronic fetal monitoring should be used only in women whose fetuses are at high risk for fetal distress.
Intrauterine growth retardation	Ultrasound examination should be performed in women whose fetuses are at high risk for intrauterine growth retardation. All pregnant women should receive counseling regarding the dangers of smoking, alcohol consumption, and use of legal and illegal drugs during pregnancy.
Preeclampsia	In pregnant women, systolic and diastolic blood pressure measurements should be taken during the first prenatal visit and periodically throughout the third trimester.
Hematologic conditions	
Anemia	Testing for anemia is recommended in pregnant women during the first prenatal visit and in infants during the first year of life. Routine testing is not recommended in other asymptomatic persons.
Hemoglobinopathies	Hemoglobin analysis is recommended in newborn infants who are of African, Mediterranean, or Southeast Asian descent and are at risk for hemoglobinopathies. Families of these infants should be counseled regarding the analysis and results.
Rh incompatibility	During the first prenatal visit, pregnant women should undergo ABO and Rh (D) blood typing and testing for anti–Rh (D) antibody. Unsensitized Rh-negative women should be given Rh (D) immune globulin between week 23 and week 29 of gestation and at delivery or termination of the pregnancy.
Infectious diseases	
Bacteriuria	Periodic dipstick testing is indicated in patients with diabetes, and urine culture is indicated in pregnant women.
Genital herpes infection	Cultures are indicated in pregnant women who have had genital herpetic lesions or whose sexual partners have had these lesions.
Gonorrhea and chlamydial infection	Newborn infants should have a topical ophthalmic antibiotic applied immediately after birth to prevent ophthalmia neonatorum. Pregnant women should have an endocervical culture for gonorrhea and chlamydial infection during their first prenatal visit, with a repeat culture during the latter part of pregnancy for those at high risk. Any person at high risk for sexually transmitted diseases should have routine cultures.
Hepatitis B	Pregnant women should be tested for hepatitis B surface antigen (HBsAg) during the first prenatal visit, and those at high risk should be tested again during the third trimester. Infants whose mothers are HBsAg-positive should receive hepatitis B immune globulin and hepatitis B vaccine immediately after birth.

Continued

BOX 17–1.   US Preventive Services Task Force Recommendations Regarding Screening for Specific Diseases, Conditions, and Risk Factors in Asymptomatic Persons* *(Continued)*

Disease, Condition, or Risk Factor	Recommendation
Infectious diseases *(continued)*	
HIV-1 infection	Persons whose sexual activity or intravenous drug use places them at high risk for type 1 human immunodeficiency virus (HIV-1) infection should be offered antibody testing and counseling.
Rubella	A serologic test for rubella antibodies is recommended for all women of childbearing age and should be performed at the first clinical opportunity. Pregnant women found to lack rubella antibodies should be immunized immediately after delivery. Nonpregnant women who lack rubella antibodies and are willing to take the necessary precautions to avoid conception during the next 3 months should be immunized.
Syphilis	Pregnant women should be tested for syphilis during the first prenatal visit and at delivery. Persons whose sexual activity places them at high risk for syphilis should be tested periodically, although the optimal screening interval has not been defined.
Tuberculosis	Persons at high risk of acquiring tuberculosis should undergo tuberculin skin testing. Bacillus Calmette-Guérin (BCG) vaccine should be used only in tuberculin-negative children who cannot take isoniazid and are in continuous contact with an infectious person.
Metabolic and genetic diseases	
Diabetes mellitus	Routine screening for hyperglycemia may be of value in high-risk groups and is recommended in pregnant women between week 24 and week 28 of gestation. It is generally discouraged in other persons.
Obesity	Periodic height and weight measurements are recommended in all children and adults.
Osteoporosis	Routine x-rays to detect low bone mineral content are not recommended.
Phenylketonuria	Newborn infants should be screened for phenylketonuria during the first week of life. Those who are tested before 24 hours of age should be retested before the third week of life.
Thyroid disease	Newborn infants should be screened for congenital hypothyroidism during the first week of life. Screening may be indicated for persons with a history of x-ray exposure to the thyroid area. Routine screening for thyroid disease in others is not recommended.
Vascular diseases	
Cerebrovascular disease	Auscultation for carotid bruits may be of value. Eliciting a history of transient ischemic attacks may be of value. Screening for the following risk factors is recommended: diet, exercise, hypertension, and smoking.
Coronary artery disease	Screening for asymptomatic coronary artery disease is not recommended. Screening for the following risk factors is strongly recommended: diet, exercise, hypertension, and smoking.
High blood cholesterol levels	Periodic measurement of total serum cholesterol is most important in middle-aged men, but it also may be wise in young men and women and in the elderly.
Hypertension	Blood pressure should be measured regularly in all persons 3 years of age and older.
Peripheral artery disease	Screening for disease is not recommended. Screening for risk factors, particularly smoking, may be of value.
Other diseases and conditions	
Alcohol and drug use	Adults and adolescents in clinical settings should be asked to describe their use of alcohol and other drugs, but routine drug testing and assays for biochemical markers are not recommended.
Dementia	Routine screening of asymptomatic persons is not recommended.
Depression and suicidal intent	The use of routine screening tests is not recommended.
Diminished visual acuity	Children should be screened for visual acuity once during the preschool period, preferably at the age of 3 or 4 years.
Glaucoma	There is insufficient evidence to recommend for or against routine screening by tonometry. However, persons 65 years or older should probably be screened periodically for glaucoma.
Hearing impairment	There is insufficient evidence to recommend for or against routine screening of asymptomatic children after the age of 3 years. However, children at high risk for hearing impairment should be screened before the age of 3 years.
Lead toxicity	Annual lead screening is recommended for children who are between 9 months and 6 years of age and are at high risk for lead toxicity.
Low back injury	Routine screening is not recommended.

Source of data: US Preventive Services Task Force (USPSTF). Guide to Clinical Preventive Services. Baltimore, Williams & Wilkins, 1989.

*Note: These recommendations are constantly being revised by the USPSTF, based on the latest research.

Without having an electronically driven HRA, the physician can make effective assessments by knowing what things to look for in each age group. The USPSTF age-related list of the leading causes of death and problems to remain alert for is presented in Box 17–2.

SUMMARY

The goal of secondary prevention is the detection of disease or risk factors in the presymptomatic stage, when medical, environmental, nutritional, and life-style interventions can be most effective. Screening is carried out in a community

BOX 17–2. Leading Causes of Death and Problems to Remain Alert for in the US Population

Age Group	Leading Causes of Death (in Order of Frequency)	Problems to Remain Alert For
0–24 months	Perinatal conditions Congenital anomalies Heart disease Injuries (non–motor vehicle) Influenza and pneumonia	Ocular misalignment Tooth decay Signs of child abuse or neglect
2–6 years	Injuries (non–motor vehicle) Motor vehicle crashes Congenital anomalies Homicide Heart disease	Vision disorders Tooth decay or misalignment Mouth breathing Signs of child abuse or neglect Abnormal bereavement
7–12 years	Motor vehicle crashes Injuries (non–motor vehicle) Congenital anomalies Leukemia Homicide Heart disease	Vision disorders Diminished hearing Tooth decay or misalignment Mouth breathing Signs of child abuse or neglect Abnormal bereavement
13–18 years	Motor vehicle crashes Homicide Suicide Injuries (non–motor vehicle) Heart disease	Symptoms of depression Suicide risk factors Abnormal bereavement Tooth decay, tooth misalignment, or gingivitis Signs of child abuse or neglect
19–39 years	Motor vehicle crashes Homicide Suicide Injuries (non–motor vehicle) Heart disease	Symptoms of depression Suicide risk factors Abnormal bereavement Tooth decay, tooth misalignment, or gingivitis Signs of physical abuse or neglect Malignant skin lesions
40–64 years	Heart disease Lung cancer Cerebrovascular disease Breast cancer Colorectal cancer Obstructive lung disease	Symptoms of depression Suicide risk factors Abnormal bereavement Signs of physical abuse or neglect Malignant skin lesions Peripheral artery disease Tooth decay or gingivitis
65+ years	Heart disease Cerebrovascular disease Obstructive lung disease Pneumonia and influenza Lung cancer Colorectal cancer	Symptoms of depression Suicide risk factors Abnormal bereavement Changes in cognitive function Medications that increase the risk of falls Signs of physical abuse or neglect Malignant skin lesions Peripheral artery disease Tooth decay, loose teeth, or gingivitis

Source of data: US Preventive Services Task Force (USPSTF). Guide to Clinical Preventive Services. Baltimore, Williams & Wilkins, 1989.

setting, whereas case finding is carried out in a clinical setting.

For community screening programs to be beneficial and cost-effective, they must fulfill various requirements concerning the health problem to be detected, the screening test to be used, and the system available to provide health care for those with positive screening results. Lead-time bias and length bias can cause health care personnel and analysts to overestimate the benefit produced by a screening program, particularly when the program is aimed at detection of cancer. Although multiphasic screening seeks to make the process more efficient by searching for many conditions at the same time, the high incidence of false-positive test results and other associated problems have made this technique less successful than was originally anticipated.

Historically, the periodic health examination has been the most common method of case finding. Because it has proved to provide disappointing benefits when examined carefully, it is now being replaced by a new approach called lifetime health monitoring. This approach focuses on monitoring individuals for the specific set of conditions and diseases that are most likely to be found in persons of the same age and gender, and its use has been advocated by experts on preventive medicine in Canada and the USA.

References Cited

Bailar, J. D., III. Mammography: a contrary view. Annals of Internal Medicine 84:77–84, 1976.

Bates, B., and J. A. Yellin. The yield of multiphasic screening. Journal of the American Medical Association 222:74–78, 1972.

Berwick, D. M. Screening in health fairs: a critical review of benefits, risks, and costs. Journal of the American Medical Association 254:1492–1498, 1985.

Boucot, K. R., and W. Weiss. Is curable lung cancer detected by semiannual screening? Journal of the American Medical Association 224:1361–1365, 1973.

Breslow, L., and A. R. Somers. The lifetime health monitoring program: a practical approach to preventive medicine. New England Journal of Medicine 296:601–608, 1977.

Brett, G. Z. The value of lung cancer detection by six-monthly chest radiographs. Thorax 23:414–420, 1968.

Canadian Task Force on the Periodic Physical Examination. The periodic health examination. Canadian Medical Association Journal 121:1193–1254, 1979.

Christopherson, W. M., J. E. Parker, and J. C. Drye. Control of cervical cancer: preliminary report on a community program. Journal of the American Medical Association 182:179–182, 1962.

Elmore, J. G., et al. Variability in radiologists' interpretations of mammograms. New England Journal of Medicine 331:1493–1499, 1994.

Foxman, B., and D. W. Edington. The accuracy of health risk appraisal in predicting mortality. American Journal of Public Health 77:971–974, 1987.

Greenberg, R. A. Mass survey detected lung cancer in Connecticut, 1949–1953. Connecticut State Medical Journal 20:857–863, 1956.

Kirscht, J. P. Process and measurement issues in health risk appraisal (editorial). American Journal of Public Health 79:1598–1599, 1989.

Krahn, M. D., et al. Screening for prostate cancer: a decision analytic view. Journal of the American Medical Association 272:773–780, 1994.

Litwin, L. S., et al. Quality of life outcomes in men tested for prostate cancer. Journal of the American Medical Association 273:129–135, 1995.

Olsen, D. M., R. L. Kane, and P. H. Proctor. A controlled trial of multiphasic screening. New England Journal of Medicine 294:925–930, 1976.

Peterson, K. W., and S. B. Hilles (editors). Society for Prospective Medicine (SPM) Directory of Health Risk Appraisals, 1992. Occupational Health Strategies, Inc., 901 Preston Ave., Suite 400, Charlottesville, VA 22903.

Potosky, A. L., et al. The role of increasing detection in the rising incidence of prostate cancer. Journal of the American Medical Association 273:548–552, 1995.

Robbins, L. C., and J. Hall. How to Practice Prospective Medicine. Indianapolis, Ind., Methodist Hospital of Indiana, 1970.

Roberts, N. J., et al. Mortality among males in periodic health examination programs. New England Journal of Medicine 281:20–24, 1969.

Schoenbach, V. J. Appraising health risk appraisal (editorial). American Journal of Public Health 77:409–411, 1987.

Schor, S. S., et al. An evaluation of the periodic health examination. Annals of Internal Medicine 61:999–1005, 1964.

Siegel, G. S. Periodic Health Examinations: Abstracts from the Literature. Washington, D. C., US Department of Health, Education, and Welfare, 1963.

Smith, K. W., S. M. McKinlay, and J. B. McKinlay. The reliability of health risk appraisals: a field trial of four instruments. American Journal of Public Health 79:1603–1607, 1989.

Smith, K. W., S. M. McKinlay, and B. D. Thorington. The validity of health risk appraisal instruments for assessing coronary heart disease risk. American Journal of Public Health 77:419–424, 1987.

Society for Prospective Medicine: Managing Health Care, Measuring Lives: Expanding the Definition and Scope of Health Risk Appraisal. Thirty-First Annual Meeting of the Society for Prospective Medicine, New Orleans, April 2–3, 1995.

Spark, R. The case against regular physicals. New York Times Magazine, July 25, 1976.

Spitzer, W. O., and B. P. Brown. Unanswered questions about the periodic health examination. Annals of Internal Medicine 83:257–263, 1975.

US Preventive Services Task Force. Guide to Clinical Preventive Services. Baltimore, Williams & Wilkins, 1989.

Selected Readings

Brownson, R. C., P. L. Remington, and J. R. Davis (editors). Chronic Disease Epidemiology and Control. Washington, D. C., American Public Health Association, 1993.

Canadian Task Force on the Periodic Physical Examination. The periodic health examination. Canadian Medical Association Journal 121:1193–1254, 1979.

US Preventive Services Task Force. Guide to Clinical Preventive Services. Baltimore, Williams & Wilkins, 1989.

CHAPTER EIGHTEEN

METHODS OF TERTIARY

PREVENTION

As discussed in Chapter 14, methods of tertiary prevention are designed to limit the physical and social consequences of an injury or disease after it has occurred or become symptomatic. There are two basic categories of tertiary prevention. The first, called **disability limitation,** has the goal of halting the progress of the disease or limiting the damage caused by an injury. In fact, this category of tertiary prevention is probably better thought of as "the prevention of further impairment" (Leavell and Clark 1965). The second category, called **rehabilitation,** focuses on reducing the social disability produced by a given level of impairment, both by strengthening the patient's remaining functions and by helping the patient learn to function in alternative ways. Disability limitation and rehabilitation should ordinarily be initiated at the same time—i.e., when the disease is detected or the injury occurs—but the emphasis on one or the other depends on factors such as the type and stage of disease, the type of injury, and available methods of treatment.

OPPORTUNITIES FOR PREVENTION

The first sign of an illness is often an excellent opportunity to initiate methods of prevention. The sooner therapy is begun, the greater the chance of preventing significant impairment. In fact, in the case of infectious diseases such as tuberculosis and sexually transmitted diseases, early treatment of a symptomatic health problem in one patient may prevent transmission of the disease and therefore constitute primary prevention of the same health problem in others. Similarly, early treatment of alcoholism or drug addiction in one family member may prevent social and emotional problems, including codependency, from developing in other family members.

Symptomatic illness can guide physicians to those persons most in need of preventive efforts. In this sense, the symptoms function in a manner somewhat similar to screening by defining especially needy individuals. People may not be convinced by a preventive message when they feel well, but when they become symptomatic, they frequently are alerted for the first time to the importance of changing their diet, behavior, or environment. For example, a person who is at risk for coronary artery disease will usually be more open to changes in diet and exercise after experiencing angina pectoris or myocardial infarction. The onset of symptoms, therefore, may provide a window of opportunity for health promotion to prevent progression of the disease. Primary health care personnel are in the most strategic position to initiate preventive measures in symptomatic patients.

DISABILITY LIMITATION

Most medical or surgical treatment of symptomatic disease is directed at preventing or minimizing impairment over the short and long run. This is true,

for example, of coronary angioplasty and coronary artery bypass grafting, which are aimed at both extending life and improving function. There is, however, a useful distinction between therapy and symptomatic stage prevention. Whereas **therapy** seeks to undo the threat or damage from an existing disease (e.g., coronary artery disease), **symptomatic stage prevention** attempts to halt or limit the future progression of disease. The strategies of symptomatic stage prevention are taken both from primary prevention (e.g., modification of diet, behavior, and environment) and from secondary prevention (e.g., frequent screening for incipient complications, followed by treatment when complications are discovered).

In this section of the chapter, coronary artery disease, hyperlipidemia, hypertension, and diabetes mellitus will be used to illustrate how methods of disability limitation can be applied to patients with chronic diseases. The emphasis will be on symptomatic stage prevention. Although a brief outline of therapy will be given, a detailed discussion of medical and surgical treatment is beyond the scope of this book.

Coronary Artery Disease

Whether the goal is to prevent the onset or the progression of coronary artery disease, efforts are aimed at assessing and reducing risk factors.

Risk Factors

Male Gender. Men are much more likely than women to show signs of atherosclerotic heart disease before the age of 60 years. In postmenopausal women, the rate of coronary artery disease rises as rapidly as that in men, but it never fully catches up on an age-specific basis.

Family History of Myocardial Infarction. If an individual has a parent or sibling who had a myocardial infarction before the age of 60 years, the individual is at increased risk for coronary artery disease.

Cigarette Smoking. Smoking accelerates blood clotting, increases blood carbon monoxide levels, and causes a reduction in the delivery of oxygen. In addition, nicotine is vasoconstrictive. The age-related risk of myocardial infarction in smokers is approximately twice as high as that in nonsmokers. For those who stop smoking, the excess risk drops fairly quickly and appears to be minimal after a year of nonsmoking.

Diabetes Mellitus. The age-related risk of myocardial infarction in diabetics is about twice as high as that in nondiabetics. There is some suggestion that low-dose aspirin therapy reduces the risk of myocardial infarction both in diabetics and in nondiabetics.

Hypertension. Severe hypertension (systolic blood pressure ≥ 195 mm Hg) approximately quadruples the risk of cardiovascular disease in middle-aged men (Breslow 1978). Lesser degrees of hypertension appear to increase the risk to a smaller degree.

Sedentary Life-Style. It appears that at least 20 minutes of vigorous exercise (fast walking or better) at least 3 times per week reduces the risk of cardiovascular disease. There is still debate regarding how large the negative impact of a sedentary life-style is on the risk of myocardial infarction. The uncertainty occurs because it is difficult to design observational studies that completely avoid the potential bias of self-selection (i.e., people with incipient heart disease may have cues that tell them to avoid such exercise).

Excess Weight. In people who are overweight, the risk for coronary artery disease depends on how the body fat is distributed. When fat is distributed in the hips and legs (giving the body the shape of a pear), there does not appear to be an increased risk of cardiovascular disease. In contrast, when fat is found primarily in the abdominal cavity (giving the body the shape of an apple, a shape more common in men than in women), the fat appears to be more metabolically active and the risk of cardiovascular disease is increased. This is not surprising, because fat mobilized from the omentum goes directly to the liver, which is the center of the body's lipid metabolism.

It is unclear what effect weight reduction per se has on the risk of heart disease. Some studies have suggested that alternating dieting and nondieting ("weight cycling") is a risk factor in itself (Lissner et al. 1991), but other studies have questioned this conclusion (Wing, Jeffery, and Hellerstedt 1995).

Hyperlipidemia. The risk of coronary artery disease is increased in patients with hyperlipidemia. As discussed below, the lipid profile is important and must be interpreted in light of the age, gender, and clinical history of the patient.

Interaction of Risk Factors

The best data on the risk factors for coronary heart disease are derived from the Framingham Study (see Dawber, Meadors, and Moore 1951; see also Breslow 1978). As discussed earlier and outlined in Table 5–2, data from the Framingham Study suggest that multiple risk factors interact in a synergistic manner. For example, the risk that a 45-year-old man will have cardiovascular disease (mostly coronary heart disease) within 8 years varies greatly, depending on whether none, one, or all of the following risk factors are present: (1) smoking, (2) glucose intolerance, (3) hypertrophy of the left ventricle, (4) severe hypertension (systolic blood pressure $\geq$ 195 mm Hg), and (5) high cholesterol level ($\geq$ 335 mg/dL).

As Table 5–2 shows, if none of these five risk factors is present, the 8-year risk is 2.2%, based on age and gender. In contrast, if all of the five risk factors are present, the risk is 77.8%—i.e., more than 35 times as high. Note that if one simply added the five individual risk percents, the expected 8-year risk would have been 3.8% + 3.9% + 6.0% + 8.4% + 8.5%, for a total of 30.6%. The observed 8-year risk, however, was 77.8%, which is more than 2.5 times as high as would be expected by simply adding the five individual risks. This suggests that the five factors (or unmeasured factors that vary with them) act synergistically to produce the final risk.

Therapy

Obviously, the immediate and long-term care of patients with symptomatic coronary artery disease will depend on the extent to which the disease has progressed when the patient seeks or is placed under medical care. Even in the presence of severe disease, there may be little or no warning before myocardial infarction occurs. After appropriate medical or surgical care is provided, efforts at symptomatic stage prevention begin.

Symptomatic Stage Prevention

The evaluation of risk factors and the development of a plan to reduce the risk of adverse cardiac events is necessary for every patient with symptomatic disease. If the patient has already had a myocardial infarction and undergone bypass surgery, the goals include preventing restenosis of the bypass grafts and slowing the progression of atherosclerosis elsewhere.

Behavior Modification. Patients should be questioned about cigarette smoking, exercise, and eating habits, all of which affect the risks of heart disease. Smokers should be encouraged to stop smoking (see Chapter 15 and Box 15–1), and all patients should receive counseling about the types and appropriate levels of exercise to pursue as well as about nutrition. Hospitalized patients should be placed on a low-fat, "heart healthy" diet and encouraged to continue this type of diet when they return home.

Other Measures. The assessment and appropriate management of other known risk factors, such as hyperlipidemia, hypertension, and diabetes mellitus, are essential for reducing the risk of adverse cardiac events in patients with symptomatic coronary artery disease. Each of these problems is the focus of a subsequent section of this chapter.

Hyperlipidemia

Hyperlipidemia is a general term used to describe an abnormal elevation in one or more of the lipids found in the blood. The **complete lipid profile** provides information on the following: total cholesterol (TC), high-density lipoprotein (HDL), low-density lipoprotein (LDL), very low density lipoprotein (VLDL), and triglycerides.

The **TC** level is equal to the sum of the HDL, LDL, and VLDL levels:

$$TC = HDL + LDL + VLDL$$

$$= (HDL) + (LDL) + (triglycerides/5)$$

HDL, the "good" cholesterol, acts as a scavenger of other types of cholesterol. **LDL** is one of the "bad" cholesterols associated with cardiovascular risk.

According to Chait, Brazg, and Tribble (1993), a high LDL level may be a necessary precursor for atherogenesis, but much of the damage may be due to oxidative modification of the LDL, making it more atherogenic. **VLDL,** another "bad" cholesterol, is carried in the **triglyceride fraction.**

Assessment

A variety of index measures have been proposed to assess the need for intervention and to monitor the success of preventive measures.

TC Level. Some screening programs measure only the TC level. The recommended diagnostic and therapeutic responses, based on the TC level alone, are summarized in Table 18–1. As indicated in the table, patients with a TC level of 200 mg/dL or greater may require testing of lipid fractions.

HDL Level. The desirable HDL level is greater than 50 mg/dL in women or greater than 35 mg/dL in men. An HDL level under 35 mg/dL is of concern if the LDL level or the triglyceride level is high (see below).

LDL Level. The desirable LDL level is often considered to be under 160 mg/dL in individuals with no symptoms of heart disease; under 130 mg/dL in patients with angina but without myocardial infarction; and under 100 mg/dL in patients with myocardial infarction. A level of 160 mg/dL or greater is undesirable, and a level of 200 mg/dL or more in anyone should cause concern. While opinions vary, a panel of experts involved in the National Cholesterol Education Program stated that medical treatment is indicated for those whose LDL level is 30 mg/dL higher than these standards (see National Cholesterol Education Program 1993). Some specialists prefer to look at the LDL level in relationship to the HDL level (see below).

Triglyceride Level. The preferred level of triglycerides is under 150 mg/dL. Levels over 200 mg/dL are reason for concern.

VLDL Level. The VLDL can be determined by dividing the triglyceride level by 5.

Total Non-HDL Cholesterol Level. Frick et al. (1987) have defined primary dyslipidemia as the presence of a non-HDL cholesterol level equal to or greater than 200 mg/dL in two successive measurements. This index is useful because it looks at the total contribution of cholesterol fractions currently considered harmful, and it would seem that minimizing the harmful types of cholesterol is a reasonable treatment goal. However, it does not consider the relationship between beneficial and harmful cholesterol fractions.

LDL/HDL Ratio. Specialists who recommend assessing and monitoring the LDL/HDL ratio believe that having a high level of HDL can compensate for having a high level of LDL. An LDL/HDL ratio under 3.5 is considered normal. A ratio greater than 4 should be of concern. One goal of atherosclerosis prevention is to increase the HDL level while decreasing the LDL level. Medical therapy, however, sometimes changes both the HDL and LDL levels in the same direction. Exercise is one way to lower the LDL level while raising the HDL level; increasing the consumption of monounsaturated fat in the diet is another way.

TC/HDL Ratio. Some investigators monitor the ratio of TC to HDL. Using this approach, Arntzenius et al. (1985) reported that angiograms in patients with a TC/HDL ratio of greater than 6.9 showed progression of coronary atherosclerosis during the study time, whereas angiograms in patients with a lower TC/HDL ratio did not show progression.

Triglyceride-HDL Relationship. Recent research suggests that the combination of an HDL level below 35 mg/dL and a triglyceride level above 200 mg/dL places an individual at high risk for coronary artery disease, and the possibility of a genetic hyperlipidemia should be considered (see Consensus Development Conference 1992).

TABLE 18–1. Recommended Diagnostic and Therapeutic Response Based on the Blood Level of Total Cholesterol (TC) Found in a Screening Program for Hyperlipidemia

Level of TC in Blood (mg/dL)	Interpretation	Recommended Response
< 200	Desirable level	Suggest that a prudent diet be followed. Repeat the TC test within 5 years.
200–239	Borderline high risk	Suggest life-style and diet modifications. Monitor with yearly TC tests. If other risk factors are present, test lipid fractions and treat on the basis of the low-density lipoprotein (LDL) level.
≥ 240	High risk	Test lipid fractions. Initiate a program for life-style and dietary modifications. Begin drug treatment if the LDL level is high.

Source of data: National Cholesterol Education Program. National Heart, Lung, and Blood Institute, Bethesda, MD.

Therapy and Symptomatic Stage Prevention

Any primary care physician must be able to treat patients with a moderately elevated TC level or abnormal lipid level and should be aware of the therapeutic options. Persons with severe lipid abnormalities, however, probably should be treated by specialists.

Except in cases of familial hyperlipidemia, pharmacologic agents probably should be reserved for use if the patient is unwilling to make life-style modifications (e.g., alter the diet and begin exercising) or if these modifications are unsuccessful in restoring the lipid patterns to normal. Box 18–1 lists the major medications for treatment of lipid abnormalities and discusses their mechanisms of action, effects, and potential side effects. The choice of medication depends on a variety of factors, including the type of lipid abnormality, the other diseases the

---

BOX 18–1.   Classification, Effects, and Potential Side Effects of Important Medications for the Treatment of Lipid Abnormalities*

Agents that suppress cholesterol production in the liver

Examples and mechanisms of action: Lovastatin is an example of a drug that reduces the liver's production of cholesterol by inhibiting the enzyme HMG-CoA reductase and thereby causing the liver to absorb more low-density lipoprotein (LDL) from the blood. *Effects:* Lovastatin may decrease the LDL level by 20–40%, increase the high-density lipoprotein (HDL) level by 5–15%, and decrease the triglyceride level by 10–20%. *Side effects:* So far, lovastatin seems to be safe over the short term, although the long-term effect on the liver must be monitored.

Bile acid sequestrants

Examples and mechanisms of action: Cholestyramine and colestipol are two examples of bile acid sequestrants. These drugs bind bile acids in the intestine, causing them to be excreted rather than reabsorbed. The liver then removes more LDL from the blood in order to make more bile acids, and this lowers the blood level of LDL. *Effects:* Bile acid sequestrants may decrease the LDL level by 15–30% and increase the HDL level by 3–5%. However, they may either increase or have no effect on the triglyceride level. They are useful in combination with other drugs. *Side effects:* Although bile acid sequestrants are safe for long-term therapy, they may interfere with the absorption of several medications, including some antibiotics, thiazide diuretics, beta blockers, and digoxin. They may also cause constipation and flatulence.

Agents that break down very low density lipoprotein (VLDL)

Examples and mechanisms of action: Gemfibrozil and fenofibrate are two examples. These fibric acid derivatives, which act by breaking down VLDL, are useful in the treatment of patients who have low HDL levels and particularly those who have a combination of low HDL and high triglyceride levels. *Effects:* These agents may decrease the triglyceride level by 20–50%, thereby decreasing the level of VLDL, which is carried in the triglyceride fraction. The agents may also decrease the LDL level by 10–15% and increase the HDL level by 10–15%. *Side effects:* General muscle aches are not common, but they are more likely to occur when gemfibrozil or fenofibrate is used in combination with an HMG-CoA reductase inhibitor. Use of an agent that breaks down VLDL may increase the likelihood of developing gallstones.

Other medications that affect blood lipid levels

Examples and mechanisms of action: Niacin (nicotinic acid) is a B complex vitamin that has a broad, positive effect on lipid metabolism. The mechanisms of action are not known, but niacin appears to work on the liver. *Effects:* Niacin may decrease the LDL level by 10–25%, decrease the triglyceride level by 20–50%, and increase the HDL level by 15–35%. *Side effects:* Itching and flushing are frequent but usually mild side effects. Niacin can have negative effects on the liver and on glucose and uric acid levels. Complications are more frequent if medication is started and stopped frequently. Nicotinic acid can be dangerous in its sustained-release form.

*Patients being treated with any of these medications should be evaluated 4–6 weeks after treatment begins and should be reevaluated every 3–4 months thereafter.

---

patient may have, the other medications the patient may be taking, and the age of the patient. A study reported by Krumholz et al. (1994) suggests that modification of blood lipid levels may not be as critical in elderly patients as it is in younger patients.

Hypertension

According to the Joint National Committee on the Detection, Evaluation, and Treatment of High Blood Pressure, hypertension is defined as an average systolic blood pressure of 140 mm Hg or higher or an average diastolic blood pressure of 90 mm Hg or higher in a person who is not acutely ill and not taking antihypertensive medications (see National Institutes of Health 1993). These are the levels that are high enough for treatment to bring proven benefits. Based on this definition, about 50 million people in the USA have hypertension. Among the groups at increased risk are pregnant women, women taking oral contraceptives, and African-Americans. Children are also at risk for hypertension.

Assessment

Hypertension may be detected by community or occupational screening, by individual case finding (e.g., when a person seeks care for dental problems or for medical problems that are unrelated to hypertension), or when a person develops one or more common complications of hypertension, such as visual problems, early renal failure, congestive heart failure, stroke, or myocardial infarction. Over the last 20 years, the risk of mortality from coronary artery disease and stroke in hypertensive individuals has dropped by 50% or more as a result of early detection and improved management of high blood pressure.

Table 18–2 provides information regarding the evaluation and staging of hypertension, based on average systolic and diastolic blood pressures. In addition to listing the ranges for optimal, normal, and high normal pressures, the table shows the ranges for four stages of hypertension.

Therapy and Symptomatic Stage Prevention

After the stage of hypertension has been determined, the Joint National Committee on Detection, Evaluation, and Treatment of High Blood Pressure recommends the following actions: individuals with **optimal or normal blood pressure** should be monitored at 2-year intervals; those with **high normal blood pressure** should be monitored at 1-year intervals; **stage 1 (mild) hypertension** should be con-

TABLE 18–2. Evaluation of Blood Pressure and Staging of Hypertension, Based on Average Systolic and Diastolic Blood Pressures in Persons Who Are Not Acutely Ill and Are Not Taking Antihypertensive Medications*

Systolic Blood Pressure (mm Hg)	Diastolic Blood Pressure (mm Hg)	Interpretation
< 120	< 80	Optimal blood pressure
120–129	80–84	Normal blood pressure
130–139	85–89	High normal blood pressure
140–159	90–99	Stage 1 (mild) hypertension
160–179	100–109	Stage 2 (moderate) hypertension
180–209	110–119	Stage 3 (severe) hypertension
≥ 210	≥ 120	Stage 4 (very severe) hypertension

Source of data: National Institutes of Health. The Fifth Report of the National Committee on Detection, Evaluation, and Treatment of High Blood Pressure. Publication No. (NIH)93-1088. Washington, D. C., Government Printing Office, 1993.

*The highest stage for which either part of the blood pressure qualifies is taken as the stage of hypertension. For example, if the systolic blood pressure is 165 mm Hg and the diastolic blood pressure is 115 mm Hg, the stage is 3 (severe).

firmed within 2 months, and evaluation and treatment, if indicated, should be done within that time; **stage 2 (moderate) hypertension** should be evaluated and treated within 1 month; **stage 3 (severe) hypertension** should be evaluated and treated within 1 week; and **stage 4 (very severe) hypertension** should be evaluated and treated immediately. During evaluation, the presence or absence of target organ damage should be noted, because any stage of hypertension is more severe if there is evidence of such damage.

Most hypertension is classified as **essential hypertension,** meaning that no known underlying specific cause exists. **Nonessential hypertension** is due to specific, treatable causes, such as renal artery stenosis or tumors of the adrenal medulla. The specific causes of hypertension should be ruled out before measures to reduce hypertension are started.

Symptomatic stage prevention and therapy are aimed at reducing the systolic blood pressure to under 140 mm Hg, reducing the diastolic blood pressure to under 90 mm Hg, and monitoring patients to make sure that these levels are maintained. The goal is to prevent damage to the organs at risk from hypertension. For patients with any stage of hypertension, the following life-style modifications are indicated: weight reduction; increased physical activity; decreased intake of sodium and fats; increased intake of potassium, calcium, and magnesium; and moderation of alcohol intake. Smokers should be encouraged to stop smoking, not because it directly influences the blood pressure but because smoking cessation will reduce the risk of damage to many of the same target organs that hypertension can damage.

For patients whose blood pressure levels remain high despite these life-style modifications, use of one or more antihypertensive medications is indicated. Because most hypertension is asymptomatic, patients must be made aware of the importance of tak-

ing medications and the risks of stopping treatment. Many of the antihypertensive medications prescribed in the past caused dizziness (because of suppression of vasal reflexes), impotence, and other side effects that discouraged patients from using them. Fortunately, medications today have relatively few side effects, are inexpensive, and are more convenient to use (e.g., need only be taken once a day).

Among the major classes of effective antihypertensive agents are diuretics, beta blockers, angiotensin-converting enzyme (ACE) inhibitors, calcium channel blockers, alpha blockers, and vasodilators. The wide range of choice should be utilized to develop a treatment plan that is satisfactory to the patient.

So far, only thiazide diuretics and beta blockers have been shown to reduce cardiovascular disease in controlled clinical trials, so there is an argument for starting with one of these first in patients with hypertension. Because the thiazide diuretics can flush out sodium and potassium, decrease blood volume, raise blood glucose levels, and raise uric acid levels, they should be used with care and monitoring, especially in older persons. Beta blockers may be the best choice for patients who have a history of myocardial infarction or angina pectoris but no history of a conduction abnormality. The use of beta blockers is contraindicated in patients with conduction abnormalities, asthma, or chronic obstructive pulmonary disease. The use of ACE inhibitors is contraindicated in patients with certain renal diseases (such as renal artery stenosis) and in pregnant women with toxemia.

Diabetes Mellitus

In the USA, about 700,000 people have insulin-dependent diabetes mellitus (IDDM), a disease that requires lifelong treatment with insulin and places them at higher risk for a variety of cardiovascular, renal, and other serious complications. An even greater number have non–insulin dependent diabetes mellitus (NIDDM), a milder form of the disease.

Programs aimed at detecting diabetes in pregnant women are the only routine screening programs for diabetes that have proved cost-effective. Nevertheless, much can be done to prevent target organ damage from diabetes, as was demonstrated in the recently completed Diabetes Control and Complications Trial (DCCT) in patients with IDDM. This trial demonstrated that improved control of blood glucose levels significantly reduced the incidence of microvascular disease (retinopathy, nephropathy, and neuropathy) and macrovascular disease (atherosclerosis of large blood vessels, myocardial infarction, angina pectoris, strokes, aneurysms, and amputations of the distal lower extremity) in patients with IDDM (see DCCT Research Group 1993 and Santiago 1993).

Members of the DCCT intervention group had to self-monitor their blood glucose levels, keep detailed records of insulin dosages and glucose levels, regulate their dietary intake and level of insulin based on the results of self-monitoring, and be actively involved in other aspects of their own care, with the supervision and support of physicians and other professionals. Although the risk of hypoglycemic episodes was 3 times as high in the intervention group as in the control group, no serious sequelae of hypoglycemia occurred in the intervention group, whereas one death from hypoglycemia occurred in the control group. Weight gain was a common side effect of tight diabetic control.

Based on the results of the DCCT, tight control (defined as control as good as that obtained in the DCCT) may be beneficial for patients who are willing to participate actively in their own care. Tight control should be supplemented with frequent examination of the eyegrounds and with laser treatment of microvascular lesions when indicated. The use of angiotensin-converting enzyme (ACE) inhibitors may be helpful in preventing or controlling hypertension and microalbuminuria, but patients taking these drugs should be watched for high potassium levels, and ACE inhibitors should not be used if there is any possibility of renal artery stenosis.

All patients with IDDM or NIDDM should be advised of the need for moderate to high levels of physical activity and should receive individual counseling about nutrition. In addition, they should be informed of the common complications of diabetes and of the importance of contacting their physician if they note early symptoms of any of these complications.

REHABILITATION

Rehabilitation, occurring as it does after disease has already caused damage, may seem to take place when there is nothing left to prevent. However, as mentioned at the beginning of the chapter, the goal of rehabilitation is to reduce the social disability produced by a given level of impairment, both by strengthening the patient's remaining functions and by helping the patient learn to function in alternative ways.

General Approach to Rehabilitation

Rehabilitation must begin in the early phases of treatment if it is to be maximally effective. For example, in patients who have suffered a stroke, head injury, hip fracture, or other problem that makes them temporarily immobile, it is important to keep the joints flexible from the beginning of the illness or injury, so that weakened but recovering muscles do not have to overcome stiffened joints. Beginning rehabilitation efforts early also tends to increase the cooperation of patients and their family members by convincing them that improvement is expected.

The most effective rehabilitation program is one tailored to meet the physical, emotional, and occupational needs of the individual patient. There is

often a **rehabilitation counselor** to coordinate the efforts of a team of specialists. **Physical therapists** work to strengthen weakened muscles, to increase joint movement and flexibility, and to teach patients ways of accomplishing routine tasks despite their disabilities. These tasks, referred to as **activities of daily living,** include feeding oneself, transferring from bed to chair and back, grooming, controlling the bladder and bowels, bathing, dressing, walking on a level surface, and going up and down stairs. **Speech therapists** seek to improve the ability of patients to articulate their thoughts following a stroke or head injury that produces aphasia. **Occupational therapists** evaluate the occupational abilities of patients, counsel them regarding suitable types of work, provide them with job training or retraining, and assist them in obtaining a suitable job. Usually, the most cost-effective efforts are those designed to help a patient return to his or her previous place of employment and obtain a new or modified job there. **Psychiatric or emotional counseling** may be important, as may **spiritual counseling** by a minister, priest, or rabbi.

Categories of Disability

Disability is a socially defined concept, but it has very practical implications in terms of financial support. There are four formal categories used in most states for reimbursement of workers who have job-related injuries or illnesses covered under a workers' compensation program: (1) **permanent total disability,** e.g., the loss of two limbs or of vision in both eyes; (2) **permanent partial disability,** e.g., the loss of one limb or of vision in one eye; (3) **temporary total disability,** e.g., a fractured arm in a truck driver; and (4) **temporary partial disability,** e.g., a fractured arm in an elementary school teacher.

A disability is temporary if it is expected that a person will return to his or her job within a time period defined by statute. The person will be partially reimbursed for lost wages, as well as the costs of medical care, from the state workers' compensation fund (see Chapters 19 and 21).

A person with a permanent disability is reimbursed at a fixed rate for the rest of his or her life. The rate varies from state to state (as stipulated by law) but is based on the type of disability and degree of function lost (as determined by a physician). In some states, permanent total disability is defined as a disease or injury that prevents a person from working at any job. In other states, it is defined as a disease or injury that prevents a person from returning to the previous job.

SUMMARY

The goal of tertiary prevention is to limit the physical and social consequences of an injury or disease after it has occurred or become symptomatic. The two major categories of tertiary prevention are disability limitation and rehabilitation.

Methods of disability limitation include therapy, which seeks to undo the threat or damage from an existing disease, and symptomatic stage prevention, which attempts to halt or limit the future progression of disease. The strategies of symptomatic stage prevention are taken both from primary prevention (e.g., modification of diet, behavior, and environment) and from secondary prevention (e.g., frequent screening for incipient complications, followed by treatment when complications are discovered). The effective management of chronic diseases such as coronary artery disease, hyperlipidemia, hypertension, and diabetes mellitus may require a combination of therapy and symptomatic stage prevention.

Rehabilitation should begin in the early stages of treatment. Depending on the needs of the patient, the rehabilitation team may include a rehabilitation counselor, physical therapist, speech therapist, occupational therapist, and psychiatric, emotional, or spiritual counselor. Under the state laws concerning workers' compensation, four categories of job-related illnesses or injuries are recognized: permanent total disability, permanent partial disability, temporary total disability, and temporary partial disability. The goal of rehabilitation for workers, whether their impairment is temporary or permanent, is to minimize the social and functional consequences of the impairment.

Although it might seem that the opportunity for prevention is lost when a disease appears or an injury occurs, this is not really the case. The appearance of symptoms or the threat of severe complications may lead patients to take an active interest in their health status, seek the health care that they need, and make positive changes in their life-style.

References Cited

Arntzenius, A. C., et al. Diet, lipoproteins, and the progression of coronary atherosclerosis: the Leiden Intervention Trial. New England Journal of Medicine 312:805–811, 1985.

Breslow, L. Risk factor intervention for health maintenance. Science 200:908–912, 1978.

Chait, A., R. L. Brazg, and D. L. Tribble. Susceptibility of small, dense, low-density lipoproteins to oxidative modification in subjects with atherogenic lipoprotein phenotype, pattern B. American Journal of Medicine 94:350–356, 1993.

Consensus Development Conference. Triglyceride, High-Density Lipoprotein, and Coronary Heart Disease. National Institutes of Health, Bethesda, Md., 1992.

Dawber, T. R., G. F. Meadors, and F. E. Moore, Jr. Epidemiologic approaches to heart disease: the Framingham Study. American Journal of Public Health 41:279–286, 1951.

Diabetes Control and Complications Trial (DCCT) Research Group. The Diabetes Control and Complications Trial. New England Journal of Medicine 329:683–689, 1993.

Frick, M. H., et al. Helsinki Heart Study: primary prevention trial with gemfibrozil in middle-aged men with dyslipidemia. New England Journal of Medicine 317:1237–1245, 1987.

Krumholz, H., et al. Lack of association between cholesterol and coronary heart disease mortality and all cause mortality in persons older than 70 years. Journal of the American Medical Association 272:1335–1340, 1994.

Leavell, H. R., and E. G. Clark. Preventive Medicine for the Doctor in His Community, 3rd ed. New York, McGraw-Hill Book Company, 1965.

Lissner, L., et al. Variability of body weight and health outcomes in the Framingham population. New England Journal of Medicine 324:1839–1844, 1991.

National Cholesterol Education Program. Expert panel on detection, evaluation, and treatment of high blood cholesterol in adults. Journal of the American Medical Association 269:3015–3023, 1993.

National Institutes of Health. The Fifth Report of the National Committee on Detection, Evaluation, and Treatment of High Blood Pressure. Publication No. (NIH)93-1088. Washington, D. C., Government Printing Office, 1993.

Santiago, J. V. Lessons from the Diabetes Control and Complications Trial. Diabetes 42:1549–1554, 1993.

Wing, R. R., R. W. Jeffery, and W. L. Hellerstedt. A prospective study of effects of weight cycling on cardiovascular risk factors. Archives of Internal Medicine 155:1416–1422, 1995.

Selected Readings

American Heart Association. Primer in Preventive Cardiology. Dallas, American Heart Association, 1994.

Diabetes Control and Complications Trial (DCCT) Research Group. The Diabetes Control and Complications Trial. New England Journal of Medicine 329:683–689, 1993.

National Cholesterol Education Program. Expert panel on detection, evaluation, and treatment of high blood cholesterol in adults. Journal of the American Medical Association 269:3015–3023, 1993.

National Institutes of Health. The Fifth Report of the National Committee on Detection, Evaluation, and Treatment of High Blood Pressure. Publication No. (NIH)93-1088. Washington, D. C., Government Printing Office, 1993.

CHAPTER NINETEEN

SPECIAL TOPICS

IN PREVENTION

MATERNAL AND CHILD HEALTH

Although efforts to prevent diseases and injuries are important throughout life, perhaps the most opportune periods for prevention are the reproductive years, infancy, and early childhood. Unfortunately, the youngest members of society act somewhat like the canaries taken into mines: they provide early warnings of health problems involving the environment, nutrition, and human behavior that ultimately will be hazardous to adults as well. This is one reason that the rates of infant mortality and deaths of children under the age of 5 years can be valuable indicators of health conditions in the general population. It is not surprising, therefore, that the first clinical specialties to emphasize preventive medicine were obstetrics and gynecology and pediatrics.

Family Planning

The opportunities for prevention begin in the preconception stage, when primary health care workers can answer questions and provide information about contraception to those who wish to plan the number of children and timing of childbirth (see Barnes 1978). The preconception period is also the time to ensure that potential mothers are in good health, are eating a healthy diet, and are taking folic acid supplements to reduce the risk for neural tube defects in the fetus (see Chapter 15).

Family planning efforts can be considered health promotion, by enabling good spacing of children, but because of the technical medical aspects of contraception, it can also be considered specific protection. Note that family planning, even if perfect, would not achieve population control (such as a zero growth rate) in a country unless the fertility goals of the people in the country were sufficiently low. Family planning, therefore, should not be equated with population control, even though family planning may contribute to population control. Such control is achieved in a country only when the policy goals of that country are in agreement with the fertility goals of its people.

Prenatal Care

Prenatal care is an accepted part of good medical care (see Institute of Medicine 1988). The benefits of prenatal care, although real, are difficult to assess because the content and the quality of prenatal care vary greatly from place to place (Klerman 1990). Ideally, prenatal care is aimed at primary, secondary, and tertiary prevention (see Barnes 1978 for guidelines).

Primary prevention includes counseling to promote good nutrition and healthful behavior, as well as referral to appropriate programs and specialists if necessary. Some women may be referred, for example, to the Women, Infants, and Children (WIC) Program, which provides food vouchers to those with low income. Others may require referral for specific programs concerning cigarette smoking, alcohol use, illegal drug use, or other behaviors that affect the health of the pregnant woman and her fetus.

Secondary prevention includes screening pregnant women for syphilis, type 1 human immunodeficiency virus (HIV-1), and other infectious diseases, followed by confirmatory diagnosis and treatment. The prevention of isoimmunization and erythroblastosis fetalis is now possible by screening for maternal antibodies to Rh (D) proteins on the fetal red blood cells, followed by the timely use of Rh (D) immune globulin when levels of these antibodies begin to rise.

Tertiary prevention includes the control of existing disease (e.g., heart disease, hypertension, and diabetes) and the control of toxemia during pregnancy.

Labor and Delivery Care

Many complications of pregnancy and delivery that can cause death or long-term damage to mother or fetus can be treated at the time of labor and delivery by expert obstetric and pediatric management. In addition, infants who are unwell at birth or whose mothers had significant risk factors can be monitored for a time and treated when necessary in a newborn special care nursery. These measures have proved their value in minimizing neonatal morbidity and mortality. While the use of new types of technology and more invasive types of procedures (such as fetal monitoring and cesarean sections) are beneficial under some circumstances, the debate continues about whether such procedures are being overused and causing unnecessary morbidity for the mother and child.

Well Child Care

Primary prevention in well child care includes immunizations (see Chapter 16 and Table 16–2) and review and counseling regarding the child's nutrition, growth, and development.

Secondary prevention includes screening for visual and hearing problems. According to the US Preventive Services Task Force (USPSTF), 2–5% of children in the USA have amblyopia ("lazy eye") and strabismus (ocular misalignment), and almost 20% have refractive errors by the time they are 16 years old. Children should be screened for these before entering school, usually by their primary care physicians. There is inadequate evidence to justify screening of children who have already reached school age, by which time therapeutic interventions are less likely to be successful. Although neonates should be screened for hearing problems, the USPSTF does not recommend routine screening of school children for hearing defects (see US Preventive Services Task Force 1989).

Day-Care and Preschool Programs

Day-care and preschool programs offer many children the opportunity to learn social skills, interact with other children and adults, and receive stimulation outside the home environment. For children enrolled in Headstart programs, there is the added benefit of involvement in a medical screening program called Healthstart, which can supplement well child visits.

Most states have regulations to promote health and safety in day-care facilities, including regulations concerning environmental sanitation, the qualifications of personnel caring for children, and the ratio of personnel to children. Specific protection as applied to day care includes the requirement that children have up-to-date immunizations and be monitored carefully for infectious diseases.

School Health

Schools can promote health by offering health education courses and programs involving a variety of participants, including teachers in the school system and representatives of the local health department and other health agencies.

Health promotion in children requires that the school setting be regularly inspected to ensure a safe water supply, sanitary food service facilities, and compliance with fire safety regulations. Specific protection is achieved through laws that make evidence of adequate immunization a prerequisite for enrolling in schools in the USA. This has helped to reduce the spread of some infections through school classrooms and from schools to younger children at home.

Secondary prevention in the school setting has historically included screening examinations of school children. These are seldom performed on a mass basis today, because of accumulated evidence that the examinations usually were not performed well and were not very productive. The emphasis now is to encourage parents to choose a primary care physician and to have their children visit the physician on a regular basis (see Well Child Care, above).

The newest role for schools in health is to provide school-based health centers that offer counseling, immunizations, and illness care. Some centers also make information about family planning available. Many students, particularly those in junior high and high school, feel more comfortable visiting school-based facilities than going to a practitioner or clinic outside the school. Although these centers have not been fully evaluated, the information so far has been encouraging.

ACQUIRED IMMUNODEFICIENCY SYNDROME (AIDS)

No new disease in modern times has had as severe a worldwide impact as acquired immunodeficiency syndrome (AIDS), which is caused by type 1 human immunodeficiency virus (HIV-1). The number of persons infected with HIV is estimated to be more than 1 million in the USA and 19 million worldwide. All of these infected persons are expected to die of AIDS eventually, if they do not die of other causes in the meantime. In the mid-1990s, between 300,000 and 600,000 persons worldwide were expected to die of AIDS per year. By the turn of the century, the number of AIDS deaths is expected to be between 1.5 and 3 million per year.

AIDS, a disease which has only been recognized since 1981 and for which there is no effective treatment to date, is now the leading cause of death in the USA for men between the ages of 25 and 44 years. Although the situation is serious in the USA, it is catastrophic in central Africa, where in some regions the prevalence of HIV infection is greater than 50% and the most productive age groups are being decimated, leaving large numbers of orphaned children. The situation is becoming very grave in Southeast Asia, with rapid increases also noted in South America and on the Indian subcontinent.

The Spread of HIV Infection

HIV-1 is spread primarily by sexual contact (both heterosexual and homosexual) and by intravenous drug use (IVDU). The spread of HIV among drug users is due to the sharing of the equipment ("works") for injecting drugs. These works include needles, syringes, cookers (for heating the drug to dissolve it), cottons (to filter the drug to be injected), and water (used for mixing the drug and cleaning the needle and syringe). HIV can also be spread by transfusions of blood and blood products, although with modern testing, this risk is vanishingly small where all of the tests are done and done correctly. Rarely, HIV is spread by accidental punctures of the skin with contaminated needles or other medical equipment. HIV is not spread by ordinary household contact that does not involve one of the above risk behaviors.

In the USA, homosexual intercourse is the most common route and IVDU is the second most common route of spread of HIV, but spread via IVDU is rising rapidly. In some countries with high rates of IVDU, sharing of drug equipment is the leading route of spread. In central Africa and Southeast Asia, however, heterosexual intercourse is the predominant route of spread. Where the rates of new HIV infections are approximately equal between men and women, heterosexual intercourse is the most important route of spread. Where the prevalence and new infections involve far more men than women, either homosexual intercourse or IVDU is likely to be the dominant route.

Primary, Secondary, and Tertiary Prevention

Despite the lack of an effective medical treatment for AIDS, the best means of preventing the spread of the causative organism have been known since soon after its discovery, even before the microorganism was identified. They consist of restricting sexual activity to a monogamous relationship and avoiding IVDU. If these two practices were followed, exposure to HIV would be limited to extremely rare events, such as might occasionally happen from a blood transfusion.

If a person chooses to have multiple sexual partners, the next best prevention is to use condoms for every act of sexual intercourse. Condoms are far from foolproof, but if used consistently, they will reduce the risk of exposure considerably. If a person chooses to use intravenous drugs, exposure can be prevented if only new, clean "works" are used for every injection. Sharing any part of the "works" with another intravenous drug user is extremely hazardous. Needle-exchange programs have been shown to reduce the rate of spread of HIV in urban areas (Kaplan 1992), but they do not eliminate it.

Infected persons may change their behaviors to protect others if they know they are infected with HIV. For this reason, HIV testing centers have been established in most parts of the USA and allow individuals to be tested anonymously.

Other than behavioral changes, the only means to prevent the spread of AIDS are (1) testing donated blood for HIV antibodies and discarding units that are infected and (2) treating HIV-positive pregnant women with azidothymidine (AZT), which reduces the proportion of infants who will be infected.

Ironically, while there is no cure for AIDS and few effective technical means of preventing the spread of HIV, the infection could be largely eliminated over time by behavioral changes alone. In the USA, the Centers for Disease Control and Prevention has played a crucial role in the surveillance of HIV infection and AIDS (see US Public Health Service 1992). Other US government agencies and representatives, however, have been criticized for their reluctance to speak out more strongly regarding AIDS prevention. Part of this reluctance is undoubtedly due to the fact that human sexuality and condom use are politically difficult issues, as is support for public needle-exchange programs.

TUBERCULOSIS

Before the process of industrialization and urbanization transformed Western civilization, tuberculosis was a known problem, but it was not a scourge in Europe and the USA. During the 19th century, however, tuberculosis became the leading cause of death in the industrialized nations. The disease killed people of all ages (but especially adolescents and young adults) and in all socioeconomic circumstances. Although it was predominantly spread within the home, it also was frequently spread in crowded working conditions. For the treatment of patients with tuberculosis, physicians prescribed rest (often in sanatoriums), exposure to fresh air, and, in some cases, lung collapse therapy or the more permanent thoracoplasty.

Despite the lack of any specific medical prevention or therapy, the tuberculosis mortality rates began to decline in the late 19th century and continued to decline steadily until the end of World War II. Dubos (1959) claimed that a crucial factor in the decline was biologic selection. Adolescents and young adults, who were particularly susceptible to infection from *Mycobacterium tuberculosis,* tended to die young from the disease, before they could produce many children. As a result, the surviving world populations derived from European stock became far more resistant to tuberculosis than other populations were. Dubos also claimed that improvements in socioeconomic conditions, including better nutrition, less crowding in homes and worksites, and improved sanitation, were important factors in the steady decline of tuberculosis in the industrialized nations.

Although control of tuberculosis was far advanced by the late 1940s, it was improved further with the introduction of streptomycin as a treatment for tuberculosis, with the subsequent discovery of the therapeutic value of isoniazid (INH) and para-amino salicylic acid (PAS), and with the availability of additional antimicrobial agents, such as rifampin, ethambutol, and pyrazinamide.

In the USA, the incidence of tuberculosis continued to decline until the mid-1980s. In 1985, the decline stopped, and a resurgence of tuberculosis was noted. Although the incidence has dropped somewhat since 1993, tuberculosis still represents a formidable threat, especially in immunocompromised patients.

Stages and Natural History of Tuberculosis

The natural history of mycobacterial infection makes the control of tuberculosis considerably more complex than the control of other bacterial diseases.

The manifestations of tuberculosis vary greatly among patients. In a small percentage of individuals who are newly infected with mycobacteria, the infection proceeds fairly rapidly either to invade lung tissue or to cause a generalized systemic disease such as miliary tuberculosis. In most persons with normal immune systems, however, lesions develop in the lung and become contained as cell-mediated immunity develops. The presence of cell-mediated immunity is revealed by a positive reaction in the tuberculin skin test using purified protein derivative (PPD).

The initial infection with tuberculosis, when it is successfully resolved, is called **primary tuberculosis,** and it often leaves a telltale radiographic picture called a primary (Gohn) complex. The resolved primary infection, however, is not necessarily the end of the story, because the mycobacteria remain alive—albeit isolated—in the body of the infected person. This person, therefore, is more correctly considered to have **inactive tuberculosis** than to be completely healed.

The inactive tuberculosis, which is noninfectious, will ultimately take one of three possible courses: (1) The tuberculosis may remain inactive for the rest of the infected person's life. In Europe and the USA, this is by far the most common course. (2) The infected person's own disease may reactivate later in life to become **active tuberculosis.** This occurs in 4–8% of infected persons and is called **reactivation**

tuberculosis or endogenous ("from within") tuberculosis. Reactivation tuberculosis is usually infectious. (3) The infected person may be exposed to a new tuberculosis infection, which may or may not become active infectious pulmonary tuberculosis. If a new exposure results in active disease, it is called **reinfection tuberculosis** or exogenous ("from without") tuberculosis.

The Incidence of Tuberculosis in the USA

From the 1960s to the mid-1980s, most new active cases of tuberculosis in the USA were due to endogenous tuberculosis, the reactivation of long-standing infection. During this period, the central goal for the US Public Health Service tuberculosis program was to minimize the spread of tuberculosis from the older population to the younger population. If this could be accomplished, over time the older people, many of whom had been infected while young, would die out, leaving the US population largely uninfected. Because of its central goal, the program was called the "child-centered" program to prevent tuberculosis (see Centers for Disease Control 1965).

The US program pursued several measures to accomplish its goal. First, school-age children were tested, and those with positive results in the tuberculin skin test were treated prophylactically with INH. Those with negative results were retested periodically. Second, efforts were made to trace the contacts of children whose skin test results recently converted from negative to positive (skin test converters) and the contacts of persons with newly discovered active tuberculosis. People who were identified as being actual sources of infection were treated to reduce the spread of mycobacteria. People who were identified as being at risk for infection were tested, and those whose results showed a recent conversion from negative to positive were given INH prophylaxis if they were under 35 years old. This age limit was imposed because of the discovery that INH use in older individuals posed a threat of severe liver damage.

The incidence of tuberculosis (often called the new active case rate) declined at approximately 5% per year from the 1950s to the mid-1980s. Indeed, by the 1970s, the proportion of school children with positive skin test results had dropped to such a low level that it was no longer cost-effective to continue skin testing in most school children. The search for the contacts of active cases continued, as did the use of INH prophylaxis for newly discovered skin test converters.

In 1985, the incidence of tuberculosis leveled off and then began to rise. Two factors appeared to be responsible for the resurgence of tuberculosis. First, an increasing proportion of newly discovered cases of tuberculosis were resistant to more than one antimicrobial agent. Much of the reason for this multiple drug–resistant tuberculosis (MDRTB) appears to be that infected persons started, but did not complete, the prescribed course of antituberculosis treatment. This allowed the mycobacteria to develop resistance to antimicrobial agents. Second, the patterns of tuberculosis were affected by the presence of type 1 human immunodeficiency virus (HIV-1) infection. In HIV-positive individuals, tuberculosis is frequently the first sign of acquired immunodeficiency syndrome, or AIDS (Selwyn et al. 1992). When HIV-positive individuals are exposed to mycobacteria, the result is often severe and sometimes overwhelming tuberculosis. Reactivation of inactive tuberculosis in HIV-positive persons tends to occur as immune deficiency progresses. Moreover, persons with HIV infection are often in a position to give their infections to other persons with immunodeficiency, thus continuing the cycle.

The problem of MDRTB has been especially severe in three types of institutions: prisons, general hospitals, and homeless shelters. Prisons and general hospitals are often overcrowded, partly because of the rise of illegal drug use, and have become important sites for the spread of tuberculosis (Bellin, Fletcher, and Safyer 1993; Edlin et al. 1992). The use of "crack" cocaine and other illegal drugs has contributed to homelessness, and homeless shelters have become sources of spread of tuberculosis (see Centers for Disease Control 1991; Brudney and Dobkin 1991). In addition, tuberculosis has been shown to spread in other public settings, such as on commercial aircraft, on occasion (see Centers for Disease Control and Prevention 1995).

Primary, Secondary, and Tertiary Prevention

The control of tuberculosis has been assisted by the discovery of methods for primary, secondary, and tertiary prevention.

The first discovery was a vaccine derived from a live, attenuated mycobacterium and called the bacillus Calmette-Guérin (BCG) vaccine after its developers. When the BCG vaccine is applied to a scratch in the skin of a previously uninfected child or adult, it stimulates the production of cell-mediated immunity, which provides some protection against a first infection with *M. tuberculosis.* Immunization with BCG can be considered a method of primary prevention. It is the least expensive approach to tuberculosis control, and although there has been considerable debate regarding its efficacy (see Clemens, Chuong, and Feinstein 1983), it is widely used in developing nations that have high rates of tuberculosis. It has the disadvantage, however, of making subsequent PPD skin test results positive.

The second discovery was that a 6-month course of isoniazid (INH) could reduce the risk of endogenous (reactivation) tuberculosis by more than 50% in people with inactive primary tuberculosis (Mount and Ferebee 1961). INH use can therefore be considered secondary prevention. The US Public Health Service chose not to recommend the use of BCG vaccine but instead to emphasize the identification of those who had positive results in the tuberculin skin test (particularly recent skin test converters) and the use of INH to reduce their risk of reactivation tuberculosis.

Subsequent discoveries have led to new strategies of secondary and tertiary prevention. Increasingly, tuberculosis control depends on the early identification and appropriate treatment of patients with MDRTB, immunodeficiency, or both. Patients with MDRTB must be treated with a combination of antituberculosis agents (Iseman 1993). To ensure compliance, therapy may be given in a setting in which patients can be directly observed while taking these agents. Although this approach is expensive in terms of personnel time, preliminary evidence indicates that directly observed therapy (DOT) can be effective in reducing the incidence of tuberculosis if it is followed consistently (Frieden et al. 1995). In addition, some hospitals have developed special negative-pressure rooms in which patients with suspected MDRTB can be tested and treated without risking the spread of drug-resistant infection to other patients (Bellin, Fletcher, and Safyer 1993).

In the presence of immunodeficiency, the tuberculin skin test using PPD often yields false-negative results (Selwyn et al. 1992). To prevent this problem in an individual who might be immunodeficient, the PPD skin test can be performed on one arm while an anergy panel is tested on the other arm. The anergy panel consists of a number of common allergens, at least one of which will elicit a reaction if the immune system is not impaired. Immunodeficient patients, however, may show no reaction, which tells the clinician that a negative result in the PPD skin test cannot be used to exclude the presence of tuberculosis.

In institutions, a variety of special precautions must be taken to prevent the spread of tuberculosis. Methods of primary prevention include the avoidance of overcrowding, the use of improved ventilation, and, when possible, the introduction of ultraviolet radiation, which kills mycobacteria in the air. Methods of secondary prevention include chest x-rays and tuberculin skin testing. Methods of tertiary prevention include combination therapy, DOT therapy, and use of negative-pressure rooms.

CHEMICAL SUBSTANCE ABUSE

Several chemical substances are frequently used to alter the mind, to elevate the mood, to modify the feelings (especially about oneself), and sometimes to improve performance temporarily. Because the chemical substances used for these purposes may cause problems even before all of the criteria for addiction are met, the broader terms "chemical dependency" and "substance abuse" have come into general use. They imply both physical dependence (including tolerance) and psychologic dependence on the use of chemicals to modify mood and performance and to escape from anxiety.

Abuse of alcohol and abuse of illegal drugs are discussed below. Cigarette smoking, which is discussed in other chapters, is also properly considered a form of chemical dependency or substance abuse, because once the use of nicotine has become regular, withdrawal symptoms occur when the substance is withdrawn for any period of time.

Abuse of Alcohol

The most commonly abused substance is alcohol. Among persons who are heavy drinkers (including alcoholics), the median estimate of the relative risk for a variety of diseases is high: almost 8 for cirrhosis of the liver; about 4 for suicides, accidents, and cancer of the upper digestive and respiratory tracts; and about 1 for stroke. The overall relative risk for mortality is slightly over 2.

The combination of a high rate of alcohol use and a relatively low rate of alcoholism in some European wine-producing countries has led some investigators to postulate that alcohol is best controlled if it is integrated into the normal pattern of food consumption and socialization. The view of alcoholism in the USA is based on the disease model: a small portion of the members of society cannot adapt successfully to alcohol use, and their failure to adapt makes them "diseased" or at least a problem to be treated.

Because alcohol abuse not only damages the body of the drinker but also affects his or her performance of tasks, it often places others at risk for serious injuries, including automobile crashes. A variety of methods of primary, secondary, and tertiary prevention have been suggested to reduce the risk of alcohol-related diseases and injuries.

Primary Prevention

The social environment in which one is raised is probably important for the primary prevention of alcohol abuse. If an individual grows up without using alcohol, he or she may avoid its use for life. The promotion of healthy life-styles in which alcohol use is avoided or controlled is largely a function of families and smaller social groups such as churches.

Reducing legal accessibility of young people to alcohol tends to reduce alcohol use, but this probably is less effective than are family values. Limiting the promotion of alcohol in the media may decrease the desire of young people to start using alcohol. Raising the tax on liquor reduces the amount of alcohol purchased, but it is not clear that it reduces rates of alcoholism.

Secondary and Tertiary Prevention

The goals of secondary and tertiary prevention are the early detection and the early treatment of alcohol problems. Unfortunately, in many cases, help is not sought for a gradually developing drinking problem until some untoward event occurs, such as injuring someone while drinking and driving. The long-term treatment of people who are alcohol abusers is difficult. There are good medications for treating the acute effects of withdrawal, but long-term success often depends on a lifetime commitment to treatment, such as is encouraged in the 12-step program of Alcoholics Anonymous. For some alcoholics, a major change in personal commitment, such as a religious conversion, may be effective.

Abuse of Illegal Drugs

The effects of psychoactive drugs such as cocaine and heroin are due as much to the rate at which the blood level of the drug is increased as they are to the blood level finally achieved (Zahler et al. 1982). A route of administration that causes a rapid rise in the blood level of a euphoria-producing drug causes more euphoria than one that delivers the same amount of drug slowly to the bloodstream. Moreover, a drug will have more psychic effect at any blood level while the level is rising than while it is falling.

An upsurge of violence began in the USA in 1986 as a result of the influx of a new form of cocaine, freebase cocaine, called "crack" because of the crackling sounds it makes when being manufactured or smoked (Allen and Jekel 1991). Crack, the most dangerous form of cocaine, is inhaled while it is heated. Inhaled crack is absorbed very rapidly, causes a strong euphoria, and is rapidly addictive.

In contrast to heroin addicts, crack addicts are at least as dangerous to others when they are high on the drug as when they are seeking money to get high. This is because crack is a stimulant, whereas heroin is a sedative. While high on crack, a user may have strong feelings of paranoia and may be in physical danger of myocardial infarction, stroke, or seizures.

Powdered cocaine (the hydrochloride) may be mixed with heroin before intravenous injection; this is an extremely dangerous mixture called a "speedball." To some extent, the stimulant effect of cocaine is counteracted by the depressant effect of heroin, but in high doses, both depress respiration.

Primary Prevention

Some experts believe that human beings have an inborn need for euphoria, whereas others believe that the desire for drugs is a learned desire for pleasure or escape. It is known that young people who smoke are more likely to experiment with drugs and eventually become drug abusers. Children are more likely to take up illegal drug use if illegal drugs are used at home. Children from religious homes have a lower risk of illegal drug use. The cost of drugs also appears to influence the rate of subsequent drug use: the cheaper a drug is, the more people will try it.

To be effective, a national illegal drug control program must be multifaceted and not rely on only one strategy. In general, one might consider the broad strategies under demand reduction, supply reduction, and the elimination of money laundering (Jekel et al. 1994). Demand reduction not only involves educating people to make them aware of the dangers of drugs but also involves the treatment of drug abusers. Supply reduction implies the reduction of the amount of drug imported, as well as the control of selling of drugs on the street. It appears that scattered drug "pushers" at isolated locations are less dangerous than are organized drug "bazaars," so that one police strategy might be to keep the selling of drugs a scattered business. It is more difficult to market large amounts of drugs if banking practices and export regulations make it problematic to "launder" the cash obtained from drug deals. In at least one experience, the use of broad strategies to reduce demand and supply and to eliminate money laundering resulted in a marked decrease in the abuse of crack cocaine following a nationwide epidemic (Jekel et al. 1994).

Secondary and Tertiary Prevention

As with alcohol abuse, with drug abuse the goals of secondary and tertiary prevention are early detection and early treatment of the problem. The treatment for illegal drug abuse may be thought of in four stages: assessment, abstinence initiation, relapse prevention, and follow-up. A careful assessment is necessary to provide the proper treatment. Abstinence initiation often involves individual psychotherapy as well as medications that suppress craving. Relapse prevention is best achieved with the help of group therapy. Long-term success depends on the individual joining support groups and developing new habit patterns. For some drug abusers, the 12-step approach to treatment, as embodied in Narcotics Anonymous, is helpful. A reorientation of the abuser's life, as with religious conversion, increases the likelihood of success.

MENTAL HEALTH

In the USA, the most direct evidence of an increase in mental health problems is seen in the rapidly rising rates of major depression. Based on their own studies and those of others, Klerman and Weissman (1989) noted that an increasing proportion of people in the USA have had one or more episodes of major depression in their lives and that the increase is occurring in younger birth cohorts. For example, 40% of the people born after 1955 have suffered from at least one episode of major depression by the age of 20 years. This represents a considerably greater incidence rate than for any prior birth cohort. The reasons for this increase are uncertain, but Klerman and Weissman suggested the following: increasing urbanization, mobility, and social anomie; changes in family structure (e.g., increases in the number of divorces and single-parent families); changing gender roles in employment and families; and increasing use of drugs and alcohol.

Although a discussion of the methods to detect and treat mental illness is beyond the scope of this book, it is important to note that a variety of methods of primary prevention have been developed with the goal of promoting mental health and providing education and emotional support during times of stress. Today, there are support groups for the families of patients with various physical, psychologic, and mental health problems, including cancer, Alzheimer's disease, alcoholism, eating disorders, and child abuse, to name only a few. There are also informal groups to provide counseling and support to new mothers, widows, widowers, retirees, and others going through major changes in life, as well as telephone "hotlines" to help people who are in a crisis and need advice about where to turn for professional help. Matthews, Larson, and Barry (1993) have reviewed the available scientific literature showing that religious belief and practice are consistently associated with better health, particularly mental health. Although more work needs to be done in this area because of the possibility of selection and detection biases, the consistency of the findings is impressive.

INJURIES

The impact of injuries is often described in terms of **years of potential life lost** (YPLL). In the USA, injuries are the leading cause of YPLL before the age of 65 (see Centers for Disease Control and Prevention 1992).

Injuries can be categorized as follows: automobile crashes; home incidents (falls, burns, poisonings, electrocutions, drownings, etc.); occupational incidents; homicides; suicides; and miscellaneous injuries (plane and train crashes, building collapses, etc.).

This section of the chapter discusses automobile crashes and home incidents, and a later section on occupational health discusses worksite incidents. Specialists in the field of injury prevention do not refer to injuries sustained from automobile crashes or incidents in the home or worksite as "accidents," because the word carries the connotation that they are not predictable. In fact, these injury-producing events are fairly predictable and therefore are preventable.

Automobile Crashes

Haddon (1972), a founder of the field of automobile injury epidemiology, developed a detailed approach to injury prevention that classifies the phases of injury and the factors involved. Haddon's approach is followed here, with the phases classified as preinjury, injury, and postinjury and with the risk factors involved in automobile injuries classified as human, vehicle, and environmental.

Risk Factors in the Preinjury Phase

Human Factors. New drivers, young drivers, and drivers suffering from alcohol intoxication, drug intoxication, fatigue, or a combination of these factors are at increased risk for automobile crashes.

In new drivers, the excess risk of automobile crashes is related to the inability to anticipate and prevent developing hazards, as well as the inability to recognize existing hazards and respond to them quickly and appropriately. For example, new drivers often do not anticipate the dangers of taking curves at high speeds, particularly when roads are wet, and they often have difficulties coordinating manual actions, such as steering and braking, when it is necessary to respond to urgent driving demands. New drivers are at increased risk, regardless of the age at which they begin driving, but the excess risk decreases to zero over a few years of driving.

People who start driving during their teenage years may be at increased risk not only because of their driving inexperience but also because of several "immaturity factors" commonly associated with adolescence: a sense of invulnerability, a refusal to be warned about hazards, and a tendency to let the mind wander and act less cautiously (including taking the eyes off the road) when friends are nearby. In the USA, the high rates of serious injuries per mile of driving for young drivers are generally attributed to a combination of inexperience and immaturity factors. However, in Canada, at least one study did not find an increased immaturity risk when the number of years of driving were controlled for in the analysis (Pierce 1977). It is not clear what factors are responsible for the differences noted between teenage drivers in the USA and those in other nations.

New proposals to reduce the injury problems from teenage driving have been advanced (see Insurance Institute for Highway Safety 1994). Among them are "graduated licensing," which would require each new teenage driver to graduate from a provisional or beginner's license to one or more intermediate licenses before receiving an unrestricted license. The major provisions of the restrictive licenses limit how late the driver can operate a vehicle (i.e., they impose various kinds of curfews). Restrictive licenses have proved to be effective in New Zealand, for example.

Driving while intoxicated (DWI) with alcohol or drugs interacts with other factors, such as fatigue, and reduces sensory input to increase the risks late at night. This is one reason for considering a curfew of 11:00 PM or midnight for new teenage drivers, who are responsible for an excess number of fatal crashes, particularly single-vehicle crashes, in the USA (Williams et al. 1995).

Although some groups have advocated driver education programs in all US high schools, Robertson and Zador (1978) showed that the rates of teenage crashes and injuries in counties where in-school driver education was given to students were as high as or higher than the rates in counties where in-school driver education was not given. The reason appeared to be that the in-school driver education programs put significant numbers of young drivers on the road at an earlier age.

Laws concerning DWI are already in place, as are regulations concerning the number of hours that professional drivers can operate trucks, buses, and other vehicles on the road per day and per week. Dozing and fatigue have been found responsible for many vehicle crashes, including many involving trucks.

Vehicle Factors.   The ability of vehicles to brake and other aspects of vehicle construction and maintenance may influence the risk of injuries. Similarly, vehicle design may play a role. For example, research has demonstrated that a tail light pattern involving two lower red lights at the sides, plus one higher red light in the center of the vehicle, catches the attention of drivers best and reduces rear-end collisions. All new vehicles sold in the USA now have this tail light pattern.

Environmental Factors.   Driving must be slowed during periods of rain, snow, or poor visibility, and this is not always done. Poor design and maintenance of roads and highways also increase the risk of vehicle crashes.

Risk Factors in the Injury Phase

Human Factors.   The ability of human beings to resist injury is influenced by the use of specific protection devices, such as seat belts in automobiles and helmets for motorcycle and bicycle riders.

Vehicle Factors.   Vehicle design has been steadily improving under the influence of federal regulations. Vehicle safety features include collapsible steering columns, energy-absorbing construction, in-door side protection, seat belts and air bags, and protected gasoline tanks.

Environmental Factors.   The object into which a vehicle crashes helps to determine the seriousness of the crash. Energy-absorbing barriers on the shoulder of the road reduce the risk of vehicles going off the road, and median strip barriers reduce injuries from head-on collisions.

Risk Factors in the Postinjury Phase

Human Factors.   The fate of crash victims may be influenced greatly by the ability of individuals at the scene of a crash to act quickly in summoning medical help and preventing other vehicles from becoming involved in the crash.

Vehicle Factors.   The construction of a vehicle, including the extent to which it absorbs energy in a crash while maintaining the integrity of the passenger cage, may determine whether or not passengers survive a crash.

Environmental Factors.   The extent of injury is influenced by the rapidity and quality of the emergency response. Unlike the older ambulance services, the advanced life support (ALS) teams seek to stabilize the condition of injured persons at the crash scene before transport. Helicopter ambulance systems appear to improve outcomes, in part because they carry injured persons to trauma centers rather than to the nearest emergency room, which may not be adequately equipped for serious trauma.

Surveillance and Prevention

One of the most important factors in prevention is improved data on the nature of injuries, the rate at which they occur, and the circumstances under which they occur. The Fatal Accident Reporting System was developed by the National Highway Traffic Safety Administration and provides valuable epidemiologic data. Other injury surveillance systems depend on the use of the E-codes in the International Classification of Diseases (ICD) and the use of hospital emergency department and admission diagnoses.

A variety of methods of primary, secondary, and tertiary prevention have been devised to prevent serious injuries from automobile crashes. Examples of primary prevention include improvements in driver training, the passage and enforcement of laws concerning driving under the influence of alcohol or drugs, the construction and maintenance of good roads and highways, and the modification of automobiles to make them easier to control under hazardous conditions and to optimize passenger safety in the event of a crash. Examples of secondary prevention include testing of each driver's skill and vision before a license is issued. And examples of tertiary prevention include developing and using effective methods of transporting and caring for victims of automobile crashes so as to limit the degree of impairment they suffer.

Because prevention focuses on human factors, as well as vehicle and environmental factors, it requires an understanding of human behavior and of the kinds of behavioral interventions that do and do not work. Regulations regarding automobile construction have had a positive effect in reducing injuries from automobile crashes. Laws regarding human behavior, such as those requiring seat belt use, have been somewhat less successful, but they have still helped to move behavior in this direction. When lack of conforming behavior is easier to detect, as it is with lack of helmet use by motorcycle riders, conforming behavior tends to be higher, but in some states laws such as the helmet law have been challenged and overturned by referendum. It is not always clear when efforts to reduce injuries and their associated costs override the sometimes necessary restrictions on behavioral freedoms. As medical care costs continue to rise, the balance may gradually shift in the direction of greater controls on behavior, especially on driving while intoxicated.

Common Injuries in the Home

Among the many types of preventable injuries in the home are poisoning, fires, falls, and drowning.

The victims of **poisoning** are usually toddlers and preschool children, who experiment with tasting or swallowing substances that they encounter while exploring. Much has been accomplished in recent decades by developing child-proof caps for containers of medicines and household products; by counseling parents to keep cleaning solutions, pesticides, medicines, and other hazardous substances out of the reach of their children; and by establishing poison control centers.

Fires are one of the most common causes of injuries in the home. Some improvement has been achieved by tightening building codes, particularly the requirement for hard-wired smoke alarms in houses. Nevertheless, many older buildings are not retrofitted with these devices. The reduction in the prevalence of cigarette smoking has reduced one source of fires, but arson is still common, either for insurance or for revenge.

Although people of all ages can be the victims of **falls,** older people are at greater risk of serious injury. In younger persons, falls are likely to be associated with activities such as climbing ladders, shoveling snow, or walking on a surface covered with ice. Among older people, falls are frequently due to failing vision, loss of equilibrium or physical strength, or use of medications that decrease stability (Tinetti, Speechley, and Ginter 1988). Architectural modifications, such as the provision of handrails in hallways and on stairs, can reduce the incidence of falls in the elderly.

Drowning occurs most often among school-age children, especially boys. Swimming lessons and water safety instruction at an early age may reduce the number of deaths and injuries associated with activities that occur in and near pools and other bodies of water.

OCCUPATIONAL HEALTH

The occupational environment is well suited for the practice of preventive medicine. There are two appropriate goals for occupational health: (1) the prevention of work-related injuries and diseases and (2) health promotion in the workplace. Occupational health is most likely to succeed when these health goals can be clearly shown to produce economic benefits for the company by increasing the productivity of its employees and reducing costs.

Surveillance of Occupational Injuries and Diseases

The surveillance of occupational injuries and diseases is as critical to their prevention as is the surveillance of infectious diseases. Federal efforts in this area were advanced when the Occupational Safety and Health Administration (OSHA) and the National Institute for Occupational Safety and Health (NIOSH) were established in 1970. Unfortunately, the surveillance of occupational diseases is far from being as adequate or as well understood as the surveillance of infectious diseases (see Centers for Disease Control 1990). There are many reasons for this, including the difficulty of recognizing many occupational diseases and an incomplete understanding by many physicians of their reporting role in occupational illness.

Surveillance of occupational diseases serves the same functions as does the surveillance of other diseases: establishing a background rate, determining significant increases in disease, setting disease control priorities, and so forth (see Chapter 3).

Currently, the majority of states have mandatory reporting requirements for occupational injuries and diseases, although these requirements, including the types of conditions that must be reported, vary somewhat from state to state.

Other sources of reporting certain occupational conditions include laboratories, workers' compensation programs, some industries, and, occasionally, death certificates. Of course, a physician may report a suspected occupational health problem directly to OSHA or to a state department of health, which will then investigate the report to determine if a problem exists and to enforce any federal regulations that may have been violated.

An important surveillance concept that has been applied to the occupational health field is the idea of **sentinel health events** (Rutstein et al. 1983). A sentinel health event is a preventable event (death, disease, or impairment) that can be used to identify a problem in the system of prevention, detection, or treatment of occupational health problems.

Work-Related Injuries

While some jobs are associated with more risks than others, no job is completely free of risks for work-related injuries. Collisions are a common risk to truck drivers, taxi drivers, and other vehicle operators; falling objects represent a frequent threat to construction workers, longshoremen, and movers; the loss of limbs or digits is a risk of working with agricultural or manufacturing machines; and explosions, fires, and discharge of firearms are threats faced by miners, firemen, and police, respectively. Less striking, but becoming increasingly more common, are repetitive motion injuries and back injuries. Repetitive motion injuries, such as carpal tunnel syndrome, can affect musicians, typists, assembly line workers, and people in various other jobs. Back injuries are a risk not only to employees whose jobs require lifting and other forms of intense physical labor but even to employees with sedentary office jobs.

Work-Related Diseases
Skin Diseases

Dermatologic diseases are the most frequent type of occupational disease. Among the causes of occupational disease are exposure to chemicals, microorganisms, and physical agents (heat, cold, vibration, etc.). A predisposing skin condition makes an occupational skin disease more likely.

According to Rosenstock and Cullen (1986), 80% of occupational skin diseases are due to exposure to chemicals. Either direct irritation or an allergic reaction to a chemical can result in contact dermatitis. Oils and greases frequently irritate the skin, causing lesions to become infected. Exposure to bacteria or fungi is a frequent cause of occupational skin diseases in persons who work with animals, fish, food, or soil. Phototoxic dermatitis and photosensitization are problems that sometimes occur in people who work outdoors without protection from the sun. Exposure to severe cold or severe vibration may result in Raynaud's phenomenon (white finger disease), and exposure to temperature extremes may also result in burns, frostbite, trenchfoot, or dermatitis. The skin is frequently abraded, penetrated, or cut by physical injury from falls or the use of tools.

Lung Diseases

Like the skin, the lung is a frequent site of work-related diseases. Occupational exposure to dusts, gases, fumes, mists, or vapors may cause acute or chronic disease, depending on factors such as the number, duration, and intensity (level) of exposures.

Obstructive Lung Disease. According to Chen-Yeung and Malo (1995), the most prevalent occupational lung disease in developed countries today is occupational asthma. There is a distinction between work-aggravated asthma and occupational asthma. The former is found in people with preexisting asthma, while the latter refers to asthma due strictly to occupational exposure. When there is no latent period in occupational asthma, it is relatively easy to determine the occupational origin of disease. It is more difficult to determine the causative agent if asthma has its onset months or years after the occupational exposure.

Among the many agents that can cause occupational asthma are animal products, plant products, wood dusts, metal dusts, soldering fluxes, drugs, and organic chemicals. Isocyanates, which are used in the manufacture of polyurethane and in many paints, are one of the most common categories of causative agent and are frequently responsible for occupational asthma in automobile painters.

Byssinosis is a respiratory disease caused by the dust formed during the processing of cotton. Although it is characterized by bronchoconstriction, with chest tightness and shortness of breath, it is not typical asthma. The symptoms are thought to be due to a toxic effect on the bronchi, rather than to an immunologic reaction; one reason for this supposition is that byssinosis can occur the first time a person is exposed to cotton dust. The symptoms of byssinosis are especially severe after a period of time away from the dust, such as after a vacation or even after a weekend, but they abate somewhat upon continued exposure during the week. Byssinosis may not result in permanent lung damage if the duration and intensity of exposure are limited. It can, however, cause severe disability in people with long-term exposure, particularly those who smoke or have chronic bronchitis. A disease similar to byssinosis sometimes occurs in workers who process flax or hemp.

Interstitial Lung Disease. Asbestosis, silicosis, and coal worker's pneumoconiosis are examples of interstitial lung diseases associated with the inhalation of dusts. Chronic inhalation of asbestos or free silica causes the gradual development of fibrosis in the lung. Inhaled asbestos can also produce two highly fatal cancers, lung cancer and mesothelioma. Coal worker's pneumoconiosis (black lung disease) can cause a massive, diffuse fibrosis, the major symptom of which is progressive shortness of breath. The degree of disease and rate of progression are related to the type of dust and to the intensity and duration of exposure.

Hypersensitivity Pneumonitis. Hypersensitivity pneumonitis is an inflammatory response of the lungs to inhaled organic agents (usually bacteria or fungi) found in a variety of work settings. One example is farmer's lung, which is associated with inhaling moldy hay dust. The names of many types of hypersensitivity pneumonitis indicate the occupation at risk (cheese handler's lung, grain handler's lung, pigeon breeder's lung, etc.). Hypersensitivity pneumonitis affects the alveoli and respiratory bronchioles, rather than the bronchi, and usually wheezing is not prominent. In the early stages, removal of the affected person usually results in complete resolution. Chronic exposure, however, may lead to permanent lung damage.

Granuloma. The most prominent occupational disease characterized by lung granuloma is berylliosis, which can be impossible to distinguish from sarcoidosis without measuring tissue levels of beryllium or performing other specialized tests.

Liver and Kidney Diseases

Because the liver is heavily involved in detoxifying absorbed substances, particularly non–water-soluble chemicals absorbed through the gastrointestinal tract, the liver is often the site of damage. Occupational exposure to chemicals such as chlorinated hydrocarbons, halogenated aromatics, nitro-aromatics, ethanol, vinyl chloride, and epoxy resins can cause acute or subacute toxic hepatitis or fibrosis. Occupational exposure to hepatitis virus, as sometimes occurs in health care workers, can cause viral hepatitis.

The kidneys are frequently damaged by water-soluble toxins and metals because of their role in the excretion of water-soluble wastes. Acute tubular necrosis can occur as a result of acute exposure to divalent metals (e.g., mercury, cadmium, and chromium), halogenated hydrocarbons, other hydrocarbons, arsine, and other compounds. Most cases of work-related chronic renal disease are caused by long-term exposure to metals (especially mercury, lead, and cadmium).

Eye Damage and Hearing Loss

Most occupational eye damage is due to chemical burns, radiation effects, or mechanical injuries, including lacerations, contusions, and damage to the eye from fractures to surrounding skull bones. Cataracts or corneal damage can result from ionizing radiation (especially to the lid) and from ultraviolet radiation. Workers exposed to the sun a great deal, such as those in the fishing trade, have an increased risk of cataracts.

Loud noise on the job may cause loss of high tone hearing, with considerable functional deafness in later life. Chronic exposure to noise at a level of 85 dB frequently results in hearing problems, and many workers are regularly exposed to a level higher than 85 dB at work. The decibel (dB) scale is a logarithmic scale of sound pressure levels; according to this scale, normal human hearing goes from near 0 to about 120 dB. The greatest hearing loss tends to occur at a frequency of 3000–4000 Hz, which is a crucial range for hearing the consonants of human speech (for example, f, p, s, and t) and therefore for understanding speech.

Prevention of Occupational Injuries and Diseases

Safety in the workplace demands control over the environment, including providing a drug-free workplace, protective equipment (safety goggles, hard hats, ear protection devices, etc.), tools and equipment in good working order, proper training for workers, and adequate rest periods. As research in the field of **ergonomics** has indicated, prevention of many occupational health problems, including repetitive motion injuries and back injuries, can be accomplished by adjusting the occupational environment to the needs of the workers. In offices, the use of properly designed computer keyboards and the correct placement of screens for each worker can reduce the risk of repetitive motion injuries. In factory warehouses, safe lifting of manufactured goods requires the proper training of individual workers, but well-designed aids to lifting, such as sturdy handles on objects to be lifted, can also help prevent back injuries.

The prevention of occupational skin diseases usually can be accomplished by eliminating the causative biologic, physical, or chemical agent or by providing barrier protection (e.g., gloves or protective uniforms) so that the causative agent does not touch the skin. Prevention of a variety of occupational diseases, including those affecting the skin, lung, liver, and kidney, requires preventing or minimizing exposures to toxic agents, including those listed in Table 19–1 and discussed below (see Exposure to Toxins).

In health care workers, the prevention of some infectious diseases, such as hepatitis, can be accomplished by the use of vaccines (see Chapter 16). If no vaccine exists, as is the case for the human immunodeficiency virus (HIV), then appropriate training and equipment for the prevention of contact with the virus should be provided to the workers.

Health Promotion in the Workplace

Workers in a company tend to be concentrated at certain places and, with the support of the company, industry, or agency, the workers can be reached for education, prevention, and health-promoting services. By the time most people reach working age, they have relatively little contact with the medical profession, except for women with fertility control needs or with pregnancies, so health promotion activities provided in the workplace are usually found to be helpful.

Activities designed to promote good health in employees often include health education about nutrition, exercise, smoking cessation, and weight reduction. In some cases, companies offer fitness programs and the use of a fitness center; limit the areas in which employees can smoke on the premises; provide immunizations (e.g., influenza and hepatitis B vaccines); and sponsor specific screening programs (e.g., for hypertension or high cholesterol levels) or the more comprehensive health risk assessments (see Chapter 17).

Mental health, including freedom from alcohol and drug abuse, is becoming increasingly important for companies. Random screening programs for alcohol or illegal drug abuse are sometimes introduced for certain critical employees, such as pilots, air traffic controllers, or railroad engineers, but it is difficult to justify such activity for all employees.

Fearing the supposedly endless costs of mental health and substance abuse treatment, some companies have developed **employee assistance programs** (EAPs) within the company or have entered a contract with an outside agency to provide employee assistance in the form of counseling and treatment services for emotional problems and substance abuse. The advantage of these programs is that they are free to the workers and usually have a high degree of confidentiality guaranteed. Their goal is to increase the attendance and productivity of the workers.

Company Support for Preventive Activities

If preventive activities can be shown to be cost-effective for a company, especially in terms of reducing worker turnover, days missed from work, and medical care costs, the company often will pay for the activities. If health promotion and disease prevention activities are sought by the workers and if provision of these activities contributes to their morale and to company loyalty, such services are more likely to be provided by companies.

There are other advantages of preventive services in the occupational setting. The health information and good health habits learned in the workplace may be carried home to improve the health of an entire family.

Occupational Health Regulations

The Occupational Safety and Health Administration (OSHA) establishes federal standards for exposure to occupational hazards, investigates complaints or reports of problems in the workplace, and enforces the federal standards and regulations in the

TABLE 19–1. Routes and Effects of Exposure to Toxins That Are Often Found in the Workplace

Toxin	Routes and Effects of Exposure
Metals*	
Arsenic	May enter via the lungs, skin, or gastrointestinal tract. Arsenic compounds are used as insecticides and weed killers. Cause respiratory and gastrointestinal symptoms and, in high doses, can cause death. Can cause lung cancer.
Beryllium	Usually enters via the lungs. Causes granulomas in the lungs; lesions appear similar to those in sarcoidosis.
Cadmium	Usually enters via the lungs. Displaces zinc in enzyme systems, often damaging the renal tubules. Causes metal fume fever.
Lead	Usually enters via the gastrointestinal tract or lungs. Displaces calcium in chemical reactions. Inorganic form of lead causes gastrointestinal and neurologic symptoms. Organic compounds of lead cause diffuse neurologic symptoms.
Mercury	May enter via the lungs, skin, or gastrointestinal tract. Used in the past by hatmakers to make felt for hats. Chronic exposure damages the central nervous system, with the elemental form of mercury tending to cause tremors ("hatter's shakes") and the organic forms tending to cause psychiatric symptoms ("mad as a hatter") and even dementia. Mercury also damages the kidneys.
Zinc	Usually enters via the lungs. Inhaling zinc oxide causes metal fume fever (a disorder that also can be caused by other metal fumes).
Insecticides, herbicides, and fungicides	
Organophosphates	Usually enter via the skin from handling, but can enter via the lungs. Block acetylcholinesterase and produce both central nervous system and peripheral nerve damage.
Pentachlorophenol	Usually enters via the skin. Used as a wood preservative. Interferes with cellular respiration. Causes anorexia and respiratory symptoms and, in high doses, can cause coma and death.
Polychlorinated biphenyls	Enter via the skin or lungs. Are teratogens and possibly also carcinogens.
Hydrocarbon solvents†	
Benzene	Absorbed through the lungs and skin. Is a lipid-soluble aromatic solvent that is used widely in industry. Chronic exposure can result in suppression of the bone marrow, with a possible end result of aplastic anemia.
Carbon tetrachloride	Absorbed readily through the lungs. Is a lipid-soluble chlorinated hydrocarbon that is not used much in industry because it is extremely toxic to kidneys and liver, but it is the prototype of this class of chemical. Damage to either the kidneys or the liver can predominate. Renal tubular necrosis may follow acute exposures, and hepatic centrilobular necrosis tends to predominate in chronic exposure, especially in the presence of ethanol or following hepatic damage by ethanol.
Toluene	Usually inhaled. Is a lipid-soluble aromatic solvent found in products such as glue. Primarily causes central nervous system effects, including hallucinations (which is why glue is sometimes sniffed).
Asphyxiants‡	
Carbon dioxide	Enters the body via the lungs and stimulates the respiratory center. Is a nonreactive asphyxiant. Begins to produce symptoms of rapid breathing when concentration reaches about 3% in the air. In high concentrations, causes coma and death.
Carbon monoxide	Enters the body via the lungs. Is a chemical asphyxiant that is ubiquitous in urban society (a product of automobile exhausts and sometimes of poorly ventilated space heaters). Combines with hemoglobin to form carboxyhemoglobin; when 50% or more of the hemoglobin is in the form of carboxyhemoglobin, fainting and death are likely. Smokers may inhale some carbon monoxide from smoking.
Hydrogen cyanide	Enters the body via the lungs or gastrointestinal tract. Is a chemical asphyxiant. Toxicity is retained in cyanide salts, because it is the reactive cyanide moiety that interferes with cytochrome oxidase. Causes headaches, rapid breathing, and, frequently, death.
Hydrogen sulfide	Absorbed through the lungs. Is a chemical asphyxiant that is as dangerous as hydrogen cyanide, but its smell tends to give warning of its presence before hazardous levels develop. Causes symptoms and effects similar to those of hydrogen cyanide.
Methane	Enters the body via the lungs. Is a nonreactive asphyxiant that is mainly a problem in mines, causing severe respiratory symptoms. The greater danger now is from explosion.
Nitrogen	Enters the body via the lungs. Is a nonreactive asphyxiant that used to be a problem in mines but now presents a hazard primarily to deep sea divers. Divers accumulate nitrogen in the fatty tissues during dives at high pressure. As divers approach the surface, nitrogen reenters their blood, and if the pressure is reduced too fast, it forms small bubbles in the blood, which interfere with circulation, especially to the brain. This process causes the "bends."
Miscellaneous organic compounds	
Resins	Usually enter via the skin, although may enter via the lungs. Produce asthma, irritation and allergic sensitization of the skin, and irritation of the eyes.
Vinyl chloride	Absorbed through the lungs and skin. Is ubiquitous in industry because it is used to make plastics. Can cause sclerodermatous skin lesions, Raynaud's phenomenon, and bone lesions in the hand, in addition to liver damage. The monomer form causes hemangiosarcoma of the liver in a small proportion of persons who are exposed.

*Metals often cause toxicity by interfering with the action of other metals as cofactors in enzyme reactions.

†Lipid-soluble hydrocarbon solvents build up in the body in tissues with high levels of lipids (e.g., the central nervous system), and they all have narcotic effects. Their central nervous system effects are exacerbated by alcohol. Exposure to more than one solvent may result in complex interactions.

‡Asphyxiants can be divided into two groups: (1) gases that have no direct toxic effect but can reduce the partial pressure of oxygen in the lungs to dangerous levels and (2) gases that interfere with respiration at the cellular level. Nonreactive asphyxiants do not enter into chemical reactions; they reduce the partial pressure of oxygen in the lungs.

workplace. OSHA has the right to issue fines or citations when it finds violations of federal laws.

Most states have occupational health units in their state health departments or elsewhere in the state government. These have the obligation to receive and investigate complaints and disease reports and, within the limits prescribed by state laws, to enforce workplace changes.

Workers' Compensation

Workers' Compensation, a mandatory insurance program in each state, provides for medical care and partial replacement of wages for workers with occupational diseases or injuries. Companies, agencies, and businesses are required to purchase a policy or to deposit premiums into a fund. For a given company, the size of the premiums is based on the amount of claims paid in recent years from Workers' Compensation to employees from that company. By this mechanism, the companies are liable without fault being assigned to the company or to the worker, and the worker's ability to sue for further damages is markedly limited.

The benefits are paid according to the severity and duration of the illness or injury, which is usually defined by law (see Chapter 18 for a discussion of the four major categories of disability). Physicians play an important role in defining the level of impairment due to the occupational injury or disease.

Medical ("Health") Insurance

In the USA, most persons under the age of 65 obtain medical insurance through their place of work. For decades, the medical insurance was a tax-free benefit to workers and, hence, was partly subsidized by the federal government. As the costs of workers' medical insurance have continued to outstrip the inflation rate, there is increasing demand on the part of companies for a limitation in their costs for such insurance. As a result, more and more companies are (1) requiring managed care plans (see Chapter 21); (2) requiring workers to pay a part of the costs of the insurance; or (3) not offering health insurance at all. The strategy of not offering health insurance is frequently used by businesses that have a rapid turnover of workers (such as restaurants) or operate on a slim profit margin. In the USA, an estimated 40 million people are without medical insurance because of unemployment or the lack of work-related medical insurance plans.

Diagnosis and Treatment of Occupational Health Problems

Traditionally, large companies had in-house physicians who, although doing some strictly preventive work, spent most of their time diagnosing and treating work-related injuries and illnesses in the company setting. These physicians were frequently in the difficult ethical position of depending on the company for their salary but believing that they were ethically responsible to advocate for the welfare of their patients. Supporting patients' claims that their illnesses were work-related could increase costs for the company and create tensions for the company physicians.

Today, many companies send their workers to outside occupational medicine practices, whose physicians can be somewhat more objective in their clinical evaluations. One advantage of employing an occupational medicine group over relying on private physicians or emergency rooms is the ability of the group practice to evaluate patients without delay.

EXPOSURE TO TOXINS
Forms of Toxins

The word "toxin" makes most people think of liquid chemicals, but toxins can be solids (such as plastics), particulate matter (such as dusts, fumes, or fibers), gases (including vapors or mists), or liquids. A **dust** consists of very fine solid particles of a larger solid (e.g., a rock or piece of coal or wood) and is created by crushing or sanding mechanisms. A **fume** consists of solid particles that develop by condensation from the gases given off by heated metals or plastics. A **gas** is a chemical that normally exists in the gaseous state at room temperature (such as oxygen or helium). A **vapor** is a gas from the evaporation of a liquid such as gasoline. A **mist** is formed when a liquid is aerosolized, as with an atomizer, forming fine droplets of the liquid.

Table 19–1 lists some of the more important toxins. Many of these are found primarily in the workplace, but some, such as carbon monoxide, are commonly encountered in everyday life. Not listed are substances that are toxic primarily if they pollute drinking water (such as gasoline, which can leak from a storage tank in a filling station and enter a nearby aquifer).

Primary Prevention

The prevention of toxic effects from a substance found in the environment or the workplace requires knowledge about what levels of the substance are considered safe, both for acute, short-term exposure and for chronic, long-term exposure. It also requires accurate measurement and surveillance of environmental or workplace levels of the substance. If the levels approach the threshold for harm, the options are (1) to reduce production or use (e.g., dry cleaners have tended to switch from using carbon tetrachloride to using less toxic solvents such as tetrachloroethylene); (2) to contain the substances within the industrial processes; (3) to remove the substances quickly from the working or living environment (e.g., by ventilation) before they can cause injury; or (4) to protect workers with special equipment (such as ventilatory masks).

Increasing knowledge of the risks of environmental exposures, particularly the possibility of fetal damage, has raised new ethical and legal liability questions. Is a company free of liability if a worker chooses to work in a potentially hazardous area and becomes ill from it? In particular, can a company prohibit pregnant women from working in an area where they might be exposed to a substance (such as lead) that could damage their fetuses? Recent court decisions have tended to say that such exclusion would be discrimination. It is not clear whether a company that initially sought to exclude pregnant women from doing certain jobs and was prohibited by law from doing so would later be liable if fetal injury occurred. The company would, however, still be liable for any violations of the Occupational Safety and Health Administration (OSHA) regulations.

Recent national laws have required that companies make public the potentially toxic substances used in the workplace. These laws have made the process of identification and control within a given area somewhat easier.

Secondary and Tertiary Prevention

It is not common for workers to be screened for asymptomatic disease referable to the environment. Nevertheless, if there is a known possible exposure, this makes sense, if the baseline measurement is known. Examples include periodic follow-up tuberculin skin tests for health care workers with negative results in the initial tuberculin test; periodic chest x-rays for health care workers with positive results in the tuberculin test; periodic pure tone audiograms to detect hearing loss in workers exposed to high levels of noise; and screening for lead in the serum of workers with unavoidable exposure to lead. Radiation-sensitive badges for workers in x-ray units or nuclear power stations are more analogous to screening for a risk factor than for a disease.

The symptoms of toxic injury and methods of treatment vary, depending on the level of exposure and the type of toxic substance to which the injured person was exposed. For persons with high-level acute exposures, emergency treatment may be necessary. For workers who have symptoms of disease and are exposed daily to toxic substances, it is important to have well-trained physicians perform a thorough evaluation and provide appropriate treatment and follow-up care. In addition, the occupational exposure should be reported, so that interventions may be made in the workplace before others are injured or poisoned.

SUMMARY

In the area of maternal and child health, efforts to promote health and well-being begin with family planning and proceed through the stages of prenatal care, labor and delivery care, and well child care. Opportunities for the prevention of injury and disease continue in day-care, preschool, and school facilities, as well as in homes and worksites.

In the area of infectious diseases, efforts to prevent the spread of the human immunodeficiency virus (HIV) and *Mycobacterium tuberculosis,* the agents responsible for acquired immunodeficiency syndrome (AIDS) and tuberculosis, have been less than successful, in part because behavioral changes are required and have been resisted by the groups most at risk. In the USA, multiple drug–resistant tuberculosis (MDRTB) has emerged and is especially severe in three types of institutions—prisons, general hospitals, and shelters for homeless people—many of which are overcrowded. The linkage between HIV infection, MDRTB, abuse of illegal drugs, and overcrowding of public institutions requires the development of strategies that address these problems jointly.

References Cited

Allen, D. F., and J. F. Jekel. Crack: The Broken Promise. London, Macmillan Academic and Professional, Ltd., 1991.

Barnes, F. E., ed. Ambulatory Maternal Health Care and Family Planning Services: Policies, Principles, Practices. Washington, D. C., American Public Health Association, 1978.

Bellin, E. Y., D. D. Fletcher, and S. M. Safyer. Association of tuberculosis infection with increased time in or admission to the New York City Jail System. Journal of the American Medical Association 269:2228–2231, 1993.

Brudney, K., and J. Dobkin. Resurgent tuberculosis in New York City: human immunodeficiency virus, homelessness, and the decline of tuberculosis programs. American Review of Respiratory Diseases 144:745–749, 1991.

Centers for Disease Control. A Child-Centered Program to Prevent Tuberculosis. Publication No. (PHS) 1280. Washington, D. C., Government Printing Office, March 1965.

Centers for Disease Control. Mandatory reporting of occupational diseases by clinicians. Morbidity and Mortality Weekly Report 39:19–28, 1990.

Centers for Disease Control. Tuberculosis among homeless shelter residents. Morbidity and Mortality Weekly Report 40:869–877, 1991.

Centers for Disease Control and Prevention. Exposure of passengers and flight crew to Mycobacterium tuberculosis on commercial aircraft, 1992–1995. Morbidity and Mortality Weekly Report 44:137–140, 1995.

Centers for Disease Control and Prevention. Years of potential life lost before age 65, by race, Hispanic origin, and sex: United States, 1986–1988. Morbidity and Mortality Weekly Report 41:13–23, 1992.

Chen-Yeung, M., and J.-L. Malo. Occupational asthma. New England Journal of Medicine 333:107–112, 1995.

Clemens, J. D., J. J. Chuong, and A. R. Feinstein. The BCG controversy: a methodological and statistical reappraisal. Journal of the American Medical Association 249:2362–2368, 1983.

Dubos, R. Mirage of Health Utopias, Progress, and Biological Change. New York, Harper and Row, 1959.

Edlin, B. R., et al. An outbreak of multidrug-resistant tuberculosis among hospitalized patients with the acquired immunodeficiency syndrome. New England Journal of Medicine 326:1514–1521, 1992.

Frieden, T. R., et al. Tuberculosis in New York City: turning the tide. New England Journal of Medicine 333:229–233, 1995.

Haddon, W., Jr. A logical framework for categorizing highway safety phenomena and activity. Journal of Trauma 12:197–207, 1972.

Institute of Medicine. Prenatal Care: Reaching Mothers, Reaching Infants. Washington, D. C., National Academy Press, 1988.

Insurance Institute for Highway Safety (IIFHS). Status Report: Slower Graduation to Full Licensing Means Fewer Teenage Deaths. Arlington, Va., IIFHS, 1994.

Iseman, M. D. Treatment of multidrug-resistant tuberculosis. New England Journal of Medicine 329:784–791, 1993.

Jekel, J. F., et al. Nine years of the freebase cocaine epidemic in the Bahamas. American Journal on Addictions 3:14–24, 1994.

Kaplan, E. Evaluating needle-exchange programs via syringe tracking and testing (STT). AIDS and Public Policy Journal 6:109–115, 1992.

Klerman, G. L., and M. M. Weissman. Increasing rates of depression. Journal of the American Medical Association 261:2229–2235, 1989.

Klerman, L. V. The need for a new perspective on prenatal care. In Merkatz, I. R., et al., eds. New Perspectives on Prenatal Care. New York, Elsevier, 1990.

Matthews, D. A., D. B. Larson, and C. P. Barry. The Faith Factor: An Annotated Bibliography of Clinical Research on Spiritual Subjects. Rockville, Md., National Institute for Healthcare Research, 1993.

Mount, F. W., and S. H. Ferebee. Preventive effects of isoniazid in the treatment of primary tuberculosis in children. New England Journal of Medicine 265:713, 1961.

Pierce, J. A. Drivers First Licensed in Ontario, October 1969 to October 1975. Toronto, Ontario Ministry of Transportation and Communication, 1977.

Robertson, L. S., and P. L. Zador. Driver education and crash involvement of teenaged drivers. American Journal of Public Health 68:959–965, 1978.

Rosenstock, L., and M. R. Cullen. Clinical Occupational Medicine. Philadelphia, W. B. Saunders Company, 1986.

Rutstein, D. D., et al. Sentinel health events (occupational): a basis for physician recognition and public health surveillance. American Journal of Public Health 73:1054–1062, 1983.

Selwyn, P. A., et al. High risk of active tuberculosis in HIV-infected drug users with cutaneous anergy. Journal of the American Medical Association 268:504–509, 1992.

Tinetti, M. E., M. Speechley, and S. F. Ginter. Risk factors for falls among elderly persons living in the community. New England Journal of Medicine 319:1701–1707, 1988.

US Preventive Services Task Force. Guide to Clinical Preventive Services. Baltimore, Williams & Wilkins, 1989.

US Public Health Service, Department of Health and Human Services. Strategic Plan to Combat HIV and AIDS in the United States. Washington, D. C., Government Printing Office, 1992.

Williams, A. F., et al. Characteristics of Fatal Crashes of Sixteen-Year-Old Drivers. Arlington, Va., Insurance Institute for Highway Safety, January 1995.

Zahler, P., et al. Kinetics of drug effect by distributed lags analysis: an application to cocaine. Clinical Pharmacology and Therapeutics 31:775–782, 1982.

Selected Readings

LaDou, J., ed. Occupational Medicine. Norwalk, Conn., Appleton and Lange, 1990.

Levy, B. S., and D. H. Wegman, eds. Occupational Health: Recognizing and Preventing Work-Related Disease, 2nd ed. Boston, Little, Brown, and Company, 1988.

Robertson, L. S. Injury Epidemiology. New York, Oxford University Press, 1992.

Rosenstock, L., and M. R. Cullen. Clinical Occupational Medicine. Philadelphia, W. B. Saunders Company, 1986.

Wallace, H. M., G. Ryan, Jr., and A. C. Oglesby. Maternal and Child Health Practices, 3rd ed. Oakland, Calif., Third Party Publishing Company, 1988.

CHAPTER TWENTY

PUBLIC HEALTH RESPONSIBILITIES

AND GOALS

DEFINITION OF PUBLIC HEALTH

The term "public health" has two meanings. The first refers to the health status of the public—that is, of a defined population. Chapter 2 provided some tools for estimating the health of a population, and Chapter 14 gave several definitions of health, including a discussion of their limitations. The second meaning, which is the focus of Chapters 20 and 21, refers to the organized social efforts made to preserve and improve the health of a defined population.

The best-known definition of public health in terms of this second meaning was written in 1920 by C.-E. A. Winslow and is still remarkably current:

Public health is the science and art of preventing disease, prolonging life, and promoting physical health and efficiency through organized community efforts for the sanitation of the environment, the control of community infections, the education of the individual in principles of personal hygiene, the organization of medical and nursing service for the early diagnosis and preventive treatment of disease, and the development of the social machinery which will ensure to every individual in the community a standard of living adequate for the maintenance of health.

This definition is profound in many ways. First, it states the central emphasis of all public health work—namely, promoting health and preventing disease. Second, it emphasizes the diverse strategies that are required to bring this about, including environmental sanitation, specific disease control efforts, health education, medical care, and an adequate standard of living. Third, it makes clear that for these goals to be achieved, organized social action is required. This action is largely expressed in the policies of the federal, state, and local government bodies and in the activities of the agencies designed to promote and protect the health of the public. As the Institute of Medicine indicated in its 1988 report entitled *The Future of Public Health,* "Public health is what we, as a society, do collectively to assure the conditions in which people can be healthy."

ADMINISTRATION OF PUBLIC HEALTH

Responsibilities of the Federal Government

In theory, the public health responsibility of the federal government in the USA is rather limited. In practice, the federal government bases its role in health on two clauses from Article 1, Section 8, of the US Constitution. One is the interstate commerce clause, which gives the federal government the right "to regulate Commerce with foreign Nations, and among the several States, and with the Indian Tribes." The other is the general welfare clause, which states that "the Congress shall have Power to lay and collect Taxes . . . for the common Defense and general Welfare of the United States." Federal responsibility is also inferred from statements about Congress having

the authority to create and support a military and the authority to deal with Indian tribes and other special groups.

Regulation of Commerce

The regulation of commerce involves controlling the entry of people and products into the USA, as well as regulating commercial relationships among the states.

People who may be excluded from entry to the USA include those with particular health problems such as active tuberculosis or human immunodeficiency virus (HIV) infection. Products excluded from entry include fruits and vegetables that are infested with certain organisms (e.g., the Mediterranean fruit fly) or have been treated with prohibited insecticides or fungicides.

The regulation of commercial relationships between states has caused much dissent in the USA in recent years. Contaminated food products that cross state lines are considered to be "interstate commerce" in harmful microorganisms. Therefore, the federal government takes the responsibility for inspection of all milk, meat, and other food products at their site of production and processing. (In contrast, the state or local government is responsible for inspection of restaurants and food stores.) Likewise, polluted air and polluted water that may flow from state to state are deemed to be "interstate commerce" in polluting agents and therefore come under federal regulation.

Taxation for the General Welfare

The power to "tax for the general welfare" is the constitutional basis for the federal government's development of most of its public health programs and agencies, including the Centers for Disease Control and Prevention (CDC) and the Occupational Safety and Health Administration (OSHA); for research programs, such as those of the National Institutes of Health (NIH); and for the payment for medical care, such as Medicare and Medicaid (see Chapter 21).

Provision of Care for Special Groups

The federal government has taken special responsibility for providing health services to active military personnel and their families through Medicare; to veterans through the Veterans' Administration hospital system; and to Native Americans and Alaska natives through the Indian Health Service of the US Public Health Service.

Coordination of Federal Agencies

In the USA, the major federal department concerned with health is the **Department of Health and Human Services** (DHHS). As outlined in Table 20–1, the DHHS has six major operating units, most of which are called "administrations."

TABLE 20–1. Major Operating Units and Subunits of the US Department of Health and Human Services

Administration on Aging
Administration for Children and Families
Health Care Financing Administration
  Medicaid
  Medicare
  Quality Assurance
Public Health Service
  Agency for Health Care Policy and Research
  Agency for Toxic Substances and Disease Registry
  Centers for Disease Control and Prevention
    Epidemiology Program Office
    International Health Program Office
    National Center for Chronic Disease Prevention and Health Promotion
    National Center for Environmental Health
    National Center for Health Statistics
    National Center for Infectious Diseases
    National Center for Injury Prevention and Control
    National Center for Prevention Services
    National Immunization Program Office
    National Institute for Occupational Safety and Health
    Public Health Practice Program Office
  Food and Drug Administration
  Health Resources and Services Administration
  Indian Health Service
  National Institutes of Health
    Fogarty International Center
    National Cancer Institute
    National Center for Human Genome Research
    National Eye Institute
    National Heart, Lung, and Blood Institute
    National Institute on Aging
    National Institute of Alcohol Abuse and Alcoholism
    National Institute of Allergy and Infectious Diseases
    National Institute of Arthritis and Musculoskeletal and Skin Diseases
    National Institute of Child Health and Human Development
    National Institute on Deafness and Other Communication Disorders
    National Institute of Dental Research
    National Institute of Diabetes and Digestive and Kidney Diseases
    National Institute on Drug Abuse
    National Institute of Environmental Health Sciences
    National Institute of General Medical Sciences
    National Institute of Mental Health
    National Institute of Neurological Disorders and Stroke
    National Institute of Nursing Research
    National Library of Medicine
Social Security Administration
Substance Abuse and Mental Health Services Administration
  Center for Mental Health Services
  Center for Substance Abuse Prevention
  Center for Substance Abuse Treatment

Source of data: Office of the Federal Register, National Archives and Records Administration. United States Government Manual 1994/1995. Washington, D. C., Government Printing Office, 1994.

Administration on Aging. This agency provides advice to the Secretary of the DHHS on issues and policies regarding aging persons in the USA. It also administers certain grant programs for the benefit of the aging population.

Administration for Children and Families. This agency is responsible for administering child welfare programs through the states, Head Start programs, child abuse prevention and treatment programs, developmental disabilities programs, and child support enforcement.

Health Care Financing Administration. This agency is responsible for administering two major programs from the Social Security Act: (1) **Medicare,** which is covered under **Title 18** and pays for medical care for the elderly; and (2) **Medicaid,** which is covered under **Title 19** and which, in cooperation with the states, pays for medical and nursing home care for the poor (see Chapter 21). The agency's duties include setting standards for programs and institutions that provide medical care, developing payment policies, contracting for third-party payers to pay the bills, and monitoring the quality of care provided.

Public Health Service. The Public Health Service (PHS) has seven constituent agencies.

(1) The **Agency for Health Care Policy and Research** is the main federal agency for research and policy development in the area of medical care organization, financing, and quality assessment.

(2) The **Agency for Toxic Substances and Disease Registry** provides leadership and direction to programs designed to protect workers and the public from exposure to and adverse health effects of hazardous substances that are kept in storage sites or are released by fire, explosion, or accident.

(3) The **Centers for Disease Control and Prevention** (CDC) has the responsibility for "protecting the public health of the Nation by providing leadership and direction in the prevention and control of diseases and other preventable conditions and responding to public health emergencies" (see Office of the Federal Register 1994). The CDC directs and enforces federal quarantine activities, works with states in disease surveillance and control activities, develops immunization and other preventive programs, is involved in research and training, works to promote environmental and occupational health and safety, provides consultation to other nations in the control of preventable diseases, and participates with international agencies in the eradication and control of diseases around the world. The CDC has 11 major operating components, as shown in Table 20–1.

(4) The **Food and Drug Administration** (FDA) is the primary agency for regulating the safety and effectiveness of drugs for use in humans and animals; vaccines and other biologic products; diagnostic tests; and medical devices, including ionizing and nonionizing radiation-emitting electronic products. The FDA is also responsible for the safety, quality, and labeling of cosmetics, foods, and food additives and colorings.

(5) The **Health Resources and Services Administration** is responsible for developing the human resources and methods to improve access to health services and improve the equity and quality of health care. Its emphasis is on promoting primary medical care.

(6) The **Indian Health Service** promotes the health of and provides medical care for American Indians and Alaska natives.

(7) The **National Institutes of Health** consists of the 18 institutes listed in Table 20–1, plus the Fogarty

International Center, the National Library of Medicine, a clinical center, and certain other support divisions. The 18 institutes perform intramural (in-house) research on particular diseases or organ systems, sponsor extramural research through competitive grant programs, and are responsible for some disease control programs and public and professional education.

Social Security Administration. This agency administers the national program of retirement payments for social security program recipients and disability payments for the disabled.

Substance Abuse and Mental Health Services Administration. This agency provides national leadership in the prevention and treatment of addictive and mental disorders, based on up-to-date science and practices. Its three major operating divisions are the Center for Mental Health Services, the Center for Substance Abuse Prevention, and the Center for Substance Abuse Treatment.

Responsibilities of States

In the USA, the fundamental responsibility for the health of the public lies with the states. This authority is clarified in the 10th amendment to the US Constitution: "The powers not delegated to the United States by the Constitution, nor prohibited by it to the States, are reserved to the States respectively, or to the people."

In each state, there is a state health department to oversee the implementation of the **public health code,** a compilation of the state laws and regulations regarding public health and safety. (While laws must be passed by the legislature, regulations are technical rules added later by an empowered body with specific expertise, such as a board of health.) Mental health services in some states are the responsibility of the health department and in other states are the responsibility of a separate department of mental health services. As a part of its duty to ensure the health of the public, every state licenses medical and other health-related practitioners, as well as medical care institutions such as hospitals, nursing homes, and home care programs.

Responsibilities of Municipalities and Counties

Although the states have the fundamental police power regarding health, they delegate much of this authority to chartered municipalities, such as cities or other incorporated areas. These municipalities accept public health responsibilities in return for a considerable degree of independence from the state in running their affairs, including matters concerning property ownership and tax levies. In this respect, they differ from counties, which are bureaucratic subdivisions of the state created for the purpose of administering (with varying degrees of local control) state responsibilities such as courts of law, educational programs, highway construction and maintenance, police and fire protection, and health services.

Local public health departments usually are administrative divisions of municipalities or counties, and their policy is established by a city or county board of health. These boards of health have the right to establish public health laws and regulations, provided that they are at least as strict as similar laws and regulations in the state public health code and that they are "reasonable." Anything that is too strict can be challenged in the courts as being "unreasonable."

The courts have generally upheld local and state health department laws and regulations when they have to do with the control of communicable diseases. For example, laws relating to safe water and subsurface sewage disposal, immunization, regulation of restaurants and food stores, quarantine or treatment of persons with an infectious disease, investigation and control of acute disease outbreaks, and abatement of complaints relating to the spread of infectious disease (e.g., via possibly rabid animals) have generally been upheld by the courts.

Neither legislatures nor courts, however, have been as supportive of laws and regulations that control human behavior when communicable diseases are not involved. For example, laws requiring motorcyclists and bicyclists to wear helmets often fail to be enacted into law or are repealed following passage, despite abundant evidence of their benefits. Recently, the federal government made recommendations for legislation and programs in this area (see Centers for Disease Control and Prevention 1995). However, if an individual risk factor for disease can be shown to have a negative public impact, such as passive smoke inhalation, legislatures are supporting increasingly strict controls.

Responsibilities of Local Public Health Departments

Beginning in the 1920s, the Committee on Administrative Practices of the American Public Health Association studied the role of local health departments and issued a series of statements about their mission (Jekel 1991). The most famous of these statements emerged in 1940, when six primary responsibilities were defined: (1) vital statistics, (2) communicable disease control, (3) maternal and child health, (4) environmental health, (5) health education, and (6) public health laboratories. These responsibilities,

TABLE 20–2. The "Basic Six" Minimum Functions of Local Health Departments as Defined by the American Public Health Association in 1940

(1) Vital statistics
(2) Communicable disease control
(3) Maternal and child health
(4) Environmental health
(5) Health education
(6) Public health laboratories

Source of data: Jekel, J. F. Health departments in the US, 1920–1988: statements of mission with special reference to the role of C.-E. A. Winslow. Yale Journal of Biology and Medicine 64:467–479, 1991.

TABLE 20–3. Types of Services Often Provided by Local Health Departments in the 1990s

Vital statistics
- Recording of birth and death certificates
- Transmittal of certificates to the state and others
- Analysis and monitoring of rates

Communicable disease control
- Immunization
- Tuberculosis control
  - Clinics for diagnosis and treatment
  - Epidemiologic follow-up, contact testing, and prophylaxis
  - Home supervision of patients and contacts (nursing)
  - Tuberculin screening programs (high-risk areas only)
- Sexually transmitted disease control
  - Clinics for diagnosis, treatment, interviewing, and prophylaxis
  - Contact tracing and cluster testing
  - Screening programs
  - Education programs
- Surveillance of disease
  - Receipt and transmittal of reports
  - Analysis of data and provision of feedback to physicians and agencies
  - Dissemination of information to physicians and clinics
- Epidemic investigation and control
  - Work with other local agencies (e.g., hospitals)
  - Work with the state health department
- Other services
  - Rabies control
  - Screening for parasites
  - Screening of food handlers and persons having extensive contact with children

Maternal and child health
- Genetic counseling
- Genetic screening programs for phenylketonuria, thyroid disorders, etc. (usually a service provided by the state health department)
- Family planning programs
- Prenatal care
- Postpartum care, usually with home nursing
- Well child care (and, in some areas, care for ill children)
- School health services
- Crippled children's services (usually provided in conjunction with the state health department)
- Medical social work

Environmental health
- Promulgation of laws, standards, and regulations
- Water and sewerage engineering
- Monitoring and control of the drilling of wells
- Testing of water safety (e.g., pools, beaches, and public supplies)
- Monitoring of sewage treatment plants and subsurface sewage disposal
- Monitoring of solid waste storage and disposal
- Insect control
- Rodent control
- Air pollution control
- Radiologic health services
- Restaurant inspection and licensing
- Facilities licensure (e.g., day-care centers, schools, hospitals, and other public buildings)
- Nuisance abatement and control
- Investigation and control of toxic waste dumping
- Housing inspection and control of health hazards in homes
- Consumer protection

Health education
- Dissemination of information (e.g., to media, schools, and organizations)
- Fostering of community action around issues
- Developing a community constituency around health department programs
- Assisting in community health planning

Laboratory services
- Support for environmental programs
- Support for disease control efforts

Chronic disease control
- Screening programs (e.g., for hypertension, cholesterol, or cervical and breast cancer)
- Home nursing programs
- Educational efforts (including behavior change programs, such as "Stop Smoking")
- Medical social work
- Lead poisoning detection and treatment programs

Occupational health
- Environmental inspections
- Health education
- Epidemic investigation
- Immunization programs
- Screening efforts (e.g., for hypertension or tuberculosis)

Dental health
- Screening and referral, especially in schools
- Primary prevention by cleaning and use of topical fluoride
- Water fluoridation advocacy
- Treatment clinics for children
- Education in nutrition and dental hygiene
- Control of vending machines in schools

Mental health
- Education
- Community mental health clinics
- Support services for deinstitutionalized patients
- Home nursing services
- Alcohol and addiction services (e.g., educational programs and halfway houses)
- Promotion of self-help groups

Emergency medical services
- Planning and development
- Coordination of community efforts
- Operation of emergency services

Nutrition services
- Women, Infants, and Children (WIC) Program
- Education and counseling programs, often in conjunction with nursing

Other programs and services
- Health planning and coordination
- Operation of medical institutions and provision of medical care
- Injury prevention
- Blindness prevention
- Substance abuse programs

which came to be known as the "basic six" functions of local health departments (Table 20–2), have continued to influence the direction of local health departments, despite the many changes in the nature of public health problems since 1940.

Because the "basic six" functions are not adequate to deal with more recent public health problems such as environmental pollution, occupational toxins and safety hazards, and the increased incidence of chronic degenerative diseases, public health leaders have continued a lively debate concerning the proper functions and responsibilities of health departments at both the local and state level (see, for example, Hanlon 1973 and Terris 1976). Table 20–3 lists functions that are now considered appropriate for local health departments.

The ability to carry out public health responsibilities depends, of course, on the allocation of funds by legislative bodies. From the 1950s to the early 1970s, the danger of infectious diseases appeared to be waning. Despite occasional warnings that communicable diseases were still major threats (Jekel 1972), legislatures saw infectious diseases as a diminishing threat and were not generous with resources for public health agencies. The appearance of legionnaires' disease and Lyme disease in the mid-1970s was soon followed by toxic shock syndrome, acquired immunodeficiency syndrome (AIDS), multiple drug–resistant tuberculosis, and the resurgence of other infectious diseases (see Institute of Medicine 1992 and Garrett 1994). Unfortunately, by the time society began to awaken to the problem of the emerging public health diseases, the Institute of Medicine and others considered the public health system to be in "disarray" (Institute of Medicine 1988). It is ironic that because of the resurgence of infectious diseases, the "basic six" functions have reappeared as the most important functions of local health departments.

The Mission of Public Health

In its 1988 committee report, the Institute of Medicine called for a new definition of the role of public health agencies: "The committee defines the mission of public health as fulfilling society's interest in assuring conditions in which people can be healthy." According to the committee, the "core functions of public health agencies at all levels of government are assessment, policy development, and assurance" (Institute of Medicine 1988).

The **assessment** role requires that "every public health agency regularly and systematically collect, assemble, analyze, and make available information on the health of the community, including statistics on health status, community health needs, and epidemiologic and other studies of health problems." The **policy development** role requires that "every public health agency exercise its responsibility to serve the public interest in the development of comprehensive public health policies by promoting the use of the scientific knowledge base in decision-making about public health, . . . by leading in developing public health policy, [and by taking] a strategic approach, developed on the basis of a positive appreciation for the democratic political process." The **assurance** role requires that "public health agencies assure their constituents that services necessary to achieve agreed upon goals are provided, either by encouraging action by other entities (private or public sector), by requiring such action through regulation, or by providing services directly" (Institute of Medicine 1988).

The Institute of Medicine's report has been generally accepted as the new directive for government functioning in public health in the USA. Administrators and others involved in the field of public health have been struggling to define how the mission

and core functions can best be fulfilled. As indicated in the statement concerning the assurance role, considerable latitude is allowed for public health agencies: they do not have to provide all of (or even most of) the services required. They do, however, need to use all their authority and resources to make sure that the policies, laws, regulations, and services exist.

It should be noted that the current view of "public health policy" in the USA is much narrower than that in the world public health scene. For example, according to the Ottawa Charter for Health Promotion (1986), which guides much of the international work in this area, health promotion requires that all policies be reviewed for their health impact and adjusted to strengthen, rather than hinder, the effort to achieve good health:

> Health promotion goes beyond health care. It puts health on the agenda of policy makers in all sectors and at all levels, directing them to be aware of the health consequences of their decisions and to accept their responsibilities for health.
>
> Health promotion policy combines diverse but complementary approaches including legislation, fiscal measures, taxation and organizational change. It is coordinated action that leads to health, income and social policies that foster greater equity. Joint action contributes to ensuring safer and healthier goods and services, healthier public services, and cleaner, more enjoyable environments.
>
> Health promotion policy requires identification of obstacles to the adoption of healthy public policies in non-health sectors, and ways of removing them. The aim must be to make the healthier choice the easier choice for policy makers as well.

An Intersectoral Approach to Public Health

Although this chapter has thus far emphasized the role of specific US public health agencies at the federal, state, and local level, many duties with public health implications are carried out by government agencies that are not usually considered health agencies (as was also emphasized by the Ottawa Charter). For example, departments of agriculture may be responsible for monitoring the safety of milk, meat, and other agricultural products, as well as controlling zoonoses (animal diseases that can be spread to human beings). Departments of parks and recreation are responsible for the safety of water and sewage disposal in their facilities. Highway departments are responsible for the safe design and maintenance of roads and highways. Education departments have the responsibility for health education, as well as for providing a safe and healthful environment in which to learn. Government departments that have to do with promoting a healthy economy are critical, because when an economy is failing, the health of the people will falter as well.

The USA is home to many voluntary health agencies, whose focus is to prevent or control certain diseases, either those of one organ system (e.g., the American Heart Association and the American Lung Association) or a related group of diseases (e.g., the American Cancer Society). Cigarette smoking is a major risk factor for heart disease, lung disease, and cancer, so these three agencies may work together to curtail smoking. Indeed, there are voluntary health agencies that focus on almost every organ system in the body and major disease type. These organizations raise money for research, public education, and preventive programs and often for direct patient care as well.

An important conclusion from this is that health is the result of the entire fabric of the environment and life of a population. Therefore, a true public health approach must be intersectoral—that is, it must consider the health impact of policies in every sector of a society and government, not just in the health sector or medical care sector.

GOALS OF PUBLIC HEALTH
US Health Goals for the Year 2000

During the 1970s, representatives from many public health and scientific organizations began to develop national health promotion and disease prevention objectives. Their efforts resulted in the publication of *Healthy People 2000* (see US Department of Health and Human Services 1990). Although the federal government acted as coordinator and facilitator of these efforts and supports the goals and objectives outlined in the publication, the document itself "is not intended as a statement of federal standards or requirements." It is, however, a national consensus strategy of the government, public health organizations, and public-spirited citizens, and it has had a major impact on the way government and other institutions in the USA are directing their resources in public health.

The first goal recommended in *Healthy People 2000* is to "increase the span of healthy life for Americans." Because a portion of the lives of many people will be spent with illness and disability, the goal is to improve the quality of remaining life and not just the length of life (see Chapter 14). The second goal is to "reduce health disparities among Americans," including disparities in life expectancy, infant mortality, and premature death due to AIDS, violence, and preventable diseases. The third goal is to "achieve access to preventive services for all Americans," especially services such as prenatal care, immunizations, primary medical care, and health insurance coverage.

Priority Objectives

The priority objectives for achieving the national health goals are divided into four main areas: **health promotion,** which requires action by individuals and by society in general (changes in individual behavior and social policy); **health protection,** which primarily requires action by industry, labor unions, legislative bodies, and government agencies; **preventive health services,** which require action by individuals, government agencies, and medical care organizations and practitioners; and **surveillance and data systems,** which focus on official health agencies, although practitioners and health care institutions are important contributors to the collection and reporting of data.

In each of the four areas, *Healthy People 2000* presents the health status and risk reduction objectives for people in different age groups (children, adolescents and young adults, adults, and older adults) and also suggests methods for achieving the objectives. The targeted activities and diseases in *Healthy People 2000* are listed in Table 20–4 and summarized briefly below.

Health Promotion

Physical Fitness and Exercise. Many Americans have a sedentary life-style. The *objective* is to increase the proportion of the population who regularly exercise to at least 30% of those who are 6 years of age or older. Regular exercise is expected to reduce the incidence of obesity, hypertension and other cardiovascular diseases, non–insulin-dependent diabetes mellitus, and osteoporosis, among other prob-

TABLE 20–4. Topics of Concern in Achieving the US National Health Promotion and Disease Prevention Objectives for the Year 2000

Health promotion
Physical fitness and exercise
Nutrition
Tobacco use
Alcohol and drug use
Family planning
Mental health
Violent and abusive behavior
Educational and community-based health programs

Health protection
Unintentional injuries
Occupational safety and health
Environmental health
Food and drug safety
Oral health

Preventive health services
Maternal and infant health
Heart disease and stroke
Cancer
Diabetes and chronic disabling conditions
Human immunodeficiency virus (HIV) infection
Sexually transmitted diseases
Vaccine-preventable and other infectious diseases
Clinical preventive services

Surveillance and data systems

Source of data: US Department of Health and Human Services, Public Health Service. Healthy People 2000: National Health Promotion and Disease Prevention Objectives. Washington, D. C., Government Printing Office, 1990.

lems. Suggested *methods* for achieving the objective include emphasizing regular exercise programs in schools, increasing the availability of employer-sponsored and community-sponsored physical fitness opportunities, and increasing the proportion of primary care providers who counsel their patients on physical activity.

Nutrition. Because many illnesses and deaths can be related either to a deficiency or to an excess of food, improving nutrition would lower the rates of many health problems, including obesity and cardiovascular diseases. The *objectives* include reducing dietary fat intake to an average of 30% or less of total calories and to no more than 10% of calories from saturated fat; increasing the intake of complex carbohydrates, fiber, calcium, and iron; and decreasing the intake of salt and other forms of sodium. Suggested *methods* for meeting these objectives include improving the labeling of food (already partly accomplished), increasing the availability of food products with reduced total and saturated fat, increasing the proportion of restaurants and school lunchrooms that offer low-fat and low-calorie alternative meals, devoting more attention to nutrition education in the schools, and increasing the proportion of primary care practitioners who regularly perform nutritional evaluation and counseling as a part of the care they provide.

Tobacco Use. The *objective* is to reduce tobacco use, particularly among teenagers. Cessation of cigarette smoking is the single most important action a smoker can take to improve his or her health. Smoking rates in general have been dropping, but recently there has been a disturbing increase in the smoking rates for teenage women. Because most smokers start the habit in their teens (very few regular smokers get started after then), the teenage period is critical for prevention of smoking. Suggested *methods* for control of the problem include establishing tobacco-free environments (particularly in schools and worksites), enacting laws to control indoor air pollution, prohibiting the sale and distribution of cigarettes to minors, restricting tobacco product advertising, and increasing the proportion of primary care and oral health providers who advise and assist with smoking cessation.

Alcohol and Drug Use. The *objective* is to reduce the incidence of substance abuse. Most use of alcohol or illegal drugs begins in the teens or 20s. It often becomes the dominant force in the life of the user and can lead to disease or death (e.g., liver disease from alcohol use, cardiovascular events from cocaine use, or hepatitis or HIV infection from the sharing of needles). Suggested *methods* for control of substance abuse include developing state plans for dealing with the problem, educating primary school children about substance abuse, adopting alcohol and drug policies in worksites, suspending or revoking the driver's license of anyone caught driving under the influence of drugs or alcohol, controlling the advertisement of alcohol, and increasing the proportion of primary care providers who look for and treat sub-

stance abuse problems. Evidence suggests that the control of cocaine, for example, cannot be achieved by a single approach, such as law enforcement alone. Rather, as illustrated by the success of the efforts to reduce cocaine use in the Bahamas (Jekel et al. 1994), a broad attack on every conceivable front is required.

Family Planning. The *objectives* include a decrease in the number of cases of infertility, unintended pregnancy, and early initiation of sexual intercourse; an increase in the effectiveness of family planning methods used; and an increase in the use of contraceptive methods by unmarried people who are sexually active. The suggested *methods* for achieving these objectives include improving education about sex and family life, improving counseling about pregnancy and adoption, and increasing the percentage of primary care providers who offer appropriate preconception care and counseling.

Mental Health. The mental health *objectives* include reductions in the rate of suicide and attempted suicide, the prevalence of mental disorders among children and adults, and the proportion of persons 18 and older who experience adverse health effects from stress. Suggested *methods* for achieving these objectives include increasing the number of states with official plans to reduce the number of suicides by prison inmates; increasing the number of worksites that provide programs to reduce employee stress; establishing mutual help clearinghouses in at least 25 states; and increasing the percentage of primary care providers who routinely review the cognitive, emotional, and behavioral functioning of their patients, especially their patients who are children and adolescents.

Violent and Abusive Behavior. The health status *objectives* include reductions in the incidence of homicide, suicide, child abuse and neglect, spouse or partner abuse, assault injury, rape, physical fighting and weapon-carrying by adolescents, and inappropriate weapon storage. Suggested *methods* for achieving these objectives include extending the surveillance and data systems to cover violent behavior, increasing the number of states that use unexplained child death review systems, providing mental health evaluations for children who have suffered from physical or sexual abuse, increasing the capacity of shelters to accept battered women and their children, teaching nonviolent conflict resolution skills in schools, increasing the number and coverage of comprehensive violence prevention programs, and increasing the number of programs seeking to prevent suicide attempts by prison inmates.

Educational and Community-Based Health Programs. Because education and health are closely linked, achieving one helps to achieve the other. In this regard, the *objectives* are to increase the expected years of healthy life (also referred to as quality-adjusted life years) to at least 65 years and to increase the high school graduation rate to at least 90 percent. Suggested *methods* for achieving these objectives include providing adequate preschool programs for disadvantaged children, including children with disabilities; increasing the percentage of primary schools that provide kindergartens; increasing the proportion of post–secondary educational institutions with health promotion programs; increasing the proportion of workplaces that offer health promotion programs and the proportion of workers who use them; increasing the number of health promotion programs for all citizens, including specific programs for senior citizens; increasing the proportion of medical care organizations (hospitals, health maintenance organizations, group practices, and so forth) that provide patient education programs; and increasing the proportion of people who are served by a full-time local health department.

Health Protection

Unintentional Injuries. Health status *objectives* include the reduction of deaths and nonfatal injuries due to motor vehicle crashes, falls, drownings, fires, poisonings, and similar events. Areas of special concern include hip fractures, head injuries, and spinal cord injuries. Suggested *methods* for achieving these objectives include increasing the use of automobile occupant protection systems (e.g., seat belts and air bags), increasing the use of helmets by motorcyclists and bicyclists, enacting laws to require the use of devices such as seat belts and helmets, developing hand gun safety methods to minimize the use of these weapons by children, increasing the use of smoke detectors and sprinkler systems, providing adequate protection for sports participants, improving highway safety signs and markers, improving trauma care networks and systems, and increasing the proportion of primary care providers who counsel about safety precautions.

Occupational Safety and Health. The *objectives* are to reduce work-related deaths and injuries. Injuries cited for special attention include cumulative trauma (e.g., repetitive motion) disorders, occupational skin disorders, and hepatitis B infections. Suggested *methods* for achieving these objectives include increasing employee use of occupant protection systems such as seat belts during vehicle travel; reducing the proportion of workers exposed to noise levels exceeding 85 decibels; reducing exposures to lead; increasing hepatitis B immunization levels among health care workers; implementing occupational safety and health plans in all 50 states; establishing standards in every state to limit exposures to safe levels of asbestos, coal dust, cotton dust, and silica; increasing the worksites with programs on worker health and safety, including back injury prevention and rehabilitation; and increasing the proportion of primary care providers who routinely elicit occupational health and safety exposures as a part of the medical history.

Environmental Health. The *objectives* include reducing the incidence of asthma, serious mental retardation, chemical poisoning, and waterborne infectious disease; reducing blood lead levels that exceed 15 µg/dL in children 6 months to 5 years of age; reduc-

ing the proportion of people who live in areas exceeding the Environmental Protection Agency (EPA) standards for air pollution; reducing the number of homes with high concentrations of radon; reducing the level of toxic agents in the air, water, and soil; and increasing the proportion of people who receive drinking water that meets the EPA standards for safety. Suggested *methods* for achieving these objectives include increasing regulations on new home construction to eliminate unsafe radon levels, increasing the number of states that require prospective buyers to be informed of radon levels, increasing testing for lead-based paint in homes built before 1950, increasing the pace of cleanup at hazardous waste sites, increasing programs for recycling materials and proper disposal of hazardous wastes, and establishing plans in at least 35 states to define sentinel environmental diseases and institute surveillance regarding these diseases.

Food and Drug Safety. The *objectives* include the reduction of infections caused by key food-borne pathogens, particularly *Salmonella enteritidis,* and the improvement of food-handling practices in homes. Suggested *methods* for achieving these objectives include increasing the proportion of states that have implemented model food codes for institutions, increasing the proportion of pharmacies that use linked systems to provide alerts of possible drug interactions among medications prescribed for individual patients, and increasing the proportion of primary care providers who routinely discuss the use of all prescribed and over-the-counter medications with their patients who are 65 years or older.

Oral Health. Health status *objectives* include a reduction in the incidence of dental caries (cavities) in children, loss of teeth in adults (especially the total loss of teeth in older adults), gingivitis and periodontal diseases in adults, and death due to cancer of the oral cavity and pharynx; an increase in the proportion of children who receive protective sealants on permanent teeth; an increase in the proportion of people who drink fluoridated water or are provided with systemic and topical fluoride treatment; and an increase in the use of feeding practices that prevent tooth decay in bottle-fed infants. Suggested *methods* for achieving these objectives include increasing the oral health screening of children in primary school and in long-term institutional facilities, increasing the proportion of people using oral health care providers, and increasing the requirement for effective head, face, and mouth protection in sports and recreational events.

Preventive Health Services

Maternal and Infant Health. The primary health status *objectives* include reducing the infant mortality rate to no more than 7 per 1000 live births; reducing the fetal death rate (death at 20 or more weeks of gestation) to no more than 5 per 1000 live births; reducing the maternal mortality rate to no more than 3.3 per 100,000 live births; reducing the incidence of fetal alcohol syndrome to no more than 0.12 per 1000 live births; reducing the incidence of low birth weight (less than 2500 g) to no more than 5% of live births and the incidence of very low birth weight (less than 1500 g) to no more than 1% of live births; reducing the cesarean section rate to no more than 15 per 1000 deliveries; increasing to 85% the proportion of mothers who achieve the minimum recommended weight gain in pregnancy; increasing to 75% the proportion of mothers who breast-feed their infants; and increasing the proportion of women who abstain from alcohol, tobacco, cocaine, and other illegal drugs during pregnancy. Suggested *methods* for achieving these objectives include increasing to 90% the proportion of pregnant women who receive prenatal care during the first trimester of pregnancy and also increasing the proportion of infants who receive regular care during the first 18 months of life.

Heart Disease and Stroke. Health status *objectives* include reducing the age-adjusted rate of deaths caused by coronary artery disease to no more than 100 per 100,000 people each year (in contrast to 135 per 100,000 in 1987) and of deaths caused by stroke to no more than 20 per 100,000 people each year (in contrast to 30.3 per 100,000 in 1987); reversing the increase in end-stage renal disease requiring dialysis or transplantation; increasing to at least 50% the proportion of hypertensive people whose blood pressure is under control (in contrast to 24% in 1984); increasing to 90% the proportion of hypertensive people who are taking steps to control their blood pressure (in contrast to 79% in 1985); reducing the mean serum cholesterol level in adults to no more than 200 mg/dL; reducing the prevalence of high blood cholesterol levels (greater than or equal to 240 mg/dL) to 20% of adults or less; reducing dietary fat intake to an average of 30% of calories or less, with 10% or less from saturated fat; reducing the prevalence of overweight adults to no more than 20%; and increasing to at least 30% the proportion of people age 6 or older who engage regularly in light to moderate physical exercise. Suggested *methods* for achieving these objectives include increasing to 90% the proportion of adults who have had a blood pressure reading within the past 2 years; increasing to 75% the proportion of adults who have had a cholesterol check within the past 5 years; increasing the proportion of primary care providers who initiate diet and other needed interventions for elevated cholesterol levels; increasing the proportion of worksites that offer education concerning high blood pressure or high cholesterol levels; and increasing to at least 90% the proportion of laboratories that meet the accuracy standard for cholesterol measurement.

Cancer. The *objectives* include reversing the recent rise in the overall cancer death rate; reducing the rate of deaths due to lung cancer (a rate that has been rising); reducing the rate of deaths due to breast cancer (a rate that has been steady); and speeding up the declines in the rates of death due to cervical cancer and colorectal cancer. Suggested *methods* for achieving these objectives include reducing cigarette smoking to no more than 15% in people age 20 years or older; reducing dietary fat intake as mentioned above; increasing the intake of complex carbohydrates and foods containing fiber and carotenoids (fruits and vegetables); limiting exposure to direct sunlight and using sunscreens when exposure to sun is not avoidable; increasing the activity of primary care providers in counseling about cessation of tobacco use, diet modification, and the need for mammography or other measures to detect the presence of cancer; increasing the proportion of women who receive a regular Papanicolaou test and the proportion of all adults who have fecal occult blood testing and skin examination; and increasing the quality standards for cytology laboratories and mammography facilities.

Diabetes and Chronic Disabling Conditions. The primary health status *objective* is increasing the healthy life expectancy (i.e., the years free of chronic disabling conditions) by reducing the prevalence of conditions causing activity limitation, such as asthma, chronic back conditions, hearing impairment, visual impairment, obesity, osteoporosis, and diabetes. Suggested *methods* for achieving these objectives include improved screening of vision and hearing in adults as well as children and improved evaluation and management of conditions such as osteoporosis.

Human Immunodeficiency Virus (HIV) Infection. The *objectives* include limiting the incidence of acquired immunodeficiency syndrome (AIDS) to no more than 98,000 cases each year and limiting the prevalence of HIV infection to no more than 800 per 100,000 people each year; reducing the proportion of adolescents who engage in sexual intercourse and reducing the proportion of sexually active unmarried adults who do not use condoms; increasing the proportion of intravenous drug users who are in treatment programs and who use only uncontaminated drug paraphernalia; reducing the risk of HIV transmission from blood products to no more than 1 per 250,000 units; increasing the proportion of HIV-infected persons who know their infection status; increasing the proportion of schools that have age-appropriate HIV education in the curriculum; and increasing both the number of training programs and the availability of protective equipment for people whose work places them at increased risk of HIV infection. Suggestive *methods* for achieving these objectives include increasing education about HIV infection and AIDS (discussed in Chapter 19).

Sexually Transmitted Diseases. The *objectives* include reducing the incidence rates of gonorrhea, genital herpes, genital warts, pelvic inflammatory disease, and sexually transmitted hepatitis B infection, as well as primary, secondary, and congenital syphilis. Suggested *methods* for achieving these objectives include increasing the number of clinics and practitioners who correctly diagnose and treat sexually transmitted diseases and also providing age-appropriate education concerning how to avoid acquiring and spreading these diseases.

Vaccine-Preventable and Other Infectious Diseases.
The *objectives* include reducing the number of cases of vaccine-preventable diseases and other infectious diseases in hospitals and in travelers, increasing national immunization levels (discussed in Chapter 16), and reducing the need for postexposure rabies treatments. Suggested *methods* for achieving these objectives include expanding immunization laws to cover children entering schools, preschools, and day-care settings; improving the financing and delivery of immunizations, so that there is no financial barrier; increasing the proportion of primary care providers and health departments that offer immunizations; and improving the compliance of patients who are undergoing treatment for tuberculosis.

Clinical Preventive Services. The health status *objective* is to increase the healthy life expectancy (as defined above) of the population by ensuring that everyone has access to preventive health services. The key *method* for achieving this objective is to remove the financial and other barriers that keep children and adults from having a primary care provider who will make sure that they receive adequate immunization, counseling, and screening services.

Surveillance and Data Systems

To measure progress toward achieving the goals outlined in *Healthy People 2000* and summarized above, one of the objectives concerning surveillance and data systems is to develop improved health status indicators that are appropriate for the use of local, state, and federal health agencies. Another is to identify—or, if necessary, create—national data sources that are not only capable of monitoring the progress in health promotion, health protection, and preventive health services but are also designed to facilitate the rapid exchange of data among the various levels of government.

SUMMARY

Public health services in the USA are provided by the federal, state, and local levels of government, although the primary authority for health lies with the states. The federal government becomes involved in health mostly by regulating international and interstate commerce and by its power to tax for the general welfare. Local governments become involved in health as the states delegate authority for health to them. The fundamental health responsibilities have

expanded greatly from the "basic six" minimum functions, which were outlined during a time when infectious diseases were the big concern, to a large and diverse set of functions that now include the control of chronic diseases, injuries, and environmental toxins. Administrators and others involved in public health services are currently moving toward a set of goals which are outlined in *Healthy People 2000* and which emphasize the need for improvements in the areas of health promotion, health protection, preventive health services, and surveillance and data systems.

References Cited

Centers for Disease Control and Prevention. Injury control recommendations: bicycle helmets. Morbidity and Mortality Weekly Report 44:1–17, 1995.

Garrett, L. The Coming Plague. New York, Farrar, Straus, and Giroux, 1994.

Hanlon, J. J. Is there a future for local health departments? Health Services Reports 88:898–901, 1973.

Institute of Medicine. Emerging Infections: Microbial Threats to Health in the United States. Washington, D. C., National Academy Press, 1992.

Institute of Medicine. The Future of Public Health. Washington, D. C., National Academy Press, 1988.

Jekel, J. F. Communicable disease control in the 1970s: hot war, cold war, or peaceful coexistence? American Journal of Public Health 62:1578–1585, 1972.

Jekel, J. F. Health departments in the US, 1920–1988: statements of mission with special reference to the role of C.-E. A. Winslow. Yale Journal of Biology and Medicine 64:467–479, 1991.

Jekel, J. F., et al. Nine years of the freebase cocaine epidemic in the Bahamas. American Journal on Addictions 3:14–24, 1994.

Office of the Federal Register, National Archives and Records Administration. United States Government Manual 1994/1995. Washington, D. C., Government Printing Office, 1994.

Ottawa Charter for Health Promotion. Report of an International Conference on Health Promotion, Sponsored by the World Health Organization, Health and Welfare Canada, and the Canadian Public Health Association, Ottawa, Ontario, Canada, November 17–21, 1986.

Terris, M. The epidemiologic revolution, national health insurance, and the role of health departments. American Journal of Public Health 66:1155–1164, 1976.

US Department of Health and Human Services, Public Health Service. Healthy People 2000: National Health Promotion and Disease Prevention Objectives. DHHS Publication No. (PHS)91-50212. Washington, D. C., Government Printing Office, 1990.

Winslow, C.-E. A. The untilled fields of public health. Science 51:22–23, 1920.

Selected Readings

US Department of Health and Human Services, Public Health Service. Healthy People 2000: National Health Promotion and Disease Prevention Objectives. DHHS Publication No. (PHS)91-50212. Washington, D. C., Government Printing Office, 1990.

CHAPTER TWENTY-ONE

MEDICAL CARE POLICY

AND FINANCING

A FRAMEWORK FOR UNDERSTANDING MEDICAL CARE SYSTEMS

Is the physician's role primarily that of master of medical technology, or is it a broad healing role, involving the physician in the lives of patients, their families, their environment and employment, and their communities? In the modern era, is the physician responsible only for giving the best possible care to individual patients, or do all physicians have an obligation to make the system in which they work operate fairly, effectively, and efficiently for everyone? What obligations do physicians owe to society beyond providing competent and ethical medical care to individuals?

Those working in preventive medicine and public health in the USA are convinced that physicians must assume a broad role of caring for individuals and that physicians are at least partly responsible for bringing about and maintaining a fair and efficient system of medical care for everyone. The first step in accepting some responsibility for the current medical care system is to understand how it functions and in what ways it currently fails to serve both the American people and the medical profession itself.

Unresolved Tensions

In the USA, there are many unresolved tensions concerning the ways in which medical care is or should be organized and financed. Different systems of care and financing emphasize different responses to the questions listed below.

(1) Should the emphasis be on prevention or cure? In general, for an insurance program or health maintenance organization to provide significant preventive services beyond immunizations, some short-term cost savings need to be demonstrated (see Chapter 14).

(2) Within prevention, should the emphasis be on health promotion or disease prevention? In general, insurance programs and medical care systems are more willing to pay for disease prevention methods (e.g., vaccines, antibiotic prophylaxis, and screening) than for health promotion programs that emphasize the improvement of nutrition, health-related behavior, and the environment. Part of the hesitancy to support health promotion comes from uncertainty about the economic benefits that health promotion will bring to the insurance programs, and part may derive from a belief that such broad issues are not the responsibility of an insurance company or the medical care system (see Chapters 15–17).

(3) What type of practice should be emphasized in medical education: primary care or specialty practice? The increasing complexity of technology and the greater financial rewards for specialty practice have encouraged specialization in medicine. The bulk of the need for medical care, however, is better served by primary care physicians, and there is increasing pressure on medical schools to emphasize this area.

(4) Should hospitals, health maintenance organizations, and group practices focus exclusively on the people who enter their institutions, or should they be actively involved in promoting the health of the entire community?

(5) To what extent should (and, indeed, to what extent can) physicians share medical decision-making with their patients?

(6) To what extent is there a tension between low cost and high quality in the care process? Depending on the circumstances, there may be no tension between these factors. The best medical care is usually the least amount of medical care that gives a good outcome. For example, the elimination of unnecessary surgery and unneeded medical procedures reduces costs and also improves care. It should be less costly to prevent hospital infections and drug errors than to pay for their negative consequences. A large proportion of medical care dollars go to caring for hopelessly ill people near the end of their lives, but there are ethical problems in knowing when to stop maximum medical effort. Nevertheless, there is no question that sometimes the best care is very costly; for example, coronary artery bypass grafts are costly but frequently improve the quality of life.

Terminology in Health Care

Health care policies and financing are influenced by distinctions between concepts such as disease and illness, impairment and disability, and needs and demands.

A **disease** is a medically definable process, in terms of pathophysiology and pathology, whereas **illness** is what the patient experiences. Several different diseases might produce similar illness experiences. For example, amebiasis, salmonellosis, shigellosis, and various other diseases can cause dysentery, which patients typically experience as gastrointestinal pain and diarrhea. On the other hand, the same basic disease process, such as diabetes mellitus, can produce different illness experiences in different patients. For example, one patient with diabetes mellitus may have a cerebrovascular accident, another may have a myocardial infarction, another may lose vision or kidney function, another may have circulatory problems in the feet, and another may experience no serious end-organ damage at all.

Impairment is defined as a limitation of capacity or functional ability, usually as determined by a licensed physician. In contrast, **disability** is a social definition of limitation, based on the degree of impairment. Disability is defined by society in laws dealing with social benefits (such as Social Security benefits) and rights for the handicapped. A physician will determine whether there is impairment in a person's eyesight, and then society determines whether or not this impairment is severe enough to prohibit a person from flying an airplane or driving a car or a bus. For purposes of social benefits, there usually are four categories of disability: (1) **temporary partial disability** (e.g., a fractured arm); (2) **temporary total**

disability (e.g., a broken back without paralysis); (3) **permanent partial disability** (e.g., permanent loss of one eye or one limb); and (4) **permanent total disability** (e.g., permanent loss of two eyes, two limbs, or an eye and a limb).

The **need for medical care** is usually considered a professional judgment. Although the term **felt need** is sometimes used to describe a patient's judgment about the need for care, more commonly this is referred to as the **demand for medical care.** Demand has both a medical and an economic definition. The medical definition of demand is the amount of care people would use if there were no barriers to care. The problem with this definition is that there almost always are barriers to care: cost, convenience, fear, lack of real availability because of distance to the care settings or because of the limited times they are open, and so forth. The economic definition of demand is the quantity of care that is purchased at a given price. For this economic definition to work, there must be an assumption of price elasticity—i.e., an assumption that as demand falls, the price for a given amount of care will also fall. This assumption sometimes proves false.

Because of the difficulties of measuring demand, what is usually studied is the effective (realized) demand, which is **utilization.** Utilization is usually less than need, so the concept of unmet need was developed. **Unmet need** can be defined by the following equation:

$$\text{Unmet need} = \text{Need} - \text{Utilization}$$

Factors Influencing Need and Demand

Demographic factors are among the most important influences on the need and demand for medical care. Foremost among these is the **age of the population,** which is defined either as the median age of persons in the population or as the percentage of persons over a certain age, such as 65 years. The median age and the percentage over 65 are both determined more by **fertility patterns** than by **mortality rates.** As the birth rate falls, the population ages because fewer young people are born to counteract the continual aging of those already in the population. The US crude birth rate (the number of births per 1000 population) and the US general fertility rate (the number of children born to women aged 15–44 divided by the population of women aged 15–44) have been declining during most of this century. The exception to this was the period immediately after World War II (the postwar "baby boom" period), when the birth rates were high. A rather sudden decline in birth rates occurred around 1970, when induced abortion became legally available. The process of aging of the population, which had been occurring somewhat gradually, accelerated after 1970.

While the reduction in the rate of children born has reduced the demand for pediatricians and, to a lesser extent, has reduced the demand for obstetrician-gynecologists, the aging of the population has increased the overall utilization of hospitals and other sources of medical care. Currently, more than 50% of the patients hospitalized at any point in time are likely to be 65 years or older, whereas only 11–12% of the population is likely to be in this age group.

Although there is currently significant unemployment in the USA, the long-term result of lowered fertility will be an extended period when the number of workers will be comparatively small. This period is expected to begin around the year 2015, when large numbers of "baby boom" children will enter retirement age. A major concern is whether the small number of workers will be able to support the large older population during its retirement with such benefits as Social Security retirement funds and medical care. The probable shortage of workers is expected to drive up wages, making medical and nursing home care more expensive than it already is. Chronic disease of the elderly, with its high demand for medical and nursing home care, will be common.

Among the other factors that influence medical needs and demands are the **advances in medical technology.** As new methods of prevention, diagnosis, or treatment become available and are found to be useful, more physicians and more patients view the use of this technology as necessary and desirable.

One might expect that the greatest unmet need for medical care would exist among the poorest members of society, but that is not always true. People below some percentage of the **poverty line** (often 125%) are eligible for Medicaid under Title 19 of the Social Security Act. In addition to providing medical care insurance, Medicaid provides coverage for nursing home stays for people who are poor. People whose incomes are too high to be eligible for Medicaid, who do not receive medical insurance in their jobs, and who are not able to pay for individual medical care insurance policies are known as **medically indigent.** They may be able to support themselves until a medical catastrophe strikes, but then they are unable to pay their bills. Many of the **medically uninsured** (i.e., those who have no health insurance) and **medically underinsured** (those who have some but inadequate health insurance) are medically indigent. They are not on welfare, but they cannot financially tolerate major medical bills. In the USA, about 37 million people (15% of the US population) were uninsured in 1993.

THE MEDICAL CARE SYSTEM
Goals of Medical Care

Different societies and different eras in a given society may emphasize one goal or another for a medical care system. Usually considered among the important goals or functions of medical care are the following (not necessarily listed in order of priority): (1) to increase the length of life, (2) to improve the function of individuals, (3) to increase the comfort of ill persons and their families, (4) to explain medical problems to patients and their families, (5) to provide a prognosis for the patient, and (6) to provide support and care for patients and their families. These goals are not always fully compatible. For example, extending biological life to the maximum may increase pain and anxiety for the patient and family.

Basic Requirements for Good Medical Care

The basic requirements for good medical care can be summarized by a list of terms called the 7 A's and the 3 C's.

Availability of medical care means that care can be obtained during the hours and days when people need it. If care is available only 5 days a week between the hours of 9 AM and 5 PM, many working people will not receive good medical care. Only if providers are available in the evenings and on weekends does care meet this criterion.

Adequacy is a sufficient volume of care to meet the need and demand of a community. In some inner-city areas, as well as in some rural areas, the limited numbers of physicians and hospital emergency departments are not able to keep pace with the demand.

Accessibility refers to both geographic and financial accessibility. Facilities that cannot be reached easily by public transportation and facilities that deny care to those without adequate insurance or financial resources are inaccessible.

Acceptability of care depends on a variety of factors, including whether the providers can communicate well with their patients (e.g., can speak the patients' languages), whether the care is seen as warm and humane and concerned with the whole person, and whether the patients believe in the confidentiality and privacy of information shared with their providers.

Appropriateness of care means that the procedures being performed are properly selected and carried out by trained personnel in the proper setting. Performing open heart surgery in a small rural hospital is probably not appropriate, since complicated procedures such as this require the resources of a major medical center where many similar operations are done each year.

Assessability means that the medical care can be readily evaluated. Care can be assessed more efficiently if the medical records are complete and if basic care information is available in linked computer data bases, allowing the facility to produce timely analyses.

Accountability has to do with public accountability. Is there public representation on the board of directors of the health care institution or facility? Are the financial records regularly reviewed by certified public accountants? Is there appropriate public disclosure of financial records and of quality of care studies?

Completeness of care requires adequate attention to all aspects of a medical problem. Complete care includes prevention, early detection, diagnosis, treatment, follow-up measures, and rehabilitation.

Comprehensiveness of care means that care is provided for all types of health problems, including dental and mental health problems. If there are major exclusions, such as for psychiatric or substance abuse care, the coverage cannot be considered comprehensive.

Continuity of care requires that the management of a patient's care over time be coordinated among providers. Is there one physician who is basically in charge of a patient's care, who sees the patient regularly and makes sure that there are no major omissions or redundancies in the care? This has become a larger issue with the increase in specialists and in referrals for high-technology procedures. Continuity of care influences quality, efficiency, and acceptability. Lack of continuity and the resultant disruption of the physician-patient relationship are thought to be significant factors in the frequency of malpractice litigation.

THE ORGANIZATION OF MEDICAL CARE
Historical Overview

In the late 1800s, most medical care was ambulatory care or care in the home, with local practitioners paid on a fee-for-service basis. The hospital tended to be viewed as a death house and a place for the sick poor, often supported by the church or other benevolent organizations. Those who could not pay for treatment were relegated to the hospital.

In the early 1900s, as medicine became more scientific and efficacious, the hospital came to be seen as the doctors' workshop. The technology and ancillary personnel and services were usually provided at no charge to the doctors and helped them to perform their craft. In turn, the doctors brought patients to the hospitals to keep the hospitals economically solvent. Thus, a mutually profitable relationship was established between hospital and physician.

Acute, general hospitals, however, did not usually offer care to the mentally ill. If mentally ill or retarded persons could not be cared for at home, they tended to be treated (often just "warehoused") in large hospitals run by the state. These mental hospitals were dismal facilities, usually built in sparsely populated areas. Eventually, the development of psychoactive medications enabled many patients with mental disorders to be treated in community settings, and state mental hospitals were progressively closed in the late 1960s and early 1970s. Unfortunately, this **deinstitutionalization** occurred without adequate community resources to receive the large numbers of mentally ill patients being discharged. Some of these patients benefited from treatment in an outpatient setting. Others, however, could not function well in society. As a result, many discharged patients became poverty-stricken and homeless, particularly if they forgot or refused to take their medications.

General hospitals in the past usually did not offer care to patients with tuberculosis. These patients were treated in special, state-run tuberculosis hospitals until after World War II, when the development of antibiotics permitted them to be treated in general hospitals or at home.

The downsizing of mental hospitals and the closing of tuberculosis hospitals considerably reduced the costs to the states for these types of medical care. However, other medical care expenses of the states increased, notably their share of Medicaid costs, particularly payments for nursing home care for the elderly.

With the founding of the National Institutes of Health in 1948 came a push for improved biomedical technology. The research done since that time has made the practice of medicine much more effective but also far more complex and costly. The increased complexity has not only resulted in increasing specialization of physicians and other health care workers but has also required an increasing rationalization of the levels of care to make the complexity of care and the resulting costs appropriate to each patient's needs.

Levels of Medical Care

In an effort to maximize the effectiveness and efficiency of the medical care process, health care professionals have proposed an integrated system of graded levels of care. As shown in Table 21–1, the levels range from treatment in a tertiary medical center (the most complex level of care) to treatment in the patient's home (the least complex level). A patient is initially assigned to an appropriate level of care and is reassigned to another level whenever there is an improvement or setback in the patient's condition. Although the movement from one level to another should be easy, rapid, and smooth, the lack of available hospital beds or lack of planning sometimes causes difficulties.

At the top of the scale of complexity are three types of **acute, general hospital facilities.** The first type is the **tertiary medical center,** which has most or all of the latest technology and which usually participates actively in medical education and even in clinical research. Within this facility there are different units offering different levels of care, including intensive care units, special units for observation of patients, and standard units for the care of patients. The second type is the **intermediate hospital,** which is a medium to large community hospital that has a considerable amount of the latest technology but less research and investigational activity. The intermediate hospital may support cardiac bypass surgery, for example, but not necessarily organ transplantation. The third type is the **local community hospital,** which provides services such as routine diagnosis, treatment, and surgery but which lacks the personnel and facilities for complex procedures.

Next on the scale of complexity are two types of **rehabilitation or convalescent care facilities.** The first type is a **special unit in a regular hospital,** and the second type is a **rehabilitation hospital.** In particular, patients recovering from trauma or from neurologic diseases or surgery may benefit from physical therapy, occupational therapy, and other methods of tertiary prevention (see Chapters 14 and 18).

If patients are not discharged from the hospital directly to their homes, they are most likely to be discharged to one of three different types of **extended care facilities** (ECFs). The first type is the **skilled nursing facility** (SNF), which is commonly called a nursing home and usually provides special kinds of care, such as intravenous fluids and medicines. The second type is the **intermediate care facility** (ICF), which is suitable if the patient's primary need is for help with the activities of daily living (eating, bathing, grooming, transferring, toileting, and so forth). Unlike an SNF, an ICF is not required to have a registered (skilled) nurse on duty at all times. Some nursing homes provide both skilled and intermediate levels of care. The third type is the **hospice,** a nursing home that specializes in providing terminal care, especially for patients with cancer or acquired immunodeficiency syndrome (AIDS).

Organized home care is necessary for patients who are discharged from the hospital to the home, where they continue to receive treatment or follow-up procedures that require specialized skills. Examples include the placement and monitoring of intravenous lines for therapy and the drawing of blood for tests. In the past, most home care was provided by not-for-profit community groups such as visiting nurse associations or by public health nurses from local health departments. More recently, hospitals have organized their own home care teams, which help smooth transitions for those going home. In addition, there are a number of proprietary (for-profit) home care organizations, many of which operate nationwide.

As shown in Table 21–1, the least complex level of medical care is **self-care** in the home. In fact, the majority of medical care decisions are not made by professionals but instead are made by people for themselves, for friends, or for members of their families. Many home diagnostic tools, such as blood

TABLE 21–1. Levels of the Medical Care System from the Most Complex (Top) to the Least Complex (Bottom)

(1) Acute, general hospital facilities
   (a) Tertiary medical center (with most or all of the latest technology)
   (b) Intermediate hospital (medium to large community hospital with a considerable amount of the latest technology)
   (c) Local community hospital
(2) Rehabilitation or convalescent care facilities
   (a) Special unit in a regular hospital
   (b) Rehabilitation hospital
(3) Extended care facilities (ECFs)
   (a) Skilled nursing facility (SNF, or "nursing home")
   (b) Intermediate care facility (ICF)
   (c) Hospice
(4) Organized home care
   (a) Public agencies (local health departments or visiting nurse associations)
   (b) Private organizations
(5) Self-care in the home

pressure cuffs and blood glucose testing equipment, have given patients greater power to monitor their own health status. One advantage of this has been improved self-care. For example, diabetic patients can monitor their blood glucose levels and more easily see for themselves the immediate results of stress and dietary indiscretions.

Some modern movements have included emphasis on the importance of people taking more control over decisions that affect their lives and bodies. Many medications that used to be by prescription only are now available over the counter. Although at one time Dr. Spock's book on infant and child care used to be practically the only available self-help book on a health care subject, now there are whole medical and health sections in bookstores, providing patients with considerably more information about (and therefore more control over) their own health and illnesses.

Medical Care Institutions

Hospitals

While the term "hospital" is generally thought to refer to an institution providing acute, general care to persons with a wide range of health problems, there are, in fact, a variety of types of hospitals. Some focus on a special group of patients (e.g., a children's hospital), while others focus on a special type of medical problem (e.g., a psychiatric hospital) or a particular type of service (e.g., a rehabilitation hospital).

Hospitals may be for-profit or not-for-profit. A for-profit hospital may be independent or part of a for-profit chain of hospitals. Not-for-profit hospitals may be sponsored by (1) the community in which they are located; (2) a church or other religious group; (3) a charitable organization (e.g., Shriners' hospitals for children); (4) a city, county, or state government; or (5) the federal government (e.g., Veterans Administration Hospitals).

Ambulatory Primary Care Systems

Solo Medical Practices.   Historically, most US physicians were in solo medical practice, although they might share night and weekend coverage with other solo practitioners. This type of practice could be quite rewarding, but it frequently was exhausting.

Partnerships.   Gradually, US physicians began to develop practice partnerships, partly to solve the problem of sharing weekend and nighttime coverage and partly to achieve efficiencies and economies by sharing the cost of office space, equipment, and staff.

Group Practices.   A logical extension of the partnership was the formation of a group practice consisting of three or more (often many more) physicians. This increased the efficiencies of sharing office space and staff and increased the free time available to physicians. It also had the advantage of providing built-in consultation with other physicians concerning complex cases.

Group practices could be of either the single-specialty or the multiple-specialty type. The physicians in some single-specialty group practices were primary care physicians (e.g., internists or pediatricians), while those in other practices were surgical specialists (e.g., neurosurgeons). Although most group practices initially operated on a fee-for-service basis, some began to develop the concept of prepaid group practice—a concept that goes at least as far back as the final report of the Committee on the Costs of Medical Care (1932). On the West Coast, the Kaiser Corporation set up its own multispecialty group practice before World War II to care for its own workers, but membership has since been opened to the general public, and it is now known as Kaiser Permanente. This was the first example of a large prepaid group practice in the USA.

Health Maintenance Organizations.   Prepaid group practices that met certain standards and contractual arrangements were named health maintenance organizations (HMOs) by the Nixon administration. The national HMO law was passed in 1973, and it encouraged the large-scale development of HMOs.

People who enrolled in an HMO were usually part of some economic group, such as workers in a company or industry, but their enrollment had to be voluntary. They paid a fixed monthly fee, which varied depending on the size of the group. In return, the HMO had the contractual obligation to provide the types of medical care specified in the contract (rather than to provide financial reimbursement, as in the case of an insurance company) or at least to ensure that the stipulated care was provided. The HMO assumed some of the risk when income was less than expenses and made a profit when income was greater than expenses.

There are three main functional parts to an HMO: the legal and fiscal entity, which does the contracting and financial transactions; the group of physicians who provide the outpatient and inpatient medical care; and the associated hospital or hospitals (Luft 1981). The manner in which each of these three functions is handled may vary considerably from one HMO to another.

Because of the many variations that are possible on the theme of prepaid group practice, no complete yet simple classification can be provided. Usually, HMOs are divided into two fundamental types: the staff model HMO and the independent (or individual) practice association.

In the **staff model HMO,** most of the physicians are salaried, full-time employees who work exclusively in the health plan or belong to a physician group that contracts to provide all of the medical services to the plan (as is typical in Kaiser Permanente). Some specialists may be retained on part-time contracts. The HMO may have its own hospitals (as does Kaiser Permanente) or may hospitalize its patients in one or more local hospitals, in which case the local hospitals are not usually a formal part of the HMO. In the staff model HMO, most physicians' time and effort are directed mainly or exclusively to the

HMO. The primary care HMO physician serves as a **gatekeeper,** controlling referrals to specialists. In theory, every patient must see a primary care physician before getting a referral to a specialist, although this may be relaxed for certain specialists, such as ophthalmologists or dermatologists, and in emergencies.

In the **independent (or individual) practice association** (IPA), the patients enrolled in the program can choose a primary care physician from a list of physicians (known as a **panel**) who have contracted to provide services for the IPA. The IPA pays each physician on a fee-for-service basis whenever an HMO member uses that physician's services. The IPA physicians limit their fees to the rates specified in the contract, and they agree to certain kinds of quality review and practice controls that are often similar to those of managed care (see below). Physicians in IPAs also serve as gatekeepers to some extent, but usually not as effectively as do physicians in staff model HMOs.

A **preferred provider organization** (PPO) is a variation on the IPA theme. The PPO is formed when a third-party payer (e.g., an insurance plan or a company) establishes a network of contracts with independent practitioners. Like the usual IPA, the PPO has a panel of physicians who have contracted to provide services at agreed rates. A major difference between the usual IPA and a PPO is that the patients in a PPO can see physicians who are not on the panel, although they will have to pay a surcharge for their services. PPOs tend not to push the gatekeeper function onto the primary care physicians, and in general the contractual arrangement is looser, with fewer controls over the physicians' practice.

Hospital Outpatient Clinics. Traditionally, many hospital outpatient clinics have served people who are poor and may not be well insured. The patients receive treatment (although often following a long wait) in return for being cared for by physicians in training, with proper supervision. Increasingly, these clinics are becoming organized into primary care centers or even HMOs. In addition, many medical schools now have group practice arrangements for the physicians on their clinical faculty to practice medicine and augment both their income and the income of the medical school.

Hospital Emergency Departments. Emergency departments are becoming increasingly complex, and because of the heavy patient loads, their staff may triage nonurgent patients to a satellite convenience clinic.

Community or Neighborhood Health Centers. Federal health programs in the 1960s and 1970s encouraged the development of community health centers. Many of these centers were supported partly through federal and state grants, and most were placed in underserved areas in big cities or rural locations.

Surgicenters. Freestanding outpatient surgical centers have become increasingly popular and may be owned by hospitals or group practice associations.

Urgent Care Centers. Urgent care centers are freestanding clinics that are conveniently located (e.g., often in shopping centers) and allow ambulatory patients to be seen on a drop-in basis not only during the usual weekday hours but also during evenings and on weekends. Most of the urgent care centers are proprietary, and many specialize in evaluating and treating injured workers promptly in order to get them back to work.

PAYMENT FOR MEDICAL CARE

A century ago, physicians were paid directly by patients for their services. If times were tight, practitioners might get paid in food or other commodities, rather than in cash. As medicine became more scientific and technical, often requiring long hospital stays, the out-of-pocket payment method became inadequate. Patients became frustrated with large bills they could not pay, and hospitals and physicians were frustrated at not being reimbursed. Today, it is not unusual for a very sick patient to be charged from $1500 to $2000 per day for a hospital stay, even if no surgery or major procedures are done. One solution to the cost problem was to have a **third-party payer,** such as an insurance company. The third-party payer collected money regularly from a large population in the form of medical insurance premiums and paid the hospitals and physicians when care was required.

Physician Payments

Physicians today are usually paid in one of three ways: by the fee-for-service method, capitation, or salary.

In the **fee-for-service method,** physicians are paid for each major item of service provided. Charges are established on the basis of the type and complexity of service (complete workup, follow-up visit, hospital visit, major surgical procedure, etc.). The amount charged by a physician may exceed the amount that a third-party payer is willing to reimburse, in which case the patient is expected to pay the difference between the charges and the third-party payment. This is the traditional form of payment, for which organized medicine has continually fought, but other payment systems are now increasingly common.

Sometimes primary care physicians are paid on a **capitation basis,** meaning on a "per head" basis. Regardless of the number of services needed by a patient, the physician receives the same amount of money per year. This method of payment has much lower administrative costs, and it is thought to promote physicians' efforts in preventive care. It may lead to poor gatekeeping, however, because it may be easier to refer a patient than to provide a service. This payment method is sometimes used in the USA to pay practitioners working in HMOs and is commonly used in Britain to pay general practitioners.

The third method of payment is a **salary.** Physicians who work full-time for HMOs, hospitals, universities, or companies may be paid this way. Productivity bonuses are sometimes added to the salary. Physicians who provide care on a part-time basis often receive a stipulated amount per clinic session.

Insurance and Third-Party Payers

About 4000 years ago, wealthy people in China were paying doctors to keep them well, and this sort of arrangement can be viewed as an early form of health insurance. However, in the Chinese system, a physician's payments ceased if the patron became sick, and the penalties if the patron died were strict, sometimes including the death of the physician (Prussin and Woods 1975).

Modern US hospital insurance had its foundation in Dallas, Texas, where a group of school teachers entered into a contract with Baylor University Hospital in 1929. The teachers paid the hospital 50 cents per person per month and, in turn, the hospital promised to cover 21 consecutive days in the hospital in a semiprivate room, along with medications, laboratory studies, the use of operating rooms, and so forth. This led to the development of Blue Cross, which is a form of insurance that covers only hospital care.

To understand how insurance companies work, it is necessary to review a few concepts concerning benefits. If an insurance policy covers **indemnity benefits,** this means that the insurance company (carrier) will reimburse the insured patient a fixed number of dollars per service, regardless of the actual charges incurred for the service. If the insurance policy states that the carrier will pay up to $300 per day toward a semiprivate hospital room and the room actually costs $500 per day, the patient must pay the difference, unless he or she has other (supplemental) insurance. In contrast, if an insurance policy covers **service benefits,** this means that the carrier will be responsible for full payment for the needed services, regardless of their costs.

Actuaries, the statisticians who estimate risks and establish premiums for insurance companies, have a standard set of **actuarial principles** that guide the process of underwriting (insuring) medical and other risks. Actuaries make sure that an insurance carrier does not collapse financially. Originally, insurance was designed to pool the risk from large groups to protect individuals from rare but devastating losses, such as those resulting from fires. The actuarial principles developed to accomplish this objective do not adapt well to medical care for two reasons. First, medical care involves frequent and fairly predictable costs as well as rare and catastrophic costs. Second, those at greatest risk of ill health and hospitalization can least afford the cost of insurance, although according to actuarial principles they should be charged the most. Therefore, other solutions are required to have a just and equitable system for financing medical care.

So far, the solution applied to this dilemma in health care has been the concept of **pooling risk.** If all of the people in a large, natural community (i.e., a community consisting of people of various ages and degrees of health) were to be insured by the same carrier and were to pay the same monthly premium rate, then the law of averages would work so as to protect the carrier from excessive loss except, perhaps, in times of disaster. In effect, the low-risk people in the population would be helping to pay the premiums for the high-risk people, because the risk would be averaged according to the "experience rating" of the entire group. This is not a complete solution, because the poor still may not be able to pay the established premium, and the plan may not be offered where they work.

Insurance companies prefer to insure groups, particularly working groups. There are several reasons. First, group insurance requires less sales effort and paperwork. Second, by insuring a large group of people, a carrier is less likely to insure a high percentage of bad risks (i.e., people who will probably require a lot of medical care). Third, by insuring a working group, the carrier benefits from the **healthy worker effect.** Because people with jobs must be in reasonably good health to work in the first place, they have a lower risk of death and illness than the population as a whole. Unfortunately, many of the individuals who need the most medical care are unemployed, and this leaves them with the multiple problems of being unable to purchase insurance because they represent undesirable risks to an insurance company, being unable to pay for the health care they need because they have no earning power, and remaining in a poor state of health that keeps them from finding employment.

Initially, the Blue Cross plans began to cover large segments of communities, and the community pooling of risk appeared to work satisfactorily. However, many insurance carriers sought to attract the business of low-risk individuals and low-risk companies by offering lower premiums. As the people with low risks were removed from the community pool (a process called **"cream skimming"**), the people remaining in the pool were, on the average, at higher risk, so they had to be charged a higher premium, making the community pool still less attractive.

Some insurance companies have sought to use epidemiologic information to undersell the Blue Plans (Blue Cross and Blue Shield). These companies offer low-cost medical insurance to individuals with low epidemiologic risk profiles, usually those who do not drink alcohol or smoke. Some justify this approach as an appropriate reward for good health behavior.

The insurance world is complex. Most Blue Cross plans cover the first several thousand dollars of their liability, but they insure themselves against disastrous medical care liability by **reinsurance.** They pay a fee to another (reinsurance) company, which then assumes the liability for Blue Cross commitments above a certain agreed-upon amount.

In order for patients to be covered for huge medical costs, many plans also include a premium for **major medical insurance.** This insurance usually pays 80% of the amount by which a hospital bill exceeds the Blue Cross maximum, and the patient is obligated to pay the other 20% of the bill for major expenses. The patient's portion is called a **copayment,** because the patient and the insurance company are sharing the total cost. The copayment is also seen as a means to enlist the patient or the family in the effort to get the patient out of the hospital as soon as possible.

Social Insurance

Compulsory insurance for a population group is often called social or public insurance. Most people employed in the USA must make payments into the Social Security Trust Fund for two national social insurance programs: Medicare and retirement benefits.

Medicare is authorized under Title 18 of the Social Security Act and is administered by the federal government, although it uses insurance carriers as fiscal intermediaries. The people eligible for Medicare include most individuals who are 65 years or older and those individuals who receive Social Security benefits due to disability.

Part A and Part B of Medicare provide partial coverage for hospital expenses and physician expenses, respectively. Although Social Security beneficiaries do not pay premiums for Part A coverage, they do pay premiums on a regular basis if they elect to have Part B coverage. Medicare also will pay for a certain amount of home care or nursing home care for a medical problem that follows directly from a Medicare-covered hospitalization.

Since Medicare does not cover all hospital expenses, patients are billed for the portion of charges not covered by Medicare. Therefore, insurance plans have developed **Medicare supplemental insurance,** so that patients have few, if any, bills after a hospital admission.

By 1948, all states in the USA had some sort of **workers' compensation program.** Workers' compensation laws stipulate that people with a job-related injury or illness have their medical and rehabilitation expenses paid and also receive a certain amount of cash payments in lieu of wages while they are recuperating. Depending on the state, companies may have the option to self-insure, to enter an agreement to insure through a private third-party carrier, or to deposit premiums into a state fund. Regardless of the method used, the size of a company's premiums depends on that company's **experience rating,** which is the amount of claims paid in recent years. This serves as a stimulus for companies to invest in safety on the job. The level of benefits that workers receive varies considerably from state to state.

Social Welfare

Medicaid is authorized under Title 19 of the Social Security Act. Unlike Medicare recipients, Medicaid recipients have not previously paid money into a trust fund. Therefore, the benefits of Medicaid are considered to be social welfare, instead of social insurance. Medicaid is paid from general tax revenues of the federal and state governments.

The people covered by Medicaid are poor and usually receive additional types of welfare assistance, such as Aid to Families with Dependent Children (AFDC). In contrast to Medicare, which is entirely federally administered, Medicaid is administered by the states, which share the costs of the program with the federal government. Although the federal government usually reimburses a state for approximately half of its Medicaid costs for a given year, poorer states get slightly more. The eligibility criteria for Medicaid, as well as the size of the benefits, vary from state to state.

Medicaid basically covers two things. First, it pays for medical care expenses, including both hospital and physician bills. The amount of reimbursement is usually far below the customary charges of physicians, making the program unpopular with many physicians. Second, Medicaid pays for long-term nursing home care, but only after people have largely exhausted their resources, a process called spend-down (see Long-Term Care, below).

THE CURRENT SITUATION IN THE USA
Historical Overview

The recent history of the struggle of organized medicine in the USA has some resemblance to the Battle of Chancellorsville, which occurred in May 1863, during the American Civil War. In the town of Chancellorsville, the Union army, under General Joseph Hooker, was braced for Confederate attacks on the left and center flanks, but its right flank was weak, almost unprotected. Confederate General Jackson took half of the Confederate army on a secret march around to the Union army's right flank and overwhelmed the troops that were there.

In like manner, organized medicine (especially the American Medical Association) has lived in fear of attacks on the primacy of private, fee-for-service medical practice from the political left flank, in the form of government programs or controls. Organized medicine spent vast amounts of money fighting government-provided medicine, national health insurance, and any form of change that would increase government control or regulation of the practice of medicine. What organized medicine did not notice was that it was entirely exposed on the political and economic right (entrepreneurial) flank.

During the past two decades, for-profit hospitals, hospital chains, nursing homes, and insurance companies have rapidly gained control of the organization and financing of medical practice and have instituted managed care to achieve cost control. The forces of organized medicine did not recognize this threat from the right until it was too late to mount a well-organized resistance. Now the managed care forces are controlling the practice of medicine as much as or more than organized medicine ever thought big government would. By guarding only its left flank, organized medicine, like General Hooker, left its right flank unprotected. As Gray and Field (1989) stated:

> With great speed and relatively little public awareness, a significant change has occurred in the way some decisions are made about a patient's medical care. Decisions that were once the exclusive province of the doctor and patient now may be examined in advance by an external reviewer—someone accountable to an employer, insurer, health maintenance organization, or other entity responsible for all or most of the cost of care. Depending upon the circumstances, this outside party may be involved in discussions about where care will occur, how treatment will be provided, and even whether some treatments are appropriate at all.

Reasons for the Rapid Increase in the Cost of Medical Care

The controls over medical practice that were developed over the last half century were largely to limit the costs of medical care. These costs were increasing much faster than the general inflation rate and in 1994 represented about 14% of the gross domestic product. Among the reasons for this rapid increase in costs were the following: increases in the demand for care, increases in the wages for personnel, reliance on complex but only partially effective medical technology, underutilization of facilities, inadequate insurance, and planning failures.

The increasing effectiveness of medical care has led to an **increased demand for care,** thereby increasing the total costs. As noted above, demographic changes, particularly the increase in the number and proportion of older persons, is one of the major reasons for increased demand.

Several decades ago, the **wages of health care workers,** particularly nursing and related personnel, fell behind the wages of workers in many other sectors of the economy. As shortages in the supply of nurses developed, hospitals and other medical care institutions had to offer better wages to lure nurses (mostly women) out of retirement to fill the needs. Nursing wages have generally kept pace with other wage increases since then. The number and wages of administrators have also increased (Woolhandler, Himmelstein, and Lewontin 1993).

Medical costs have been and continue to be increased by the use of complex but only **partially effective technology** for the diagnosis and treatment of disease. Before polio vaccines were developed, for example, iron lungs were used to extend the lives of paralytic poliomyelitis victims. In con-

trast to the polio immunization program, which has proved to be highly cost-effective, the iron lung was an expensive and ineffective ("halfway") technology. Two current examples of "halfway" technologies are renal dialysis and coronary artery bypass grafts, which are more costly and less effective than implementing programs to prevent renal damage and coronary atherosclerosis.

As medical care increasingly is dependent on technology, the cost of medical education increases. Medical education is now so expensive that many new physicians begin practice with more than $100,000 of educational debt. The median debt of graduating US physicians exceeds $60,000.

Medical care facilities need to be properly utilized to be efficient and effective. **Underutilization of hospitals,** in particular, hurts the financial stability of the institutions. Hospitals need to have a steady bed occupancy rate of greater than 80% to remain solvent over the long run. Many hospitals, especially in rural areas, have closed in recent years because of low occupancy rates.

Not providing medical insurance for everyone is more costly than providing it. **Lack of insurance** leads to inappropriate utilization of emergency departments and to delayed care, with resulting increased expense because disease is found at a later and less treatable stage and in a more costly setting. The costs of this care eventually must be borne by society, and often this is done by shifting the costs in some hidden fashion from those who cannot pay to those who can.

Planning failures have contributed to the problem of increasing costs of medical care. One could argue that health care planning began with the Hill-Burton Act of 1946, which encouraged hospital construction. Beginning in the mid-1960s and continuing for almost 20 years, the federal government supported official health planning strategies, largely in an effort to control costs. Among the primary strategies it supported were the appointment of rate-setting authorities within states and the issuance of certificates of need (CON) for the construction of new hospitals or purchase of expensive equipment in particular locales.

Because many of the planning efforts were underfunded or difficult to enforce, they were often ineffective in preventing the duplication of facilities and expensive equipment. In some areas, however, the regulatory efforts were reasonably effective. For example, research has shown that Medicare hospital admission and readmission rates for given diseases are considerably lower in New Haven, Connecticut, than in Boston, Massachusetts, despite similar medical outcomes (Wennberg, Freeman, and Culp 1987; Fisher et al. 1994). The number of beds per 1000 population is considerably lower in Connecticut as a result of decades of aggressive state regulatory efforts at cost control. If there is an empty hospital bed, there is a tendency to fill it.

To ensure that cost-cutting efforts did not decrease the quality of care, regulations were instituted to control the medical care institutions and the process of care. The effects of these regulations on quality is uncertain, but they add considerably to the costs of care by increasing all of the following: the amount of paperwork to be completed, the complexity of the administrative process, and the number of managers and administrators required. Sweet (1993) predicted that if the present trends in health care management and utilization continue, by the year 2026 there will be over two million administrators and no patients.

Because all of the methods noted above have either added to the costs of medical care or failed to contain the rising costs, there has been increasing use of new cost-containment strategies, many of which are lumped under the general term "managed care" (see below). Managed care has so changed the practice of medicine during the past decade that no physician is adequately prepared to enter residency, to say nothing of medical practice, without a basic understanding of it. Managed care techniques will be around in one form or another for the foreseeable future.

Traditional Cost-Containment Strategies

The cost of medical care has been a topic of concern for a long time in the USA. The first committee focusing on this topic was established in 1929 and was called the Committee on the Costs of Medical Care. It published its landmark report in 1932. Until recent decades, the most common forms of cost containment were simple and straightforward.

The first and most basic method of discouraging the overuse of medical care has been to create **deductibles,** which are out-of-pocket payments made by the patient, often at the beginning of the care process. Medical deductibles work in much the same way as current automobile or home insurance deductibles: they discourage the use of insurance for "unimportant" problems and reduce the amount of paperwork for the insurance companies. Deductibles could be applied for an entire year (the patient might have to pay the first $500 of yearly costs) or to each physician visit (the patient might have to pay $5 or $10 for each visit), with the insurance company paying the remainder of the eligible charges. In general, physicians have worried that deductibles might discourage patients from coming in for early symptoms of serious disease. Most HMOs have not had deductibles.

The second basic cost-control method has been **copayments,** as discussed in the section entitled Insurance and Third-Party Payers (see above). Copayments were thought to "encourage" patients not to stay in hospitals longer than necessary.

The third common method has been **exclusions** in the insurance. Some insurance policies totally excluded psychiatric care and dental care from coverage, while others severely restricted the reimbursement for these types of care. Psychiatric care, in particular, was perceived by third-party payers as a potentially bottomless pit that could consume large amounts of money in endless visits.

Another cost-control method used in the 1960s, that of requiring hospitalization for most diagnostic procedures, seemed counterproductive, even at the time. Most insurance plans required all major diagnostic workups to be done in hospitals, even though there often was no medical reason that they could not be done on an outpatient basis. This can only be understood from the insurance companies' viewpoint. They worried that there might be no end to ambulatory diagnostic testing and that the actuaries could not determine the true liability. If diagnostic testing were only reimbursed while the patient was in the hospital, there was a known maximum liability for all of the insurance companies in an area: the total number of inpatient beds multiplied by the average cost per bed-day, plus ancillary costs. Illogical though it seems now, this kind of thinking enabled the insurance companies to set a finite and predictable limit to their financial liability.

During this time, there was considerable discussion about **health care markets,** based on assumptions of the free market economic model. Such a model requires many things to be true that are untrue in the world of medical care. First, there must be many sellers and many buyers for the buyers to have free choice. Second, the buyers must have good information regarding the products from which they choose. Third, there must not be monopolies; that is, no seller and no buyer should be able to dominate the market (Kropf 1990). The health care market usually does not meet any of these characteristics. First, in many areas, there are few choices of provider, either physician or hospital, and the federal government is often the dominant purchaser of care in the market. Second, patients usually do not have enough information about the quality and cost of medical care for them to make a valid market-based decision concerning their medical needs. Third, increasingly large market forces, such as hospital chains or huge HMOs, dominate the market in their primary regions. Market forces are inadequate to maximize efficiency and control the costs of medical care, because of the complexity of the care.

New Cost-Containment Strategies

If resources for medical care are inadequate to meet demand, there are three basic methods of responding: (1) increase resources; (2) decrease demand (or at least utilization); and (3) increase efficiency. Although efforts are generally made in all three areas, the recent emphasis is on decreasing demand and increasing efficiency through two relatively new cost-containment strategies. One is the prospective payment strategy based on diagnosis-related groups, and the other is managed care.

Prospective Payment System Based on Diagnosis-Related Groups

Developed in the 1970s but first applied nationally in the USA to Medicare reimbursement in 1983, the prospective payment system (PPS) based on diagnosis-related groups has changed the way hospitals are reimbursed and the way hospitals and physicians think about the provision of care. Each hospital admission is classified into one of 23 major diagnostic categories based on organ systems, and then these diagnostic categories are further subdivided into diagnosis-related groups (DRGs). A DRG may consist of a single diagnosis or procedure, or it may consist of several diagnoses or procedures that, on average, have similar hospital costs per admission. An uncomplicated delivery of an infant, for example, is coded as DRG #313, and a nonradical hysterectomy in a woman who is under the age of 70 and has no complicating condition is coded as DRG #355.

DRGs were first developed to enable hospitals to look for cost "outliers." For example, hospitals could analyze and identify those physicians who regularly generated greater than average costs for care coded as DRG #313. The hospitals could then try to find out why these physicians generated excess costs and to devise methods to control these costs in the future. The federal government, however, decided to use the DRG system to pay hospitals on the basis of a prospectively determined average cost for each of the more than 470 DRGs. This system began to be used in the treatment of Medicare patients in October 1983. Although there is no federal requirement that hospital payers other than Medicare use the DRG system for reimbursement, several states requested and received federal permission to incorporate DRGs into their own prospectively determined rate-setting programs. When this happened, all third-party payers in the state had to conform to the same prospectively determined rates. This is referred to as an **all-payer system.**

Note that the hospital is actually reimbursed *after* a specific type of care is given; however, the amount of payment for the specific type of care is decided prospectively (in advance). The average cost for each of the more than 470 DRGs is set prospectively for each region of the country. Although extra amounts are added for tertiary hospitals and for hospitals engaged in medical education, these adjustments have failed to cover fully the costs of hospital-based medical education. Medicare reimburses hospitals with the predetermined fixed amount for the entire hospital stay of a Medicare patient, based on his or her DRG, regardless of whether it actually cost the hospital more or less than the prospectively determined DRG-specific payment to provide that care. If a hospital can find a way to reduce the costs and provide the care for less than the amount reimbursed by the PPS, it can retain the excess amount. If a hospital is inefficient and has higher than average costs for a hospital admission, it will lose money on that admission. Because hospitals with the strongest administrative teams and data systems are best able to keep costs below PPS reimbursements, there is a tendency for the strong hospitals to get stronger and the weak hospitals to get weaker.

There have been some good results from the PPS. For example, there are now more and better data than before, and hospitals have a greater ability than before to find unnecessary costs. Initially, because of efficiencies introduced in response to the PPS and because of the more rapid discharge of some patients, the PPS reduced hospital utilization (and therefore costs) considerably. After a period of reduced costs, however, the upward pressure on the cost of medical care has resumed.

The full impact of the PPS on the quality of medical care has not been determined. There is evidence that some patients are being discharged sooner than desirable, but no major change in medical care quality has been clearly discernible. Often, early discharge merely passes the medical care problems (and therefore costs) down the line to the care institutions receiving the patients from the hospital: the home, home care agencies, and nursing homes.

The PPS added urgency to an already-growing trend to move as much medical care as possible out of acute, general hospitals and into ambulatory surgery and diagnostic centers. Because the PPS does not apply to ambulatory procedures, providers in ambulatory settings could set their own rates. In addition, many hospitals and staff model HMOs began to develop infirmaries, where patients who did not need acute, intensive care could be given moderate supervision and some treatment at a much lower cost than if they were in hospitals.

Managed Care

In an analysis of the social structure of medical care, Freidson (1970) claimed that the characteristic which uniquely defines the "professions," including medicine, is autonomy in practice. With the advent of managed care, also known as **utilization management,** the trend appears to be away from physician autonomy in some aspects of medical practice, such as deciding which patients can be admitted to the hospital and how long they may remain there. Managed care is a system of administrative controls, the goal of which is to reduce the costs of medical care. According to Gray and Field (1989),

> Such "utilization management" is part of a complex balancing act created by society's struggles with two important questions. First, how do we ensure that people get needed medical care without spending so much that we compromise other important social objectives? Second, how do we discourage unnecessary and inappropriate medical services without jeopardizing necessary high-quality care?

Managed care, which consists of some combination of the strategies that are discussed in this section, is thought to reduce medical care costs to the payer (usually a third-party payer) over the short run.

Preadmission Review and Certification. Some designated person in the managed care office (usually a nurse) must approve a nonemergent hospital admission before the admission occurs. Otherwise, the hospital is not guaranteed payment from the patient's third-party payer. Using the emergency department for a nonemergent condition is not a way to bypass preadmission certification, as can be seen below.

Emergency Department Admission Review. An admission from the emergency department must have a case review within a day to be sure it is a justified admission. If the reviewer does not consider the admission justified, the hospital will not be paid, so the patient will receive the bill.

Concurrent (Continued Stay) Review. The attending physician must justify keeping a patient in the hospital longer than the number of days expected for that patient's DRG.

Discharge Planning. To avoid discharging patients to inappropriate places for their needs and to avoid delays in outplacement, planning for discharge should begin the day the patient is admitted to the hospital.

Second Opinions. A second physician's opinion concerning the patient's need for surgery must be obtained before a major elective invasive procedure is performed. Requiring a second opinion markedly reduces the rates for certain types of surgery, such as hysterectomy.

Gatekeepers. Many managed care plans, particularly staff model HMOs, require that all referrals to specialists be approved by the patient's primary care practitioner. In this role, the primary care practitioners are functioning as "gatekeepers."

High-Cost Case Management. If the hospital care for a particular patient is costing or potentially will cost the third-party payer a large amount of money, an administrator is appointed to look hard for a less costly alternative, such as ambulatory care or home care. This strategy tends to work best in cases in which the patient has complex or multiple medical problems.

Benefit Design. Every benefit plan offered by a third-party payer, including HMOs of various types, seeks provisions to attract the patients they want to recruit to the plan while at the same time limiting the financial exposure of the insurer. First, the plan may try to reduce premiums and costs by enlisting the patients themselves in reducing costs by means of such traditional methods as deductibles and copayments. Second, a common practice is to exclude or at least limit the amount of certain benefits from the policy. Plans frequently limit or exclude mental health and dental health benefits. Where it is legal to do so, some plans limit the coverage of costs related to human immunodeficiency virus (HIV) infection or substance abuse.

Financial Incentives for Physicians. If physicians are paid on a salary or capitation basis rather than on a fee-for-service basis, they have no incentive to provide unnecessary services to their patients. In theory, there should be an incentive for preventive measures when a physician or a health plan is paid on a capitation basis, because effective prevention may reduce the time and effort the physician must spend on the average patient. A strategy that may be pursued to reduce unnecessary care is a system of bonuses for physicians if they use efficient practice techniques or if their group practice makes a sufficient profit in a given year.

National Health Insurance

The financial problems created by "cream skimming" (see above) and other techniques for enticing low-risk populations into third-party payer networks could be reduced by taking any large natural population (either the entire US population or each state's population) as a risk pool. If this were done for the entire US population, it would be a form of nationwide (national) health insurance. National health insurance has been vigorously opposed by much of organized medicine, which still fears government control over medical practice as well as possible limitations of physician charges. The irony, as mentioned above, is that physicians now may be controlled as much or more from the "free enterprise" side of medical care than they probably would have been under national health insurance.

National health insurance is unlikely to be enacted unless a reliable way is found to control the costs of medical care. Given the economic problems of the USA and the size of the national debt, some members of Congress tend to view the passage of national health insurance as equivalent to writing a blank check. In light of the Congress members' experiences with the rapidly rising cost of the Medicare program, which really is a kind of federally administered national health insurance for the beneficiaries of Social Security, Congress is not likely to want to undertake a much larger version of it.

In 1994, President Clinton had proposed a new system designed to ensure coverage of everybody and yet give people freedom of choice of health plans and physicians. The President's plan was based on ideas formulated by a "think tank" of individuals. The centerpiece of this plan was the development of **health insurance purchasing cooperatives** (HIPCs), which the President termed **health alliances.**

Within defined regions, each of which could be as large as a state, the health alliances would (with minor exceptions) be the sole organizations to receive the health insurance premium payments from companies, individuals, and the government. In turn, the health alliances would have the responsibility for approving a number of providers (mostly HMOs or IPAs) who met certain criteria. Individuals or families could then choose one of the health plans approved by the health alliance in their area, and their premiums would be channeled through the health alliance to the health plan of their choice, which would provide their care. Because the providers would be in competition with one other to attract people but would also be regulated by the government through the health alliances, the entire process was called **managed competition.** This plan had some attractive aspects, but it appeared so complex that the public and Congress were generally swayed by the arguments of opponents, and the plan failed politically.

The prospects for the foreseeable future are for continuing reform from within the medical care system. Strategies for reform include (1) efforts by the states to create their own state solutions; (2) efforts by the federal government to modify Medicare, Medicaid, and third-party insurance; (3) efforts to develop some form of national health insurance for pregnant women and young children; and (4) efforts to develop some form of catastrophic health insurance plan.

Long-Term Care

A fairly high proportion (about 43%) of people who reach the age of 65 years eventually will spend some time in a nursing home (Kemper and Murtaugh 1991). Medicare (Title 18) will cover nursing home costs for a limited period (up to 100 days) only if two conditions are met: the patient is released from a hospital directly to the nursing home, and this immediate posthospital nursing home care is considered likely to improve the patient's condition. Medicare will not pay for nursing home care beyond the 100 days after discharge from a hospital. Medicare will not pay for nursing home care if a nonhospitalized person requires nursing home care because of failing strength or inability to care for himself or herself in the activities of daily living.

After Medicare coverage of nursing home (or home care) services is used up, the patient must assume the costs for these services until his or her financial resources have been "spent down" to a prescribed level (e.g., ownership of a home may be maintained as long as a spouse or dependent survives, and up to about $4000 in personal resources may be maintained). When the spend-down is complete, Medicaid (Title 19) begins to cover the costs, and in essence the patient is a welfare recipient.

Because part of the Medicaid costs are borne by the state in which the patient enters a nursing home, the state could put a lien on the patient's house and property, although it would not be taken until the patient's spouse had died. Some elderly people, suspecting that they would likely need a long stay in a nursing home soon, gave their wealth to their children to avoid having their property and savings used to pay nursing home costs. For this reason, state governments have stipulated that if the gift giver is placed in a nursing home and requires Medicaid within a certain number of years of giving the gift, the gift recipient must reimburse the state for the nursing home costs, up to an amount equal to the gift.

A number of experiments with long-term care insurance have been initiated. Long-term care insurance will pay all or part of the costs of a nursing home but will not pay for an acute hospitalization or for physicians' charges. This type of insurance tends to be very costly and has not gained general acceptance thus far. Long-term care insurance is expensive because good nursing home care now costs more than $1000 per week in many areas of the USA and the need for nursing home care can extend for many years.

Assessment of the Quality of Medical Care

The quality of medical practice has been a major concern since early in this century. In 1910, for example, the Flexner Report was especially concerned with the need to improve medical education. Quality of medical care became a bigger issue after World War II, when Donabedian and other investigators began to define more clearly the dimensions of quality. In 1969, Donabedian indicated that quality should be examined in terms of **structure** (the physical resources and human resources that a hospital or HMO possessed for providing care), **process** (the way in which the physical and human resources were joined in the activities of physicians and other health care providers), and **outcome** (the end results of care, such as whether the patients actually did as well as would be expected, given the severity of their problems).

State accreditation of facilities usually focuses on structural issues, with some evaluation of process. Quality review programs of the past, including the programs of professional review organizations, tended to focus on particular aspects of process called **procedural end points** and offered a detailed review of the methods of care provided and an analysis of how well certain disease-specific criteria were met.

Measuring the quality of medical outcomes in a fair manner is a significant methodologic problem. Unless outcomes are adjusted for the severity of the patients' illnesses, hospitals treating the sickest patients would be at an unfair disadvantage. The process of adjusting for the severity of illness is usually referred to as **case-mix adjustment.** Moreover, the question arises as to whose judgment of outcome—the judgment of patients or that of professionals—should be used to evaluate outcomes.

The federal government now rates hospitals by giving a **case-mix adjusted mortality rate** for each hospital. Although controversial, this process has generally provided reproducible results. Hospitals that have initiated measures to improve medical care have been successful in lowering their case-mix adjusted mortality rates.

One major concern about the current efforts to reduce costs is whether quality will be reduced as well. Clinicians and epidemiologists continue to address this question in ongoing studies.

Current Trends in Medical Care

Because US companies are paying huge amounts for the medical care insurance they provide to their workers, they are exploring a variety of means to reduce their costs. These include self-insuring, re-packaging their insurance policies, and requiring their employees to pay a portion of the medical care premiums. In many cases, cost-saving packages often come through special financial arrangements with providers in a preferred provider organization (see above).

In the USA, current medical care policy is largely determined by what care is reimbursed. Because reimbursement regulations vary from state to state, from year to year, from insurance plan to insurance plan, and even from person to person depending on the type of coverage that a person has, medical care policy is always in flux. Care that is reimbursed by HMOs, insurance programs, federal government programs, or a combination of these sources is part of the medical care policy; what is not reimbursed is not policy.

Many of the current trends in medical care have evolved from efforts to reduce costs. One trend is the increasing use of ambulatory (outpatient) facilities for hernia repair, cataract removal, and a whole host of operative procedures that would have been unthinkable to perform on an outpatient basis a decade or two ago. Another trend is the increase in the amount of care provided by medical personnel other than physicians. Experiences with medical corpsmen in World War II led to the development of the **physician assistant,** who could provide some primary care and could monitor ongoing care of more complex diseases once the diagnosis and treatment had been established. Today, through intensive clinical programs, **nurse practitioners** are trained to provide primary care and to recognize when the care of a physician is needed. **Certified nurse midwives** are licensed to provide prenatal care, labor and delivery care, and postpartum care for uncomplicated pregnancies and deliveries. **Alternative practitioners,** particularly chiropractors, have become more common in the USA and are consulted by a larger proportion of the population. Recently, Congress established a new national program to study alternative medicine approaches.

For-profit, investor-owned hospital chains (e.g., the Hospital Corporation of America), nursing homes, diagnostic laboratories, radiologic facilities, home care programs, urgent care facilities, and renal hemodialysis units now represent a significant proportion of provider institutions. According to Gray (1991), 14% of community hospitals in 1985 were for-profit institutions, and if other hospitals (such as public hospitals managed by for-profit organizations) were included, the figure would rise to 20%. In addition, as reported by Gray, the percentages of other types of medical care institutions run by for-profit organizations were as follows: 34% of psychiatric hospitals in 1984; 81% of nursing homes in 1980; 66% of HMO plans in 1987; 57% of PPOs in 1985; 32% of Medicare-certified home health agencies in 1985; 90% of freestanding surgery centers in 1986; 93% of primary care centers in 1986; and 63% of blood banks in 1986.

It is not always easy to distinguish for-profit from not-for-profit hospitals, because many not-for-profit community hospitals are becoming large multifaceted medical care corporations providing a complex mix of services, including home care, long-term care, HMOs, and even some for-profit ventures under holding companies. Arnold Relman, former editor of the *New England Journal of Medicine,* has strongly criticized the morality of the "new medical-industrial complex" that has resulted from an increasing intrusion of for-profit ventures into the world of medical care (Relman 1991).

THE PROBLEM OF THE "MEDICAL COMMONS"

In 1968, Garrett Hardin wrote "The Tragedy of the Commons," perhaps the most famous contribution to the population control debates of the 1960s. Pointing out that the shared resources of the earth (the commons) are limited, Hardin argued that the attempt by one individual or group to maximize its own welfare by using more than its fair share of the commons would necessarily diminish the good that others can derive from it. This logic can be applied to the use of medical resources in the USA. Unless Americans are able and willing to organize, finance, and regulate medical care in light of the needs of the entire population, then various individual groups (e.g., industries, hospitals, hospital chains, HMOs, insurance companies, nursing homes, and home care programs) will continue to seek to maximize their benefits (their share of the commons) at the expense of others.

Apportioning resources from the medical commons is not simple, but a satisfactory resolution will not be achieved by piecemeal approaches. It is tempting to postulate that a single-payer system will improve the ability to achieve an ethical and rational allocation, but this method also has hazards. Health promotion and disease prevention will help, but they are not panaceas either. Efficiency will play a role, but what is needed now is more medically directed efficiency and possibly less emphasis on managerial and cost efficiency. A close monitoring of quality is essential, or the result may be a loss of the benefits that all are striving to achieve.

SUMMARY

In the USA, the medical care system has developed without strong direction from the local, state, or federal government. The result is a confusing mix of ways in which services are organized and paid for. The per capita cost of medical care and the proportion of the gross domestic product used for medical care are higher in the USA than anywhere else in the world, yet approximately 15% of Americans still have no financial protection from the costs of medical care. Moreover, the medical care cost inflation rate is one of the highest in the world.

Because of the high costs of medical care, a variety of cost-containment strategies have been developed. Two that are used extensively today in the USA are the prospective payment system and managed care. In the prospective payment system, the third-party payer reimburses hospitals for care at a predetermined rate, depending on the average duration and complexity of the medical care provided for each condition. In managed care, hospitalizations will be reimbursed by a third-party payer only if the payer has approved the admission beforehand (preadmission review and certification). If a patient is admitted through the emergency department, this admission is reviewed the next day and if not approved by the third-party payer, reimbursement may not be paid (emergency department admission review). Once a patient is in the hospital, the length of stay is closely monitored, and the patient may be forced to leave the hospital as soon as possible (concurrent review and discharge planning). Other aspects of managed care include second opinions before elective surgery; use of primary care physicians as gatekeepers; high-cost case management; benefit design; and the provision of financial incentives for physicians to practice economically.

The current medical care system in the USA has many costly inefficiencies, which may not be able to be corrected without major changes, such as national or regional health insurance, a single-payer system, or a combination of both. Nevertheless, the possibly high initial costs of shifting to a new system, the uncertainty of its benefits, and the complex political compromises that would probably be required suggest that in the immediate future, there will be no major, rapid change in the organization or financing of medical care in the USA.

References Cited

Committee on the Costs of Medical Care. Medical Care for the American People. Chicago, University of Chicago Press, 1932.

Donabedian, A. A Guide to Medical Care Administration. Vol. 2, Medical Care Appraisal. New York, American Public Health Association, 1969.

Fisher, E. S., et al. Hospital readmission rates for cohorts of Medicare beneficiaries in Boston and New Haven. New England Journal of Medicine 331:989–995, 1994.

Flexner, A. Medical Education in the United States and Canada: A Report to the Carnegie Foundation for the Advancement of Teaching. Buffalo, N. Y., Heritage Press, 1910.

Freidson, E. Professional Dominance: The Social Structure of Medical Care. New York, Atherton Press, 1970.

Gray, B. H. The Profit Motive and Patient Care. Cambridge, Mass., Harvard University Press, 1991.

Gray, B. H., and M. J. Field, eds. Controlling Costs and Changing Patient Care? The Role of Utilization Management. Washington, D. C., National Academy Press, 1989.

Hardin, G. The tragedy of the commons. Science 162:1243–1248, 1968.

Kemper, P., and C. M. Murtaugh. Lifetime use of nursing home care. New England Journal of Medicine 324:595–600, 1991.

Kropf, R. Planning for health services. *In* Kovner, A. R., ed. Health Care Delivery in the United States, 4th ed. New York, Springer Publishing Company, 1990.

Luft, H. S. Health Maintenance Organizations. New York, John Wiley and Sons, 1981.

Prussin, J. A., and J. C. Woods. Development of Health Insurance. Topics in Health Care Financing 2:1–12, 1975.

Relman, A. S. The health care industry: where is it taking us? New England Journal of Medicine 325:854–859, 1991.

Sweet, V. Letter to the editor. New England Journal of Medicine 329:1655, 1993.

Wennberg, J. E., J. L. Freeman, and W. J. Culp. Are hospital services rationed in New Haven or overutilized in Boston? Lancet 1:1185–1189, 1987.

Woolhandler, S., D. U. Himmelstein, and J. P. Lewontin. Administrative costs in US Hospitals. New England Journal of Medicine 329:400–403, 1993.

Selected Readings

Gray, B. H. The Profit Motive and Patient Care: The Changing Accountability of Doctors and Hospitals. Cambridge, Mass., Harvard University Press, 1991.

Jonas, S. An Introduction to the US Health Care System, 3rd ed. New York, Springer Publishing Company, 1992.

Luft, H. S. Health Maintenance Organizations. New York, John Wiley and Sons, 1981.

APPENDIX

TABLE A.   Random Numbers*

53872	34774	19087	81775	71440	12082	75092	34608	75448	13148
04226	62404	71577	00984	56056	32404	87641	53392	92561	33388
28666	44190	75524	62038	21423	46281	92238	96306	72606	80601
63817	30279	14088	86434	16183	06401	90586	80292	54555	47371
22359	16442	83879	47486	19838	32252	39560	95851	36758	36141
50968	28728	83525	16031	77583	65578	84794	51367	32535	83834
39652	24248	96617	91200	10769	52386	39559	75921	49375	22847
35493	00529	69632	29684	80284	87828	72418	80950	86311	34016
75687	53919	80439	20534	96185	72345	96391	52625	50866	45132
31509	93521	10681	44124	88345	84969	88768	48819	22311	41235
40389	76282	37506	60661	23295	67357	95419	10864	87833	09152
59244	54664	63424	97899	44153	69251	08781	18604	02312	21658
99876	17075	40934	08912	96196	58503	63613	24486	98092	45672
06457	50072	18060	71023	84349	40984	59487	77782	32107	53770
14297	07687	05517	10362	35783	62236	63764	45542	68889	03862
51661	57130	97442	29590	21634	79772	73801	70122	46467	47152
53455	41788	16117	09698	24409	05079	76603	57563	33461	46791
48086	31512	62819	27689	63744	11023	11184	87679	22218	70139
19108	01602	96950	41536	39974	88287	83546	69187	45539	78263
39001	77727	33095	58785	29179	45421	71416	20418	38558	78700
72346	55617	14714	21930	14851	38209	52202	03979	05970	74483
19094	64359	89829	10942	53101	37758	29583	26792	42840	45872
82247	77127	01652	50774	04970	83300	33760	22172	67516	62135
75968	18386	31874	52249	21015	20365	57475	32756	58268	75739
01963	38095	99960	91307	99654	74279	80145	53303	11870	50485
64828	15817	80923	55226	51893	93362	15757	47430	84855	95822
64347	61578	44160	06266	35118	52558	56436	96155	10293	67506
54746	52337	84826	39012	59118	19851	10156	78167	41473	99025
22241	41501	02993	99340	91044	67268	51088	12751	74008	33773
11906	20043	10415	44425	31712	54831	85591	62237	88797	14382
76637	07609	95378	95580	86909	50609	99008	99042	50364	36664
93896	47120	98926	30636	28136	49458	84145	79205	79517	93446
75292	88232	14360	12455	13656	65736	70428	66917	64412	38502
98792	29828	10577	48184	29433	98278	22543	76155	82107	22066
65751	91049	94127	47558	99880	79667	86254	72797	67117	44699
72064	62102	39155	79462	82975	02638	00302	79476	72656	84003
01227	35821	80607	61734	02600	45564	72344	71034	48370	96826
44768	56504	13993	59701	88238	92483	09497	66058	36651	37927
69838	91226	85736	72247	64099	86305	49877	76215	66980	30228
01800	39313	57730	84410	47637	81369	51830	43536	58937	91901
11756	45441	59948	57975	92422	70057	50210	30345	55912	31638
39056	86614	53643	62909	27198	04454	33789	86463	66603	48083
88086	93172	68311	39164	42012	10447	45933	28844	36844	57684
12648	27948	76750	19915	66815	34015	43011	27150	94264	89516
16254	87661	66181	68609	58626	58428	75051	27558	49463	66646
69682	19109	94189	94626	09299	10649	55405	54571	57855	54921
61336	86663	13010	40412	50139	30769	13048	61407	41056	60510
65727	66488	12304	70011	93324	58764	87274	43103	96002	06984
55705	34418	99410	32635	42984	40981	91750	27431	05142	77950
95402	51746	98184	38830	97590	00066	82770	42325	28778	83571
79228	94510	57711	64366	89040	43278	69072	22003	89465	61483
48103	56760	82564	33649	35176	32278	51357	05489	47462	55931
70969	27677	99621	63065	73194	70462	19316	77945	45004	39895
69931	20237	75246	59124	12484	22012	79731	82435	56301	99752
37208	22741	41946	74109	03760	24094	40210	76617	52317	50643
60151	92327	85150	27728	64813	47667	66078	03628	95240	03808
46210	47674	53747	95354	67757	75477	26396	09592	96239	50854
55399	48142	12284	95298	56399	61358	87541	12998	79639	63633
23677	64950	97041	43088	80143	34294	91468	01066	90350	78891
41947	70066	90311	17133	11674	00826	75760	37586	33621	14199

Source of data: RAND Corporation. A Million Random Digits with 100,000 Normal Deviates. New York, Free Press, 1955. Copyright 1955 and 1983 by the RAND Corporation. Used by permission.

*Instructions for use of the table: Decide in advance how many table columns will be used and in what direction the numbers will be assigned after the starting point is identified. Then blindly put a pencil on the table, and start with the numbers nearest the pencil point, moving in the predetermined direction (e.g., moving up the columns).

TABLE B. Standard Normal-Tail Probabilities (Table of z Values)*

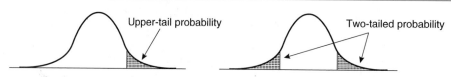

z	Upper-Tail Probability	Two-Tailed Probability	z	Upper-Tail Probability	Two-Tailed Probability
0.00	0.5000	1.0000	0.36	0.3594	0.7188
0.01	0.4960	0.9920	0.37	0.3557	0.7114
0.02	0.4920	0.9840	0.38	0.3520	0.7039
0.0251	0.49	0.98	0.3853	0.35	0.70
0.03	0.4880	0.9761	0.39	0.3483	0.6965
0.04	0.4840	0.9681	0.40	0.3446	0.6892
0.05	0.4801	0.9601	0.41	0.3409	0.6818
0.0502	0.48	0.96	0.4125	0.34	0.68
0.06	0.4761	0.9522	0.42	0.3372	0.6745
0.07	0.4721	0.9442	0.43	0.3336	0.6672
0.0753	0.47	0.94	0.4399	0.33	0.66
0.08	0.4681	0.9362	0.44	0.3300	0.6599
0.09	0.4641	0.9283	0.45	0.3264	0.6527
0.10	0.4602	0.9203	0.46	0.3228	0.6455
0.1004	0.46	0.92	0.4677	0.32	0.64
0.11	0.4562	0.9124	0.47	0.3192	0.6384
0.12	0.4522	0.9045	0.48	0.3156	0.6312
0.1257	0.45	0.9	0.49	0.3121	0.6241
0.13	0.4483	0.8966	0.4959	0.31	0.62
0.14	0.4443	0.8887	0.50	0.3085	0.6171
0.15	0.4404	0.8808	0.51	0.3050	0.6101
0.1510	0.44	0.88	0.52	0.3015	0.6031
0.16	0.4364	0.8729	0.5244	0.3	0.6
0.17	0.4325	0.8650	0.53	0.2981	0.5961
0.1764	0.43	0.86	0.54	0.2946	0.5892
0.18	0.4286	0.8571	0.55	0.2912	0.5823
0.19	0.4247	0.8493	0.5534	0.29	0.58
0.20	0.4207	0.8415	0.56	0.2877	0.5755
0.2019	0.42	0.84	0.57	0.2843	0.5687
0.21	0.4168	0.8337	0.58	0.2810	0.5619
0.22	0.4129	0.8259	0.5828	0.28	0.56
0.2275	0.41	0.82	0.59	0.2776	0.5552
0.23	0.4090	0.8181	0.60	0.2743	0.5485
0.24	0.4052	0.8103	0.61	0.2709	0.5419
0.25	0.4013	0.8026	0.6128	0.27	0.54
0.2533	0.40	0.80	0.62	0.2676	0.5353
0.26	0.3974	0.7949	0.63	0.2643	0.5287
0.27	0.3936	0.7872	0.64	0.2611	0.5222
0.2793	0.39	0.78	0.6433	0.26	0.52
0.28	0.3897	0.7795	0.65	0.2578	0.5157
0.29	0.3859	0.7718	0.66	0.2546	0.5093
0.30	0.3821	0.7642	0.67	0.2514	0.5029
0.3055	0.38	0.76	0.6745	0.25	0.50
0.31	0.3783	0.7566	0.68	0.2483	0.4956
0.32	0.3745	0.7490	0.69	0.2451	0.4902
0.33	0.3707	0.7414	0.70	0.2420	0.4839
0.3319	0.37	0.74	0.7063	0.24	0.48
0.34	0.3669	0.7339	0.71	0.2389	0.4777
0.35	0.3632	0.7263	0.72	0.2358	0.4715
0.3585	0.36	0.72	0.73	0.2327	0.4654

Continued

TABLE B.   Standard Normal-Tail Probabilities (Table of z Values)* *(Continued)*

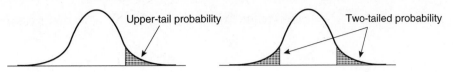

z	Upper-Tail Probability	Two-Tailed Probability	z	Upper-Tail Probability	Two-Tailed Probability
0.7388	0.23	0.46	1.13	0.1292	0.2585
0.74	0.2296	0.4593	1.14	0.1271	0.2543
0.75	0.2266	0.4533	1.15	0.1251	0.2501
0.76	0.2236	0.4473	1.16	0.1230	0.2460
0.77	0.2206	0.4413	1.17	0.1210	0.2420
0.7722	0.22	0.44	1.175	0.12	0.24
0.78	0.2177	0.4354	1.18	0.1190	0.2380
0.79	0.2148	0.4295	1.19	0.1170	0.2340
0.80	0.2119	0.4237	1.20	0.1151	0.2301
0.8064	0.21	0.42	1.21	0.1131	0.2263
0.81	0.2090	0.4179	1.22	0.1112	0.2225
0.82	0.2061	0.4122	1.227	0.11	0.22
0.83	0.2033	0.4065	1.23	0.1093	0.2187
0.84	0.2005	0.4009	1.24	0.1075	0.2150
0.8416	0.20	0.40	1.25	0.1056	0.2113
0.85	0.1977	0.3953	1.26	0.1038	0.2077
0.86	0.1949	0.3898	1.27	0.1020	0.2041
0.87	0.1922	0.3843	1.28	0.1003	0.2005
0.8779	0.19	0.38	1.282	0.10	0.20
0.88	0.1894	0.3789	1.29	0.0985	0.1971
0.89	0.1867	0.3735	1.30	0.0968	0.1936
0.90	0.1841	0.3681	1.31	0.0951	0.1902
0.91	0.1814	0.3628	1.32	0.0934	0.1868
0.9154	0.18	0.36	1.33	0.0918	0.1835
0.92	0.1788	0.3576	1.34	0.0901	0.1802
0.93	0.1762	0.3524	1.341	0.09	0.18
0.94	0.1736	0.3472	1.35	0.0885	0.1770
0.95	0.1711	0.3421	1.36	0.0869	0.1738
0.9542	0.17	0.34	1.37	0.0853	0.1707
0.96	0.1685	0.3371	1.38	0.0838	0.1676
0.97	0.1660	0.3320	1.39	0.0823	0.1645
0.98	0.1635	0.3271	1.40	0.0808	0.1615
0.99	0.1611	0.3222	1.405	0.08	0.16
0.9945	0.16	0.32	1.41	0.0793	0.1585
1.00	0.1587	0.3173	1.42	0.0778	0.1556
1.01	0.1562	0.3125	1.43	0.0764	0.1527
1.02	0.1539	0.3077	1.44	0.0749	0.1499
1.03	0.1515	0.3030	1.45	0.0735	0.1471
1.036	0.15	0.3	1.46	0.0721	0.1443
1.04	0.1492	0.2983	1.47	0.0708	0.1416
1.05	0.1469	0.2937	1.476	0.07	0.14
1.06	0.1446	0.2891	1.48	0.0694	0.1389
1.07	0.1423	0.2846	1.49	0.0681	0.1362
1.08	0.1401	0.2801	1.50	0.0668	0.1336
1.080	0.14	0.28	1.51	0.0655	0.1310
1.09	0.1379	0.2757	1.52	0.0643	0.1285
1.10	0.1357	0.2713	1.53	0.0630	0.1260
1.11	0.1335	0.2670	1.54	0.0618	0.1236
1.12	0.1314	0.2627	1.55	0.0606	0.1211
1.1264	0.13	0.26	1.555	0.06	0.12

Continued

TABLE B.   Standard Normal-Tail Probabilities (Table of z Values)* *(Continued)*

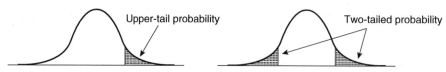

z	Upper-Tail Probability	Two-Tailed Probability	z	Upper-Tail Probability	Two-Tailed Probability
1.56	0.0594	0.1188	2.03	0.0212	0.0424
1.57	0.0582	0.1164	2.04	0.0207	0.0414
1.58	0.0571	0.1141	2.05	0.0202	0.0404
1.59	0.0559	0.1118	2.054	0.02	0.04
1.60	0.0548	0.1096	2.06	0.0197	0.0394
1.61	0.0537	0.1074	2.07	0.0192	0.0385
1.62	0.0526	0.1052	2.08	0.0188	0.0375
1.63	0.0516	0.1031	2.09	0.0183	0.0366
1.64	0.0505	0.1010	2.10	0.0179	0.0357
1.645	0.05	0.10	2.11	0.0174	0.0349
1.65	0.0495	0.0989	2.12	0.0170	0.0340
1.66	0.0485	0.0969	2.13	0.0166	0.0332
1.67	0.0475	0.0949	2.14	0.0162	0.0324
1.68	0.0465	0.0930	2.15	0.0158	0.0316
1.69	0.0455	0.0910	2.16	0.0154	0.0308
1.70	0.0446	0.0891	2.17	0.0150	0.0300
1.71	0.0436	0.0873	2.18	0.0146	0.0293
1.72	0.0427	0.0854	2.19	0.0143	0.0285
1.73	0.0418	0.0836	2.20	0.0139	0.0278
1.74	0.0409	0.0819	2.21	0.0136	0.0271
1.75	0.0401	0.0801	2.22	0.0132	0.0264
1.751	0.04	0.08	2.23	0.0129	0.0257
1.76	0.0392	0.0784	2.24	0.0125	0.0251
1.77	0.0384	0.0767	2.25	0.0122	0.0244
1.78	0.0375	0.0751	2.26	0.0119	0.0238
1.79	0.0367	0.0734	2.27	0.0116	0.0232
1.80	0.0359	0.0719	2.28	0.0113	0.0226
1.81	0.0352	0.0703	2.29	0.0110	0.0220
1.82	0.0344	0.0688	2.30	0.0107	0.0214
1.83	0.0336	0.0672	2.31	0.0104	0.0209
1.84	0.0329	0.0658	2.32	0.0102	0.0203
1.85	0.0322	0.0643	2.326	0.01	0.02
1.86	0.0314	0.0629	2.33	0.0099	0.0198
1.87	0.0307	0.0615	2.34	0.0096	0.0193
1.88	0.0301	0.0601	2.35	0.0094	0.0188
1.881	0.03	0.06	2.36	0.0091	0.0183
1.89	0.0294	0.0588	2.37	0.0089	0.0178
1.90	0.0287	0.0574	2.38	0.0087	0.0173
1.91	0.0281	0.0561	2.39	0.0084	0.0168
1.92	0.0274	0.0549	2.40	0.0082	0.0164
1.93	0.0268	0.0536	2.41	0.0080	0.0160
1.94	0.0262	0.0524	2.42	0.0078	0.0155
1.95	0.0256	0.0512	2.43	0.0075	0.0151
1.960	0.025	0.05	2.44	0.0073	0.0147
1.97	0.0244	0.0488	2.45	0.0071	0.0143
1.98	0.0239	0.0477	2.46	0.0069	0.0139
1.99	0.0233	0.0466	2.47	0.0068	0.0135
2.00	0.0228	0.0455	2.48	0.0066	0.0131
2.01	0.0222	0.0444	2.49	0.0064	0.0128
2.02	0.0217	0.0434	2.50	0.0062	0.0124

Continued

TABLE B. Standard Normal-Tail Probabilities (Table of z Values)* *(Continued)*

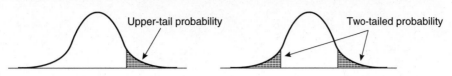

z	Upper-Tail Probability	Two-Tailed Probability	z	Upper-Tail Probability	Two-Tailed Probability
2.51	0.0060	0.0121	2.90	0.0019	0.0037
2.52	0.0059	0.0117	2.95	0.0016	0.0032
2.53	0.0057	0.0114	3.00	0.0013	0.0027
2.54	0.0055	0.0111	3.05	0.0011	0.0023
2.55	0.0054	0.0108	3.090	0.001	0.002
2.56	0.0052	0.0105	3.10	0.0010	0.0019
2.57	0.0051	0.0102	3.15	0.0008	0.0016
2.576	0.005	0.01	3.20	0.0007	0.0014
2.58	0.0049	0.0099	3.25	0.0006	0.0012
2.59	0.0048	0.0096	3.291	0.0005	0.001
2.60	0.0047	0.0093	3.30	0.0005	0.0010
2.61	0.0045	0.0091	3.35	0.0004	0.0008
2.62	0.0044	0.0088	3.40	0.0003	0.0007
2.63	0.0043	0.0085	3.45	0.0003	0.0006
2.64	0.0041	0.0083	3.50	0.0002	0.0005
2.65	0.0040	0.0080	3.55	0.0002	0.0004
2.70	0.0035	0.0069	3.60	0.0002	0.0003
2.75	0.0030	0.0060	3.65	0.0001	0.0003
2.80	0.0026	0.0051	3.70	0.0001	0.0002
2.85	0.0022	0.0044	3.75	0.0001	0.0002
			3.80	0.0001	0.0001

Source of data: National Bureau of Standards. Applied Mathematics Series—23. US Government Printing Office, Washington, D. C., 1953. Abstracted by Shott, S. Statistics for Health Professionals. Philadelphia, W. B. Saunders Company, 1990. Used by permission.

*Instructions for use of the table to determine the *p* value that corresponds to a calculated z value: In the left-hand column (headed z), look up the value of z found from calculations. Look at the first column to the right (for a one-tailed *p* value) or the second column to the right (for a two-tailed *p* value) that corresponds to the value of z obtained. For example, a z value of 1.74 corresponds to a two-tailed *p* value of 0.0819. **Instructions for use of the table to determine the z value that corresponds to a chosen *p* value:** To find the appropriate z value for use in confidence limits or sample size determinations, define the one-tailed or two-tailed *p* value desired, look that up in the second or third column, respectively, and determine the z value on the left that corresponds. For example, for a two-tailed alpha at 0.05, the corresponding z is 1.960; and for a one-tailed beta of 0.20, the corresponding z is 0.8416.

TABLE C. Upper Percentage Points for *t* Distributions*

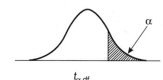

$t_{\alpha,df}$

	Upper-Tail Probability						
df	0.40	0.30	0.20	0.15	0.10	0.05	0.025
1	0.325	0.727	1.376	1.963	3.078	6.314	12.706
2	0.289	0.617	1.061	1.386	1.886	2.920	4.303
3	0.277	0.584	0.978	1.250	1.638	2.353	3.182
4	0.271	0.569	0.941	1.190	1.533	2.132	2.776
5	0.267	0.559	0.920	1.156	1.476	2.015	2.571
6	0.265	0.553	0.906	1.134	1.440	1.943	2.447
7	0.263	0.549	0.896	1.119	1.415	1.895	2.365
8	0.262	0.546	0.889	1.108	1.397	1.860	2.306
9	0.261	0.543	0.883	1.100	1.383	1.833	2.262
10	0.260	0.542	0.879	1.093	1.372	1.812	2.228
11	0.260	0.540	0.876	1.088	1.363	1.796	2.201
12	0.259	0.539	0.873	1.083	1.356	1.782	2.179
13	0.259	0.537	0.870	1.079	1.350	1.771	2.160
14	0.258	0.537	0.868	1.076	1.345	1.761	2.145
15	0.258	0.536	0.866	1.074	1.341	1.753	2.131
16	0.258	0.535	0.865	1.071	1.337	1.746	2.120
17	0.257	0.534	0.863	1.069	1.333	1.740	2.110
18	0.257	0.534	0.862	1.067	1.330	1.734	2.101
19	0.257	0.533	0.861	1.066	1.328	1.729	2.093
20	0.257	0.533	0.860	1.064	1.325	1.725	2.086
21	0.257	0.532	0.859	1.063	1.323	1.721	2.080
22	0.256	0.532	0.858	1.061	1.321	1.717	2.074
23	0.256	0.532	0.858	1.060	1.319	1.714	2.069
24	0.256	0.531	0.857	1.059	1.318	1.711	2.064
25	0.256	0.531	0.856	1.058	1.316	1.708	2.060
26	0.256	0.531	0.856	1.058	1.315	1.706	2.056
27	0.256	0.531	0.855	1.057	1.314	1.703	2.052
28	0.256	0.530	0.855	1.056	1.313	1.701	2.048
29	0.256	0.530	0.854	1.055	1.311	1.699	2.045
30	0.256	0.530	0.854	1.055	1.310	1.697	2.042
40	0.255	0.529	0.851	1.050	1.303	1.684	2.021
60	0.254	0.527	0.848	1.045	1.296	1.671	2.000
120	0.254	0.526	0.845	1.041	1.289	1.658	1.980
∞	0.253	0.524	0.842	1.036	1.282	1.645	1.960

Continued

TABLE C. Upper Percentage Points for *t* Distributions* *(Continued)*

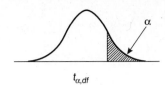

$t_{\alpha,df}$

	Upper-Tail Probability						
df	0.02	0.015	0.01	0.0075	0.005	0.0025	0.0005
1	15.895	21.205	31.821	42.434	63.657	127.322	636.590
2	4.849	5.643	6.965	8.073	9.925	14.089	31.598
3	3.482	3.896	4.541	5.047	5.841	7.453	12.924
4	2.999	3.298	3.747	4.088	4.604	5.598	8.610
5	2.757	3.003	3.365	3.634	4.032	4.773	6.869
6	2.612	2.829	3.143	3.372	3.707	4.317	5.959
7	2.517	2.715	2.998	3.203	3.499	4.029	5.408
8	2.449	2.634	2.896	3.085	3.355	3.833	5.041
9	2.398	2.574	2.821	2.998	3.250	3.690	4.781
10	2.359	2.527	2.764	2.932	3.169	3.581	4.587
11	2.328	2.491	2.718	2.879	3.106	3.497	4.437
12	2.303	2.461	2.681	2.836	3.055	3.428	4.318
13	2.282	2.436	2.650	2.801	3.012	3.372	4.221
14	2.264	2.415	2.624	2.771	2.977	3.326	4.140
15	2.249	2.397	2.602	2.746	2.947	3.286	4.073
16	2.235	2.382	2.583	2.724	2.921	3.252	4.015
17	2.224	2.368	2.567	2.706	2.898	3.222	3.965
18	2.214	2.356	2.552	2.689	2.878	3.197	3.922
19	2.205	2.346	2.539	2.674	2.861	3.174	3.883
20	2.197	2.336	2.528	2.661	2.845	3.153	3.849
21	2.189	2.328	2.518	2.649	2.831	3.135	3.819
22	2.183	2.320	2.508	2.639	2.819	3.119	3.792
23	2.177	2.313	2.500	2.629	2.807	3.104	3.768
24	2.172	2.307	2.492	2.620	2.797	3.091	3.745
25	2.167	2.301	2.485	2.612	2.787	3.078	3.725
26	2.162	2.296	2.479	2.605	2.779	3.067	3.707
27	2.158	2.291	2.473	2.598	2.771	3.057	3.690
28	2.154	2.286	2.467	2.592	2.763	3.047	3.674
29	2.150	2.282	2.462	2.586	2.756	3.038	3.659
30	2.147	2.278	2.457	2.581	2.750	3.030	3.646
40	2.123	2.250	2.423	2.542	2.704	2.971	3.551
60	2.099	2.223	2.390	2.504	2.660	2.915	3.460
120	2.076	2.196	2.358	2.468	2.617	2.860	3.373
∞	2.054	2.170	2.326	2.432	2.576	2.807	3.291

Source of data: Shott, S. Statistics for Health Professionals. Philadelphia, W. B. Saunders Company, 1990. Used by permission.

***Instructions for use of the table:** To determine the *p* value that corresponds to a calculated *t* value, first find the line that corresponds to the column of degrees of freedom *(df)* on the left. Then in the center of the table find the value that most closely corresponds to the value of *t* found from calculations. **(1) For a paired (one-tailed) *t*-test:** Look at the top row to find the corresponding probability. For example, a *t* value of 2.147 on 30 *df* corresponds to a *p* value of 0.02. If the observed value of *t* falls between values given, state the two *p* values between which the results of the *t*-test fall. For example, if a *t* of 2.160 is found on 30 *df*, the probability is expressed as follows: $0.015 < p < 0.02$. **(2) For the Student's (two-tailed) *t*-test:** The procedure is the same as for a one-tailed test, except that the *p* value obtained must then be *doubled* to include the other tail probability. For example, if the Student's *t*-test gives a *p* value of 2.147 on 30 *df*, the *p* value of that column (0.02) must be doubled to give the correct *p* value of 0.04.

TABLE D. Upper Percentage Points for Chi-Square Distributions*

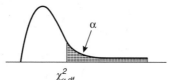

	Probability								
df	0.9995	0.995	0.99	0.975	0.95	0.90	0.80	0.70	0.60
1	0.000000393	0.0000393	0.000157	0.000982	0.00393	0.0158	0.0642	0.148	0.275
2	0.00100	0.0100	0.0201	0.0506	0.103	0.211	0.446	0.713	1.022
3	0.0153	0.0717	0.115	0.216	0.352	0.584	1.005	1.424	1.869
4	0.0639	0.207	0.297	0.484	0.711	1.064	1.649	2.195	2.753
5	0.158	0.412	0.554	0.831	1.145	1.610	2.343	3.000	3.655
6	0.299	0.676	0.872	1.237	1.635	2.204	3.070	3.828	4.570
7	0.485	0.989	1.239	1.690	2.167	2.833	3.822	4.671	5.493
8	0.710	1.344	1.646	2.180	2.733	3.490	4.594	5.527	6.423
9	0.972	1.735	2.088	2.700	3.325	4.168	5.380	6.393	7.357
10	1.265	2.156	2.558	3.247	3.940	4.865	6.179	7.267	8.295
11	1.587	2.603	3.053	3.816	4.575	5.578	6.989	8.148	9.237
12	1.934	3.074	3.571	4.404	5.226	6.304	7.807	9.034	10.182
13	2.305	3.565	4.107	5.009	5.892	7.042	8.634	9.926	11.129
14	2.697	4.075	4.660	5.629	6.571	7.790	9.467	10.821	12.078
15	3.108	4.601	5.229	6.262	7.261	8.547	10.307	11.721	13.030
16	3.536	5.142	5.812	6.908	7.962	9.312	11.152	12.624	13.983
17	3.980	5.697	6.408	7.564	8.672	10.085	12.002	13.531	14.937
18	4.439	6.265	7.015	8.231	9.390	10.865	12.857	14.440	15.893
19	4.912	6.844	7.633	8.907	10.117	11.651	13.716	15.352	16.850
20	5.398	7.434	8.260	9.591	10.851	12.443	14.578	16.266	17.809
21	5.896	8.034	8.897	10.283	11.591	13.240	15.445	17.182	18.768
22	6.404	8.643	9.542	10.982	12.338	14.041	16.314	18.101	19.729
23	6.924	9.260	10.196	11.689	13.091	14.848	17.187	19.021	20.690
24	7.453	9.886	10.856	12.401	13.848	15.659	18.062	19.943	21.652
25	7.991	10.520	11.524	13.120	14.611	16.473	18.940	20.867	22.616
26	8.538	11.160	12.198	13.844	15.379	17.292	19.820	21.792	23.579
27	9.093	11.808	12.879	14.573	16.151	18.114	20.703	22.719	24.544
28	9.656	12.461	13.565	15.308	16.928	18.939	21.588	23.647	25.509
29	10.227	13.121	14.256	16.047	17.708	19.768	22.475	24.577	26.475
30	10.804	13.787	14.953	16.791	18.493	20.599	23.364	25.508	27.442
35	13.787	17.192	18.509	20.569	22.465	24.797	27.836	30.178	32.282
40	16.906	20.707	22.164	24.433	26.509	29.051	32.345	34.872	37.134
45	20.137	24.311	25.901	28.366	30.612	33.350	36.884	39.585	41.995
50	23.461	27.991	29.707	32.357	34.764	37.689	41.449	44.313	46.864
60	30.340	35.534	37.485	40.482	43.188	46.459	50.641	53.809	56.620
70	37.467	43.275	45.442	48.758	51.739	55.329	59.898	63.346	66.396
80	44.791	51.172	53.540	57.153	60.391	64.278	69.207	72.915	76.188
90	52.276	59.196	61.754	65.647	69.126	73.291	78.558	82.511	85.993
100	59.896	67.328	70.065	74.222	77.929	82.358	87.945	92.129	95.808
120	75.467	83.852	86.923	91.573	95.705	100.624	106.806	111.419	115.465
140	91.391	100.655	104.034	109.137	113.659	119.029	125.758	130.766	135.149
160	107.597	117.679	121.346	126.870	131.756	137.546	144.783	150.158	154.856
180	124.033	134.884	138.820	144.741	149.969	156.153	163.868	169.588	174.580
200	140.660	152.241	156.432	162.728	168.279	174.835	183.003	189.049	194.319

Continued

TABLE D. Upper Percentage Points for Chi-Square Distributions* (Continued)

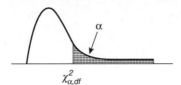

$$\chi^2_{\alpha, df}$$

					Probability					
df	0.50	0.40	0.30	0.20	0.10	0.05	0.025	0.01	0.005	0.0005
1	0.455	0.708	1.074	1.642	2.706	3.841	5.024	6.635	7.879	12.116
2	1.386	1.833	2.408	3.219	4.605	5.991	7.378	9.210	10.597	15.202
3	2.366	2.946	3.665	4.642	6.251	7.815	9.348	11.345	12.838	17.730
4	3.357	4.045	4.878	5.989	7.779	9.488	11.143	13.277	14.860	19.997
5	4.351	5.132	6.064	7.289	9.236	11.070	12.833	15.086	16.750	22.105
6	5.348	6.211	7.231	8.558	10.645	12.592	14.449	16.812	18.548	24.103
7	6.346	7.283	8.383	9.803	12.017	14.067	16.013	18.475	20.278	26.018
8	7.344	8.351	9.524	11.030	13.362	15.507	17.535	20.090	21.955	27.868
9	8.343	9.414	10.656	12.242	14.684	16.919	19.023	21.666	23.589	29.666
10	9.342	10.473	11.781	13.442	15.987	18.307	20.483	23.209	25.188	31.420
11	10.341	11.530	12.899	14.631	17.275	19.675	21.920	24.725	26.757	33.137
12	11.340	12.584	14.011	15.812	18.549	21.026	23.337	26.217	28.300	34.821
13	12.340	13.636	15.119	16.985	19.812	22.362	24.736	27.688	29.819	36.478
14	13.339	14.685	16.222	18.151	21.064	23.685	26.119	29.141	31.319	38.109
15	14.339	15.733	17.322	19.311	22.307	24.996	27.488	30.578	32.801	39.719
16	15.338	16.780	18.418	20.465	23.542	26.296	28.845	32.000	34.267	41.308
17	16.338	17.824	19.511	21.615	24.769	27.587	30.191	33.409	35.718	42.879
18	17.338	18.868	20.601	22.760	25.989	28.869	31.526	34.805	37.156	44.434
19	18.338	19.910	21.689	23.900	27.204	30.144	32.852	36.191	38.582	45.973
20	19.337	20.951	22.775	25.038	28.412	31.410	34.170	37.566	39.997	47.498
21	20.337	21.991	23.858	26.171	29.615	32.671	35.479	38.932	41.401	49.011
22	21.337	23.031	24.939	27.301	30.813	33.924	36.781	40.289	42.796	50.511
23	22.337	24.069	26.018	28.429	32.007	35.172	38.076	41.638	44.181	52.000
24	23.337	25.106	27.096	29.553	33.196	36.415	39.364	42.980	45.559	53.479
25	24.337	26.143	28.172	30.675	34.382	37.652	40.646	44.314	46.928	54.947
26	25.336	27.179	29.246	31.795	35.563	38.885	41.923	45.642	48.290	56.407
27	26.336	28.214	30.319	32.912	36.741	40.113	43.195	46.963	49.645	57.858
28	27.336	29.249	31.391	34.027	37.916	41.337	44.461	48.278	50.993	59.300
29	28.336	30.283	32.461	35.139	39.087	42.557	45.722	49.588	52.336	60.735
30	29.336	31.316	33.530	36.250	40.256	43.773	46.979	50.892	53.672	62.162
35	34.336	36.475	38.859	41.778	46.059	49.802	53.203	57.342	60.275	69.199
40	39.335	41.622	44.165	47.269	51.805	55.758	59.342	63.691	66.766	76.095
45	44.335	46.761	49.452	52.729	57.505	61.656	65.410	69.957	73.166	82.876
50	49.335	51.892	54.723	58.164	63.167	67.505	71.420	76.154	79.490	89.561
60	59.335	62.135	65.227	68.972	74.397	79.082	83.298	88.379	91.952	102.695
70	69.334	72.358	75.689	79.715	85.527	90.531	95.023	100.425	104.215	115.578
80	79.334	82.566	86.120	90.405	96.578	101.879	106.629	112.329	116.321	128.261
90	89.334	92.761	96.524	101.054	107.565	113.145	118.136	124.116	128.299	140.782
100	99.334	102.946	106.906	111.667	118.498	124.342	129.561	135.807	140.169	153.167
120	119.334	123.289	127.616	132.806	140.233	146.567	152.211	158.950	163.648	177.603
140	139.334	143.604	148.269	153.854	161.827	168.613	174.648	181.840	186.847	201.683
160	159.334	163.898	168.876	174.828	183.311	190.516	196.915	204.530	209.824	225.481
180	179.334	184.173	189.446	195.743	204.704	212.304	219.044	227.056	232.620	249.048
200	199.334	204.434	209.985	216.609	226.021	233.994	241.058	249.445	255.264	272.423

Instructions for use of the table: Determine the degrees of freedom *(df)* appropriate to the chi-square test just calculated, and go to the line that most closely corresponds, using the left-hand column (headed *df*). On that line, move to the right in the body of the table and find the chi-square value that corresponds to what was calculated. The corresponding *p* value is found at the top of that column. For example, on 6 *df*, a calculated chi-square of 12.592 corresponds to a *p* value of 0.05. If the calculated chi-square value falls between two columns in the table, state the two *p* values between which the results of the chi-square test fall. For example, on 6 *df*, the probability of a chi-square of 13.500 is expressed as follows: $0.025 < p < 0.05$.

INDEX

Note: Page numbers in *italics* indicate figures; those followed by t indicate tables; those followed by b indicate boxes.